Critical Care Nursing

Monitoring and Treatment for Advanced Nursing Practice

Critical Care Nursing

Monitoring and Treatment for Advanced Nursing Practice

EDITED BY

Kathy J. Booker, PhD, RN, CNE

Professor, School of Nursing Millikin University Decatur, Illinois, USA

WILEY Blackwell

CHAPTER 1

Philosophy and treatment in US critical care units

Kathy J. Booker

School of Nursing, Millikin University, Decatur, IL., USA

In this chapter, the evolution of critical care practice and advanced nursing roles are explored. An examination of factors that contribute to safe monitoring and treatment in critical care units includes certification processes and national support for critical care nursing practice, perspectives on patient and family-focused care, and the evolution of rapid response team (RRT) roles in hospital settings.

US critical care units

Critical care units were formally developed in the United States in the years following World War II. Common elements driving the origin of critical care units remain important even today, including close patient monitoring, application of sophisticated equipment, and surveillance-based interventions to prevent clinical deterioration or health complications. Today's critical care units are often diverse, specialized areas of care for patients at high risk or those undergoing critical health events requiring nursing attention. The critical care team is generally quite complex, including medical management increasingly supported by intensivists, residents, acute care nurse practitioners (ACNPs), clinical nurse specialists (CNSs), and other nursing personnel. Additional vital practitioners include respiratory therapists, dietitians, pharmacists, social workers, and physical/occupational therapists. Over the last 50 years, sophisticated treatment modalities, technology, and care philosophies have evolved to promote a strong patient-centered care ethic coupled with technological complexity.

The cost of delivering care to the critically ill continues to rise. The Society of Critical Care Medicine (2013a) identified increasing costs of critical care medicine in the United States, with current projections of $81.7 billion (13.4% of hospital costs) in the care delivery of over 5 million patients annually in the nation's critical care units.

Organization of critical care delivery

Haupt *et al.* (2003) published guidelines for delivering critical care based on a multidisciplinary review of the literature and writing panelists with representation from important critical care providers including physicians, nurses, pharmacists, respiratory therapists, and other key critical care team representatives. A three-level system of intensive care unit (ICU) care was promoted in these guidelines, acknowledging various ICU care systems based on the availability of key personnel, educational preparation, certification, and fundamental skill requirements. These general guidelines for hospitals in establishing and maintaining critical care services assigned levels of care as follows:

1 Level I care: units that provide medical directorships with continual availability of board-certified intensivist care and appropriate minimal preparation recommendations for all key and support personnel.

2 Level II care: comprehensive care for critically ill but unavailability of selected specialty

Critical Care Nursing: Monitoring and Treatment for Advanced Nursing Practice, First Edition. Edited by Kathy J. Booker.
© 2015 John Wiley & Sons, Inc. Published 2015 by John Wiley & Sons, Inc.

care, requiring that hospitals with units at this level have transfer agreements in place.

3 Level III care: units that have the ability to provide initial stabilization and/or care of relatively stable, routine patient conditions. Level III units must clearly assess limitations of care provision with established transfer protocols (Haupt *et al.*, 2003, p. 2677).

Emphasis on intensivist medical management, diagnostic testing availability, and specialty interventional availability guides hospitals to provide optimal care to the critically ill. This has also been supported by the Society of Critical Care Medicine (SCCM, 2013a). Haupt *et al.* (2003) also made recommendations for graduate education and/or certification by critical care nursing managers within the leadership structure. Transfer protocols for higher levels of care were recommended if selected life-saving services were unavailable, suggesting that protocols be incorporated into patient management systems in all hospitals without the full range of service based upon these guidelines. Despite the fact that these guidelines were advanced over 10 years ago, critical care practice remains diverse across the nation due in part to the availability of key personnel, state emergency system organization, system restrictions due to population and area coverage, and cost constraints. Emergency management and trauma support guidelines have been advanced by the American College of Surgeons (ACS) though the Advanced Trauma Life Support courses and guidelines for the transfer of patients in rural settings are also published on the ACS web site (Peterson and the Ad Hoc Committee on Rural Trauma, ACS Committee on Trauma, 2002).

Monitoring and surveillance in critical care

In the care of critically ill patients, the use of monitoring technology to support care is central to evidence-based practice. Research on the frequency and types of monitoring that affect the best patient outcomes is growing. Selected technologies, such as the use of pulmonary artery catheters in the critically ill, have been studied extensively. But the rapid growth of new technologies for monitoring at the bedside are often labor-intensive, requiring considerable nursing time to set up and manage to ensure good outcomes. In addition, ethical, humane application of technology must be continually considered so that the effect of intrusive or invasive technology is continually monitored in individualized care (Funk, 2011). Effective monitoring requires familiarity with the patient's condition and preferences, the equipment, the processes inherent in obtaining the data, and the interpretation of monitored data, all affected by potential error in acquisition and management. Monitoring allows for the calculation of critically ill patients' physiological reserve and effectiveness of interventions but also carries the caveat that practitioners must be familiar with the pitfalls associated with data interpretation commonly found in all areas of acute and critical care practice (Andrews and Nolan, 2006).

Young and Griffiths (2006) reviewed clinical trials monitoring acutely ill patients and observed that "to display data which cannot influence the patient's outcome might increase our knowledge of disease processes but does not directly benefit the monitored patient. Nor is it harmless, more information brings with it more ways to misunderstand and mistreat" (p. 39). More monitoring may not be the answer to improving the treatment of critically ill persons but individualized monitoring of the right parameters to guide therapy and improve patient outcomes is the goal of the critical care team. Revolutionary changes in patient outcomes have been obtained with the development of selected technology, including pulse oximetry, bispectral index for depth of anesthesia, and noninvasive measurement of cardiac output and stroke volume (Young and Griffiths, 2006). Despite the expansiveness of monitoring, many have noted the paucity of evidence of its effectiveness. Particularly in the arena of hemodynamic monitoring, studies have been equivocal regarding the effectiveness of monitoring data to influence patient outcomes (see Chapter 5).

Surveillance

Kelly (2009) studied nursing surveillance and distinguished monitoring from surveillance by noting that surveillance informs decision making and involves action steps that stem from more passive monitoring. Kelly (2009) defined surveillance as "a process to identify threats to patients' health and safety through purposeful and ongoing acquisition, interpretation, and synthesis of patient data for clinical decision making in the acute care setting" (p. 28). Surveillance is a core role of critical care; while not unique to nursing, surveillance is applied continuously in critical care units worldwide. Henneman, Gawlinski, and Giuliano (2012) identified surveillance as a nursing intervention critical to patient safety. In a review of practices recently studied in acute and critical care nursing, Henneman, Gawlinski, and Giuliano (2012) examined the use of checklists, interdisciplinary rounds, and other clinical decisional support and monitoring systems important to surveillance and prevention of errors.

The need for monitoring systems that produce reliable and accurate data has never been more urgent. Monitoring systems should be designed to foster action and supportive care to improve patient and family experience and physiological outcomes for patients. Practices that do not improve patient outcomes should be eliminated. In addition, clinicians need to help patients and family members understand monitoring systems. Continual assessment of changing conditions, critical reflection, critical reasoning, and clinical judgment are all supported with the use of appropriate technology (Benner, Hughes, and Sutphen, 2008). Safe care practices depend on these habits of the mind as well as reliable and accurate technology. The potential for error is evident at many junctures in today's complex hospital systems and the critical care unit is the hub of such concentrated complexity, making surveillance essential for safe patient care.

Research on monitoring and surveillance is increasing. Schmidt (2010) studied the concepts of surveillance and vigilance, and identified the basic social process of nursing support for patients in a critical care environment, ensuring continual vigilance and protective action to ensure safety. Yousef *et al.* (2012) examined continuous monitoring data in 326 surgical trauma patients to determine parameters associated with cardiorespiratory instability. These were defined as heart rate less than 40/min or greater than 140/min; respirations less than 8/min or greater than 36/min; SpO_2 less than 85%; and blood pressure less than 80 mmHg, greater than 200 mmHg systolic, or greater than 110 mmHg diastolic. Patients who remained clinically stable versus those who had even one period of instability were more likely to have more comorbidities, as measured by the Charlson Comorbidity Index. In earlier work, these authors found that 6.3 h ensued between periods of cardiorespiratory instability and activation of a rapid response team (RRT) (Hravnak *et al.*, 2008). In these studies, automated, continuous monitoring recorded and validated in the clinical monitoring system strengthened the data validity, including automated blood pressure measurements measured at least every 2 h. Clear consideration for technology advancement and the effects on both nursing practice and patient outcomes is needed.

Nursing certification and competency in critical care units

One method of moving toward more consistent and safe practice involves certification in critical care practice. All nurses practicing in the ICU environment have curricula and orientation programs, the ability to become certified in the care of the critically ill, and, in the case of the ACNPs and CNSs, the ability to attain national certification and advanced practice licensure. Does national certification ensure quality care? Kaplow (2011) identified the value associated with nursing certification, including the value to patients and families, employers, and individual nurses, noting that certification validates specialty practice and competency. Research is insufficient in linking certification to improved patient outcomes but denotes a level of professionalism and recognition for increasing education and competency (Kaplow, 2011). Coverage of the many contributions of advanced practice nurses to patient outcome measures will be explored in the following sections.

Studies have shown links between nursing certification and patient satisfaction with care as well as nurses' job satisfaction (Wade, 2009). Fleischman, Meyer, and Watson (2011) reviewed and highlighted best practices to create a culture of certification across institutions in the United States including fostering supportive environments, recognition, and improved research utilization as identified best practices in critical care environments. Wade (2009) identified a sense of increased collaborative practice and empowerment among certified nurses. Further work is needed to validate patient outcomes associated with certification.

Overcoming barriers to integration of research at the bedside remains a challenge to all providers concerned with improved quality of critical care delivery (Leeman, Baernholdt, and Sandelowski, 2007; Penz and Bassendowski, 2006). The use of improved educational strategies to better prepare practitioners for evidence-based practice guidance (Penz and Bassendowski, 2006) and more refined change strategies, including coordination across disciplines, outcome-focused change, and methods to increase behavioral control, such as change leaders or champions, is recommended (Leeman, Baernholdt, and Sandelowski, 2007). In rapidly changing environments such as critical care units, sustained change is difficult to maintain and improved systems are needed for better integration of evidence-based care.

Professional organizations often lead the way in research to practice innovation. The American Association of Critical Care Nurses (AACN, 2013a) has developed a series of practice alerts, available as easy pdf file downloads with selected power point slides for teaching care providers. These are frequently updated by leading researchers in the field and incorporate current evidence for application to practice. Mallory (2010) reported on strategies used by the Oncology Nurse Society (ONS) to promote evidence-based practices for translational research (see Fig. 1.1). Adoption of clinical practice guidelines is not a simple process and often requires the attention of advanced practice nurses and other team members dedicated to attaining a high standard of care and a strong method to ensure sustainable change.

Identify clinical problem or
New research knowledge emerges
↓
Primary research/Systematic reviews are accessed
↓
Research evidence is critically appraised
↓
Evidence is synthesized
↓
Guidelines and/or protocols are developed
↓
Strategies for implementation into practice are formulated
↓
Evaluation of the impact of change is planned

Figure 1.1 Knowledge transformation processes. Adapted from Mallory (2010, pp. 280–284).

Explosive growth has occurred in the application of evidence-based models to guide education and practice. While too numerous to highlight within this book, selected models applied frequently to critical care practice include the Iowa Model (Titler *et al.*, 2001) and the Johns Hopkins Model (Newhouse *et al.*, 2007).

US national critical care organizations

The AACN and the SCCM have a long history fostering collaborative practice and improvement of outcomes for critically ill patients. Vibrant and patient-centered, these organizations work to further the science and practice of members and share a commitment to the advancement of the art and science of critical care practice, including the role of nurses in improving patient outcomes and treatment modalities.

American Association of Critical Care Nurses

The AACN promulgates nursing standards and is affiliated with a certification corporation dedicated to certification of nurses in critical care (AACN, 2013b). With a focus on promotion of patient-centered care and support for critical care nursing practice, the AACN endorses three major advocacy initiatives, including healthy work environments, end-of-life care, and staffing/workforce development. Current certifications available through the AACN certification program include specialty certifications in acute/critical care nursing (adult, neonatal, or pediatric), earning critical care registered nurse (CCRN) certification; CCRN-E, a tele-ICU version; adult progressive care certified nurse (PCCN) credential; and a certified nurse manager and leader (CNML) credential. Subspecialty certifications are also available in Certification in Cardiac Medicine (CMC) and adult cardiac surgery (cardiac surgical certification, CSC). Advanced practice certifications are transitioning to the consensus model certifications of Adult-Gerontology Acute Care Nurse Practitioner Certification (ACNPC-AG) and ACCNS, CNSs (wellness through acute care), available as gerontology, pediatric, and neonatal designations. Adult advanced practice certification is currently available as adult ACNPC or adult, neonatal, or pediatric versions of the acute care certification of clinical nurse specialist (CCNS) exam (AACN, 2013b). The latter two certifications will continue to be available for renewal but candidates should see the AACN web site for guidance concerning certification eligibility. Certification programs are evaluated every 5 years and are based on competency assessments.

Society of Critical Care Medicine

The SCCM promotes excellence in patient care, education, research, and advocacy in the care of critically ill patients. The SCCM self-identifies as the only organization to represent all professional members of the critical care team and has a membership of nearly 16 000 in over 100 countries (SCCM, 2013b). The SCCM web site includes a compilation of evidence-based guidelines directly applicable to the care of critically ill patients. There are also podcasts and webinars available at no charge along with other practitioner resources.

Acute care advanced practice nursing

As the role of the advanced practice nurse has evolved over the past several decades, implementation of the role differs worldwide. Mantzoukas and Watkinson (2006) sought to clarify generic features of advanced nursing practice through a review of the international literature. In their summary, consistent features included (i) the use of knowledge in practice, (ii) critical thinking and analytical skills, (iii) clinical judgment and decision-making skills, (iv) professional leadership and clinical inquiry, (v) coaching and mentoring skills, (vi) research skills, and (vii) changing practice (Mantzoukas and Watkinson, 2006, p. 28).

Implementation of nurse practitioners (NPs) and CNSs in critical care varies across the United States. While growth in these advanced practice roles is expected, care delivery and role implementation often vary regionally and are often driven by physician and nurse practice patterns, hospital initiatives, and financial support. Kleinpell and Hudspeth (2013) reviewed terminology and organizational frameworks for scope of practice in critical care advanced practice roles. Competencies and national models are reviewed with clarification on the scope of practice of an advanced practice registered nurse (APRN), particularly for ACNPs.

Becker *et al.* (2006) reported on the national task force survey for delineation of the work of advanced practice critical care nurses in an effort to clarify roles of the ACNPs and CNSs. The specific aims of this study were to reveal criticality and frequency ratings for 65 APRN activities and to compare spheres of influence distinctive to each role. Significant distinctions included a focus on individual patients in the role of ACNP (74 versus 25.8% for CNS) and relatively small amount of advanced practice nursing time spent on interventional skills in both APRN roles. Eight activities were reported with greater frequency by ACNPs compared with CNSs: developing/implementing and modifying the plan of care; prescribing medications and therapeutics; comprehensive history and physical examinations; differential diagnoses; ordering diagnostic studies; making referrals; performing invasive procedures; and empowering patients and families as own advocates (Becker *et al.*, 2006, p. 142).

Clinical nurse specialists

The CNS's role is focused on three spheres of influence advanced by the National Association of Clinical Nurse Specialists (NACNS): patients and families, nurses/nursing practice, and organization/systems. It incorporates the AACN Synergy Model (AACN, 2013b), and the competencies of advanced practice nursing presented by Hamric, Spross and Hanson (2009). Outcome assessment in complex environments has become an important part of advanced practice for CNSs and integral to graduate programs.

The NACNS (2009) developed the *Core Practice Doctorate Clinical Nurse Specialist Competencies* in collaboration with other stakeholders. These have been endorsed by a number of national organizations (NACNS, 2009). In this document, expansion of advanced practice competencies to the doctoral level includes emphasis on expanded translational research, interprofessional collaboration, and many other competencies identified by national organizations to advance clinical nursing practice (NACNS, 2009). The competencies that were advanced included client sphere of influence, nurse and nursing practice competencies, and organizational systems competencies (NACNS, 2009).

Altmiller (2011) applied a framework of quality and safety education for nurse competencies using these spheres of influence for CNS preceptors designed to bring transparency to the many contributions made by CNSs to hospital systems that improve care at the bedside but are often difficult to track. These include the influence of skilled CNSs in precepting other nurses, building teamwork and collaboration, implementing evidence-based practice, quality improvement practices, safety promotion through system effectiveness, and informatics applications to ensure effective communication, management of knowledge, and foundational decision making. These competencies were promulgated by the Quality and Safety Education for Nurses (QSEN) project, funded by the Robert Wood Johnson Foundation in response to the initial Institute of Medicine report targeting the education of health professionals to improve safety (Institute of Medicine, 2001; Hughes, 2008).

Acute care nurse practitioners

The evolution the ACNP's role has been attributed to workforce issues related to restrictions in the hours medical students were able to work during residencies (D'Agostino and Halpern, 2010; Kleinpell, Ely, and Grabenkort, 2008; Weinstein, 2002). Among the newest NP roles, ACNPs were first certified in 1975 (Becker *et al.*, 2006). Over time, advanced practice nursing programs emerged with significant variability across the United States. In the past decade, significant progress has been made in promoting standard terminology and educational guidelines for advanced practice nurses (APRN Joint Dialogue Group Report, 2008). In these guidelines, endorsed by most national nursing organizations, the four roles of APRNs are confirmed (clinical nurse specialist, certified registered nurse anesthetist, nurse practitioner, and nurse midwife) and educational guidelines have broadly changed to an educational focus on patient population rather than specialty tracks. APRN regulatory standards encompass guidelines on licensure, accreditation, certification, and education (APRN Joint Dialogue Group Report, 2008), addressed through established standards for guidance on advanced nursing educational program content in the United States. In these guidelines, the specialty role is not distinguished as a broad NP practice categorization (e.g., ACNP, Oncology). The APRN guidelines have evolved so that widespread changes in certification are planned for 2015 (National Task Force on Quality Nurse Practitioner Education, 2012). ACNPs will obtain certification as advanced practice nurses (APRNs) with an adult/gerontology focus or a pediatric focus through selected examinations offered by the American Nurses Certification Corporation (ANCC, 2013). The ANCC identifies December 31, 2014, as the last date for applications for certification as an ACNP. As the NTF guidelines (2012) are implemented, certification will move the ACNP role to an APRN title with specialty exams focused on adult/gerontology or pediatrics. Most ACNP and Oncology educational programs have strengthened the adult/gerontological or pediatric population focus with continued unique coursework to guide specialty practice. Certification is currently required to obtain state licensure as APRNs. Many current ACNP programs require registered nurse licensure and clinical experience in critical care prior to entry into the NP track although a number of programs nationally allow second baccalaureate or higher degree entry and accelerated progress over several years to graduation. Students interested in becoming safe practitioners must recognize the complexity of the critical care environment and give careful consideration to their own skills and capabilities when examining educational options. The richness of multiple learners with a variety of experience adds value to the learning environment and promotes multidisciplinary communication, an important factor in critical care safe practices, although this is an area that remains understudied.

Kleinpell and Goolsby (2006) evaluated ACNP practice identified by 635 national ACNPs from survey data associated with the 2004 American Academy of Nurse Practitioner database. The majority of studies reviewed the impact of ACNPs and physician assistants in acute and critical care, ranging from evaluating specific patient care and disease management outcomes to communication, compliance with guidelines, and other process management strategies. Studies demonstrate similar patient outcomes delivered by ACNPs and physician assistants (PAs) in critical care settings although few large-scale, randomized studies have been done (Kleinpell, Ely, and Grabenkort, 2008). As the ACNP role evolves and additional research clarifies outcomes, integration within the healthcare team will be better elucidated.

As a relatively new role in critical care, the ACNP role integration into systems has generally enhanced patient satisfaction and collaborative care practices (Cobb and Kutash, 2011; Howie and Erickson, 2002). Hoffman *et al.* (2005) compared outcomes of care managed in a subacute medical ICU to that provided by resident physicians and found no differences in length of stay, readmissions to critical care, or number of patients weaned prior to discharge.

A growing role for APRNs is on hospitalist teams (Kleinpell *et al.*, 2008). Another relatively recent addition to hospital practice, hospitalist medicine generally represents coverage of care for inpatients by internal medicine, family practice, or pediatric specialties. Over 40 000 hospitalists practice in US and Canadian hospitals and continued growth is expected (Society of Hospital Medicine, 2012).

Critical care and ACNP outcomes research

Within acute care environments, ACNPs may practice in areas beyond the traditional ICU environment. D'Agostino and Halpern (2010) studied the integration of ACNPs into an oncology practice, reviewing educational and support programs for staff to aid transitions to specialty practice. Using a multidisciplinary model, including departments of nursing, anesthesiology, and critical care medicine, the authors provide a structure for planned implementation of the role. Due to regional shortages of ACNPs, other NP specialists, including family NPs and adult NPs may enter NP programs with experience in areas of traditional nursing such as critical care. Following graduation, these NPs may practice in acute care environments or specialty office practices, making it difficult to track practice patterns among ACNPs nationally.

Kleinpell, Ely, and Grabenkort (2008) analyzed research on nonphysician providers in acute and critical care settings, focusing on PAs and NPs. In a systematic review of 145 manuscripts, only two randomized control trials (RCTs) were found by Cooper *et al.* (2002) and Sakr *et al.* (1999). Both of these RCTs were conducted in the emergency department setting. While support for the contributions of NPs and PAs to critical care delivery was found among other strong prospective studies, the level of evidence remains weak and further studies are needed. Further studies targeting dissemination of practice models for advanced practice roles; ICU patient outcome impact of advanced roles; research regarding supply and demand of staffing needs in the ICU, including intensivist and midlevel providers; and studies on billing of services are recommended (Kleinpell, Ely, and Grabenkort, 2008).

Kleinpell (2013) extensively reviewed outcome research in advanced practice nursing, comparing studies across APRN roles. This text provides a strong contribution to the literature on effectiveness of APRNs, summarizing patient and care-related outcomes including studies on economic effectiveness. Overwhelmingly, APRN contributions to care are demonstrated to be strong and equal or superior to the care of other practitioners such as physicians or PAs. In many studies, the addition of an NP team member resulted in improved care delivery, shorter lengths of hospital stay, and reduced costs (Kleinpell, 2013). As the role of the ACNP remains relatively new and evolving, further outcome studies are needed that highlight the cost-effectiveness of these roles such as those attained in specific settings (e.g., cardiac catheterization laboratories, surgical or transplant services) to broader patient treatment lines (e.g., care of congestive heart failure patients and patients on prolonged ventilator management).

As critical care settings evolve, advanced practice nurses and researchers continue to examine changing health-care systems. Burman et al. (2009) recommend a reconceptualization of the core elements of NP education and practice, emphasizing stronger classroom and clinical coursework in health promotion and disease prevention. Emerging programs for patients with chronic diseases such as heart failure and chronic obstructive pulmonary disease (COPD) are potentially life-changing as chronic diseases account for 60% of all deaths worldwide. Advanced practice nurses, particularly those with strong education and practice in critical care settings, may contribute significantly to these evolving models of care.

Evolution of families in the critical care unit

In the early days of critical care units, an ethic of isolation of patients emerged, attributable to the beliefs on rest and healing. Familes were often considered a distraction with the potential to interfere rather than support the healing process. AACN and SCCM have joined in promoting less restrictive visiting privileges in the

critical care arena. In 2007, Davidson et al. promulgated clinical practice guidelines for support of the family in the patient-centered ICU based on an extensive literature review. Categories of studies reviewed and clinical practice recommendations were offered in 10 areas: decision-making, family coping, staff stress related to family interactions, cultural support of the family, spiritual and religious support, family visitation, family environment of care, family presence on rounds, family presence at resuscitation, and palliative care. Most recommendations are based on case series or expert opinion rather than controlled studies but further research needs are highlighted. Of the 43 recommendations given within these guidelines, supportive references and overviews of current practice are analyzed carefully, making these important to new and seasoned practitioners in the critical care environment (Table 1.1).

Research has demonstrated improvements in patient comfort and enhanced support when family presence is less restrictive, including family presence during resuscitation and ventilator weaning (Doolin et al., 2011; Happ et al., 2007). The team must always seek to balance the presence of families and others who are significant in the patient's life with patient's care needs. The context of family presence must be carefully evaluated since prior relationships with family members may drive whether patients view family presence as helpful or harmful. In their ethnographic research of family presence during weaning from mechanical ventilation, Happ et al. (2007) noted that clinicians reported that calming or soothing presence including touch and gentle talk was supportive to patients undergoing weaning trials, while a "tense demeanor, hovering, being overly close, and asking the patient about symptoms, activity tolerance, or weaning progress were considered a hinderance" (p. 56). Many studies have confirmed the needs of families as well as patient-identified desire to have family and/or significant others present in the ICU. Henneman and Cardin (2002) offered a 10-step approach to improve family-centered care in the ICU with a focus on multidisciplinary involvement and inclusion of the philosophy from orientation of

Table 1.1 Family support in the ICU.

Recommendations (Davidson *et al.*, 2007)	Sample recommendation	Evidence grade
1 Decision-making	Decision making in the ICU is based on a partnership between the patient, his or her appointed surrogate, and the multiprofessional team (p. 608)	B
2 Family coping	ICU staff receives training in how to assess family needs and family members' stress and anxiety levels (p. 609)	C
3 Staff stress related to family interactions	The multiprofessional team is kept informed of treatment goals so that the messages given to the family are consistent, thereby reducing friction between team members and between the team and the family (p. 610)	C
4 Cultural support of the family	On request or when conflict arises due to cultural differences in values, when there is a choice of providers, the provider's culture is matched to the patient's (p. 610)	C
5 Spiritual and religious support	Spiritual needs of the patient are assessed by the health-care team, and findings that affect health and healing incorporated into the plan of care (p. 612)	C
6 Family visitation	Open visitation in the adult intensive care environment allows flexibility for patients and families and is determined on a case-by-case basis (p. 613)	B
7 Family environment of care	Improve patient confidentiality, privacy, and social support by building ICUs with single-bed rooms that include space for the family (p. 613)	B
8 Family presence on rounds	Parents or guardians of children in the ICU are given the opportunity to participate in rounds (p. 614)	B
9 Family presence at resuscitation	Institutions develop a structured process to allow the presence of family members during cardiopulmonary resuscitation of their loved one that includes a staff debriefing (p. 615)	C
10 Palliative care	Assessments are made of the family's understanding of the illness and its consequences, symptoms, side effects, functional impairment, and treatments and of the family's ability to cope with the illness and its consequences. Family education should be based on the assessment findings (p. 616)	D

Adapted from Davidson *et al.* (2007).
Evidence grades: B, systematic reviews or strong cohort studies; C, case series or weak cohort studies; D, expert opinion.

new staff members to initial encounters with family members of patients admitted to the ICU. They suggest that clarity be first reached among the multidisciplinary team with endorsement of a family-centered philosophy that should be systematized in a unit. Family-centered care is much more than simple visitation policies and involves true trust and collaboration between patients, their families, and the care team.

Doolin and colleagues. (2011) credit Foote Hospital in Jackson, Michigan, as the first to implement a formal hospital policy supporting family presence during resuscitation. They offer a strong review of the literature guiding family presence, including a review of attitudes and beliefs of patients, caregivers, and family members and historical issues associated with hospital policies concerning family presence. A strong advocacy role for APRNs in promoting policies that support family presence and other evidence-based interventions in critical care areas is needed.

Progression and development of rapid response teams

RRTs have emerged over the past 10 years as a means to improve patient safety and reduce failure to rescue situations. Sonday, Grecsek, and Casino (2010) reviewed the role of NPs in the application of RRTs, describing an approach driven by an ACNP model. The authors observed that this approach provides for patient-centered care by relying on expert assessment, critical thinking, and medical management skills rather than static protocol-driven management. In a primary physician/ICU nurse mode, Buist *et al.* (2002) retrospectively analyzed the patient outcomes associated with the implementation of a medical emergency team following unexpected cardiac arrests in hospitals. Examining data from 1996 compared with 1999, they found significant reductions in cardiac arrests and reductions in mortality from 77 to 55% following the introduction of medical emergency teams within the hospital. Comparative odds ratio for cardiac arrest with the team in place was 0.50 (0.35–0.73) (Buist *et al.*, 2002).

The use of integrated systems has grown in the intensive care environment. Tarassenko, Hann, and Young (2006) examined the use of integrated monitoring systems for early warning of patient deterioration and activation of RRTs. In one evaluation of a system designed to trigger activation of the team, an early warning system trended five vital sign measures and data fusion to create a single status measure. Patients' heart rate, blood pressure, oxygen saturation, skin temperature, and respiratory rate were combined to produce this single measure. Most alerts were found to be valid but other important measures of evaluation, including mental status and urine output, remained dependent on regular assessments.

Cherry and colleagues (2009) examined a response team designed to activate for a series of patient conditions, including changes in vital signs, cardiac rhythm, mental status, oxygenation decline, altered fluid status, and symptoms such as chest pain, dyspnea, or stroke signs. After implementation, improved outcomes included timeliness of response of the team within 10 min and significant reductions in non-ICU cardiac arrests.

Critical care practice continues to evolve and the role of advanced practice nursing in patient care continues to grow and be refined. While practice patterns and financial issues often dictate the implementation of these roles at the bedside, advanced practice nurses will increasingly play a role in surveillance, treatment, and safety of critically ill patients in the future.

References

Altmiller, G. (2011) Quality and safety education for nurses competencies and the clinical nurse specialist role: implications for preceptors. *Clinical Nurse Specialist*, **25** (1), 28–32.

American Association of Critical-Care Nurses (AACN) (2013a) *Website for Clinical Practice Alerts and Evidence-Based Practice*, http://www.aacn.org/wd/practice/content/practicealerts.pcms?menu=practice (accessed July 12, 2014).

American Association of Critical-Care Nurses (AACN) (2013b) *Website for Certification Information*, http://www.aacn.org/wd/certifications/content/selectcert.pcms?menu=certification&lastmenu (accessed July 12, 2014).

American Nurses Certification Corporation (ANCC) (2013) *Certification Overview*, http://www.nursecredentialing.org/Certification (accessed July 12, 2014).

Andrews, F.J. and Nolan, J.P. (2006) Critical care in the emergency department: monitoring the critically ill patient. *Emergency Medicine Journal*, **23**, 561–564.

APRN Joint Dialogue Group Report (2008) *A Consensus Model for APRN Regulation: Licensure, Accreditation, Certification & Education*. APRN Consensus Work Group & the National Council of State Boards of Nursing APRN Advisory Committee, https://www.ncsbn.org/Consensus_Model_Report.pdf (accessed July 12, 2014).

Becker, D., Kaplow, R., Muenzen, P.M., and Hartigan, C. (2006) Activities performed by acute and critical care advanced practice nurses: American Association of Critical-Care Nurses study. *American Journal of Critical Care*, **15**, 130–148.

Benner, P., Hughes, R.G., and Sutphen, M. (2008) Clinical reasoning, decisionmaking, and action: thinking critically and clinically, in *Patient Safety and Quality: An Evidence-Based Handbook for Nurses* (ed. R.G. Hughes), Agency for Healthcare Research and Quality, Rockville, pp. 103–125.

Buist, M.D., Moore, G.E., Bernard, S.A. *et al.* (2002) Effects of a medical emergency team on reduction of incidence and mortality from unexpected cardiac arrests in hospital: preliminary study. *British Medical Journal*, **324**, 387–390.

Burman, M.E., Hart, A.M., Conley, V. *et al.* (2009) Reconceptualizing the core of nurse practitioner education and practice. *Journal of the American Academy of Nurse Practitioners*, **21**, 11–17.

Cherry, K., Martinek, J., Esleck, S. *et al.* (2009) Developing and evaluating a trigger response system. *Joint Commission Journal on Quality and Patient Safety*, **35** (6), 331–338.

Cobb, S.E. and Kutash, M. (2011) A study to describe perceptions of ARNP roles in an acute care setting. *The Journal for Nurse Practitioners*, **7** (5), 378–384.

Cooper, M.A., Lindsay, G.M., Kinn, S., and Swann, I.J. (2002) Evaluating emergency nurse practitioner service: a randomized controlled trial. *Journal of Advanced Nursing*, **40** (6), 721–730.

D'Agostino, R. and Halpern, N.A. (2010) Acute care nurse practitioners in oncologic critical care: the Memorial Sloan-Kettering Cancer Center experience. *Critical Care Clinics*, **26**, 207–217.

Davidson, J.E., Powers, K., Hedayat, K.M. *et al.* (2007) Clinical practice guidelines for support of the family in the patient-centered intensive care unit: American College of Critical Care Medicine task force 2004–2005. *Critical Care Medicine*, **35**, 605–622.

Doolin, C.T., Quinn, L.D., Bryant, L.G. *et al.* (2011) Family presence during cardiopulmonary resuscitation: using evidence-based knowledge to guide the advanced practice nurse in developing formal policy and practice guidelines. *Journal of the American Academy of Nurse Practitioners*, **23**, 8–14.

Fleischman, R.K., Meyer, L., and Watson, C. (2011) Best practices in creating a culture of certification. *AACN Advanced Critical Care*, **22** (1), 33–49.

Funk, M. (2011) As health care technology advances: benefits and risks. *American Journal of Critical Care*, **20**, 285–291.

Hamric, A.B., Spross, J.A., and Hanson, C.M. (2009) *Advanced Practice Nursing: An Integrative Approach*, Saunders Elsevier, St. Louis.

Happ, M.B., Swigart, V.A., Tate, J.A. *et al.* (2007) Family presence and surveillance during weaning from prolonged mechanical ventilation. *Heart & Lung*, **36** (1), 47–57.

Haupt, M.T., Bekes, C.E., Brilli, R.J. *et al.* (2003) Guidelines on critical services and personnel: recommendations based on a system of categorization of three levels of care. *Critical Care Medicine*, **31**, 2677–2683.

Henneman, E.A. and Cardin, S. (2002) Family-centered critical care: a practical approach to making it happen. *Critical Care Nurse*, **22**, 12–19.

Henneman, E.A., Gawlinski, A., and Giuliano, K.K. (2012) Surveillance: a strategy for improving patient safety in acute and critical care units. *Critical Care Nurse*, **32**, e9–e18.

Hoffman, L.A., Tasota, F.J., Zullo, T.G. *et al.* (2005) Outcomes of care managed by an acute care nurse practitioner/attending physician team in a subacute medical intensive care unit. *American Journal of critical Care*, **14**, 121–130.

Howie, J.N. and Erickson, M. (2002) Acute care nurse practitioners: creating and implementing a model of care for an inpatient general medical service. *American Journal of Critical Care*, **11**, 448–458.

Hravnak, M., Edwards, L., Clontz, A. *et al.* (2008) Defining the incidence of cardiorespiratory instability in patients in step-down units using an electronic integrated monitoring system. *Archives of Internal Medicine*, **168** (2), 1300–1308.

Hughes, R.G. (ed) (2008) *Patient Safety and Quality: An Evidence-Based Handbook for Nurses*, Agency for Healthcare Research and Quality, Rockville.

Institute of Medicine (2001) *Crossing the Quality Chasm: A New Health System for the 21st Century*, The National Academies Press, Washington, DC.

Kaplow, R. (2011) The value of certification. *AACN Advanced Critical Care*, **22**, 25–32.

Kelly, L.A. (2009) *Surveillance in the Acute Care Setting: Latent Variable Development and Analysis*. Unpublished dissertation, http://www.nursing. arizona.edu/Library/Kelly_Lesly_Dissertation. pdf (accessed July 12, 2014).

Kleinpell, R.M. (ed.) (2013) *Outcome Assessment in Advanced Practice Nursing*, 3rd edn, Springer Publishing Company, New York.

Kleinpell, R.M. and Goolsby, M.J. (2006) 2004 American Academy of Nurse Practitioner National Nurse Practitioner Sample Survey: focus on acute care. *Journal of the American Academy of Nurse Practitioners*, **18**, 393–394.

Kleinpell, R.M. and Hudspeth, R.S. (2013) Advanced practice nursing scope of practice for hospitals, acute care/critical care, and ambulatory care settings: a primer for clinicians, executives, and preceptors. *AACN Advanced Critical Care*, **24**, 23–29.

Kleinpell, R.M., Ely, E.W., and Grabenkort, R. (2008) Nurse practitioners and physician assistants in the intensive care unit: an evidence-based review. *Critical Care Medicine*, **36** (10), 2888–2897.

Kleinpell, R.M., Hanson, N.A., Buchner, B.R. *et al.* (2008) Hospitalist services: an evolving opportunity. *The Nurse Practitioner*, **33** (5), 9–10.

Leeman, J., Baernholdt, M., and Sandelowski, M. (2007) Developing a theory-based taxonomy of methods for implementing change in practice. *Journal of Advanced Nursing*, **58** (2), 191–200.

Mallory, G.A. (2010) Professional nursing societies and evidence-based practice: strategies to cross the quality chasm. *Nursing Outlook*, **58**, 279–286.

Mantzoukas, S. and Watkinson, S. (2006) Review of advanced nursing practice: the international literature and developing the generic features. *Journal of Clinical nursing*, **16**, 28–37.

National Association of Clinical Nurse Specialists in Collaboration with Other Stakeholders/Partners (NACNS) (2009) *Core Practice Doctorate Clinical Nurse Specialist (CNS) Competencies*, http://www. nacns.org/docs/CorePracticeDoctorate.pdf (accessed July 12, 2014).

National Task Force on Quality Nurse Practitioner Education (2012) *Criteria for Evaluation of Nurse Practitioner Programs*, National Organization of Nurse Practitioner Faculties, Washington, DC.

Newhouse, R.P., Dearholt, S.L., Poe, S.S. *et al.* (2007) *Johns Hopkins, Nursing Evidence-Based Practice Model*, Sigma Theta Tau International, Indianapolis.

Penz, K.L. and Bassendowski, S.L. (2006) Evidence-based nursing in clinical practice: implications for nurse educators. *The Journal of Continuing Education in Nursing*, **37** (6), 250–254.

Peterson, S.R. and the Ad Hoc Committee on Rural Trauma, ACS Committee on Trauma (2002) *Interfacility Transfer of Injured Patients: Guidelines for Rural Communities*, http://www.facs.org/trauma/publications/ ruralguidelines.pdf (accessed July 12, 2014).

Sakr, M., Angus, J., Perrin, J. *et al.* (1999) Care of minor injuries by emergency nurse practitioners or junior doctors: a randomised controlled trial. *Lancet*, **354**, 1321–1326.

Schmidt, L.A. (2010) Making sure: registered nurses watching over their patients. *Nursing Research*, **59**, 400–406.

Society of Critical Care Medicine (SCCM) (2013a) *Critical Care Statistics*, http://www.sccm.org/Communications/Pages/CriticalCareStats.aspx (accessed July 12, 2014).

Society of Critical Care Medicine (SCCM) (2013b), http://www.sccm.org/About-SCCM/Pages/default.aspx (accessed July 12, 2014).

Society of Hospital Medicine (2012) *Hospital Focused Practice*, http://www.hospitalmedicine.org/Content/NavigationMenu/Membership2/HospitalFocusedPractice/Hospital_Focused_Pra.htm (accessed July 12, 2014).

Sonday, C., Grecsek, E., and Casino, P.D. (2010) Rapid response teams: NPs lead the way. *The Nurse Practitioner*, **35** (5), 40–45.

Tarassenko, L., Hann, A., and Young, D. (2006) Integrated monitoring and analysis for early warning of patient deterioration. *British Journal of Anaesthesia*, **97**, 64–68.

Titler, M.G., Kleiber, C., Steelman, V.J. *et al.* (2001) The Iowa model of evidence-based practice to promote quality care. *Critical Care nursing Clinics of North America*, **13**, 497–509.

Wade, C.H. (2009) Perceived effects of specialty nurse certification: a review of the literature. *AORN*, **89** (1), 183–192.

Weinstein, D.F. (2002) Duty hours for resident physicians—tough choices for teaching hospitals. *The New England Journal of Medicine*, **347** (16), 1275–1278.

Young, D. and Griffiths, J. (2006) Clinical trials of monitoring in anaesthesia, critical care and acute ward care: a review. *British Journal of Anaesthesia*, **97**, 39–45.

Yousef, K., Pinsky, M.R., DeVita, M.A. *et al.* (2012) Characteristics of patients with cardiorespiratory instability in a step-down unit. *American Journal of Critical Care*, **21** (5), 344–350.

CHAPTER 2

Vital measurements and shock syndromes in critically ill adults

Kathy J. Booker[1] and Laura Kierol Andrews[2]

[1] School of Nursing, Millikin University, Decatur, IL., USA
[2] Yale School of Nursing, Orange, CT., USA

Monitoring basic vital signs

Analysis of vital signs is a cornerstone of management of the critically ill adult patient. Subtle changes that might represent normal shifts in a healthy person may signal early decline for those in critical states. Monitoring vital signs is one of the most common techniques employed continuously in critical care units and careful attention should be given to setting alarms so that they are informative and not overly sensitive. Alarms that continually discharge have a negative influence on care and may be turned off as a nuisance, placing patients at increased risk. Due to the complexity of direct care needs, nurses may find it difficult to be attentive to monitoring systems at all times even when caring for patients one-on-one. An American Association of Critical Care Nurses (AACN) practice alert on alarm management was issued in 2013, recommending careful attention to appropriate skin preparation for electrodes, customization of alarms in bedside monitoring systems to patient condition and surveillance needs (AACN, 2013).

Interestingly, how often to monitor and record vital signs has been studied infrequently. In addition, the use of continuous monitoring and trending capabilities of bedside systems requires considerable foresight and evaluation due to errors in monitoring from patient movement, loose electrodes, and other technical issues. In a systematic review of vital sign measurement in hospitalized patients, Evans, Hodgkinson, and Berry (2001) noted that most recommendations for frequency are based on expert opinion and tradition with little research-based support for monitoring frequency linked to patient outcomes. Schumacher (1995) studied 766 postoperative patients' vital sign monitoring and recommended measurements 15 min after return from postanesthesia units, followed by 30 min × 2, 1 h, then every 4 h × 4. These recommendations continue to be employed in postoperative management today and further research is needed, particularly evaluations of frequency of intermittent methods as harbingers of patient decline.

Evans, Hodgkinson, and Berry (2001) also reviewed the literature support for the addition of a fifth vital sign, including the potential addition of nutritional status, body mass index, spirometry, orthostatic blood pressure (BP) changes, pulse oximetry, and smoking status. Of these, pulse oximetry showed considerable promise as an addition that may influence patient outcomes (Evans, Hodgkinson, and Berry, 2001; Mower et al., 1995). Pulse oximetry is also continuously monitored in most intensive care unit (ICU) settings today and is often a key driver of respiratory interventions. Others have suggested that pain assessment should comprise the fifth vital sign (Merboth and Barnason, 2000).

Future research should examine the effectiveness of increasingly integrated monitoring systems used for critically ill patients to reveal best practices for stronger surveillance and prevention of physiological decline. In addition to the rapid growth of interventional protocols, technology has allowed for most vital measures to be continuously displayed but accuracy is not always ensured. With thousands of devices and specialized equipment in use in ICUs across the nation, safety and error prevention must be a priority (Mattox, 2012). Device safety involves many important aspects and clinicians must also master technology evaluation skills and continuously question the accuracy produced by bedside and clinical evaluation systems (Henneman, 2010). Implementation of new technologies should always require careful system analysis and involvement of nurses caring for patients.

In this chapter, standard vital sign measurement and monitoring for shock states will be reviewed. Overall, the level of evidence for frequency of standard vital measures, while ubiquitous to critical care, remains relatively low. Overuse of technology increases staff workload while not necessarily improving patient outcomes. Selected elements of shock management and the growth of care bundling have moved evidence-based practices to moderate to high levels. Monitoring and surveillance in shock conditions will also be reviewed.

Temperature monitoring

In general, the most accurate methods of measuring temperature include the use of pulmonary artery thermistor, urinary bladder probes, esophageal probes, and rectal probes (O'Grady et al., 2008). The Heart and Stroke Foundation of Canada (2004) issued a position statement recommending bladder probe or pulmonary artery thermistor monitoring as the most reliable in therapeutic hypothermia patient monitoring. Most ICU monitoring systems have probe connectors so that core temperature may be continuously trended with other bedside vital signs data although today pulmonary artery catheters are used less frequently in medical ICU settings.

Temperature monitoring options range from standard intermittent oral, skin, and tympanic measurements to more invasive continuous monitoring with sensors placed in the bladder or bloodstream as part of indwelling catheters

or centrally introduced lines, respectively. Accuracy varies considerably by site. Generally, lines placed internally in core areas such as the bladder or bloodstream are more reflective of core temperature than those measured externally; however, accuracy ranges should be evaluated carefully through a review of manufacturing guidelines and confirmed by multiple techniques when temperature change is in question. O'Grady et al. (2008) published guidelines for the evaluation of new temperature elevations in critically ill patients, recommending that assessment findings rather than automatic blood testing should guide management of temperature elevations. Blood culture techniques and interventions should be implemented when noninfectious causes for temperature elevation have been ruled out (O'Grady et al., 2008) (see Table 2.1).

Schey, Williams, and Bucknall (2010) reviewed the use of core–peripheral temperature gradients and the research linking this measure to cardiac output changes. This technique has been studied for decades but well-designed definitive studies have not been conducted. In the largest study of over 1000 patients in cardiogenic shock, distal skin temperature was not prospectively obtained; cold periphery and oliguria served as comparisons to cardiac output and no direct correlation was found (Menon et al., 2000). Schey, Williams, and Bucknall (2010) noted that confounding factors, small enrollments, and the use of multiple methods precludes firm conclusion on the use of core–peripheral temperature comparative research and requires further prospective trials. Frequency outcome of vital sign monitoring remains understudied.

Hypothermia

Over the last decade, the use of hypothermia protocols following cardiac arrest has evolved as an evidence-based practice (Nolan et al., 2003; Nunnally et al., 2011; Peberdy et al., 2007; Sasson et al., 2011). Improved neurological outcomes have been associated with the use of hypothermia protocols initiated as soon as possible following successful return of spontaneous circulation (ROSC) (Kagawa et al., 2010; Nunnally et al., 2011; Peberdy et al., 2007; see

Table 2.1 Recommendations for measuring temperature.

Elements	Monitoring recommendation
Method and site	Temperature measurements are most accurate using intravascular, esophageal, or bladder measurements (Nonose et al., 2012; O'Grady, 2008); Tympanic measurement should be avoided in adults and children (Frommelt, Ott, & Hays, 2008; Nonose et al., 2012). Rectal, oral, and tympanic may be used, in that order if IV, esophageal or bladder monitoring not available (O'Grady et al., 2008). Axillary measurements, temporal artery estimates, and chemical dot thermometers should not be used in the ICU (level 2). Rectal thermometers should be avoided in neutropenic patients (O'Grady et al., 2008) (level 2).
Monitoring device	Safe practices of calibration and manufacturer's guidelines should be followed (O'Grady et al., 2008) (level 2).
Infection control	All practices associated with temperature monitoring must employ safe instrument usage and handwashing to limit microorganism spread (O'Grady et al. 2008) (level 2).
Site	The site of temperature measurement should be recorded with the temperature in the chart (level 1).
Further diagnostics	A new onset of temperature >/= 38.8 °C or < 36 °C <36 °C is a reasonable trigger for a clinical assessment but not necessarily a laboratory or radiologic evaluation for infection (O'Grady et al., 2008) (level 3).

Adapted from Frommelt et al., 2008; Nonose et al., 2012; O'Grady et al., 2008.
Society of Critical Care Medicine recommendation levels: level 1, convincingly justifiable on scientific evidence alone; level 2, reasonably justifiable by available scientific evidence and strongly supported by expert critical care opinion; level 3, adequate scientific evidence is lacking but widely supported by available data and expert critical care opinion (O'Grady et al., 2008), p. 1331–1332.

Table 2.2). The targeted temperature for hypothermia is 32–34°C for 12–24 h post cardiac arrest following ROSC (Nunnally et al., 2011; Peberdy et al., 2007). While no specific method of hypothermia induction is endorsed, the published guidelines support the use of cooled isotonic fluid administration and external cooling devices and monitoring of core temperature during the cooling phase. Prospective trials have also validated cooling patients using ice packs, intravascular cooling devices, and selected treatments such as cooling helmets or cool air tents (Australian Resuscitation Council, New Zealand Resuscitation Council, 2011). Additional critical monitoring elements include prevention and detection of shivering and early management and treatment of seizures.

Since cardiac arrest often accompanies acute myocardial infarction, rapid assessment of electrocardiogram (ECG) changes and rapid percutaneous intervention are recommended if indicated following ROSC. While outcomes have improved with the use of hypothermia treatment, implementation of rapid hypothermia protocols is not consistent across the nation and research is still needed for optimal treatment protocols for managing patients following cardiac arrest.

Complications of cooling

Hypothermia treatment can be risky and has been associated with arrhythmias, infection, and coagulopathies (Heart and Stroke Foundation of Canada, 2004). During hypothermia, shivering is a frequent complication and must be treated to prevent increased cerebral oxygen consumption, which is estimated to be elevated by 40–100% during shivering episodes (Sinclair and Andrews, 2010). In alert patients, progressive symptoms that can be expected include the following:

- 36 °C: Increased activity attempting to warm up, skin pale, numb, and waxy, muscles tense, fatigue, and signs of weakness.
- 34–35 °C: Uncontrolled intense shivering, still alert but movements uncoordinated, and pain and discomfort due to coldness.
- 31–33 °C: Shivering slows or stops, muscles stiffen, mental confusion, apathy, speech slowed and slurred, breathing slower and shallow, drowsiness.
- <31 °C: Skin cold, pupils dilated, extreme weakness, slurred speech, exhausted, denies problems, resists help, gradual loss of consciousness, and progressive respiratory arrest and arrythmias (Nunnally et al., 2011, p. 1116).

Table 2.2 Beneficial effects of hypothermia.

Possible mechanisms underlying the beneficial effects of hypothermia

Secondary injury	Explanation	Time frame after injury
Prevention of apoptosis*	Ischaemia can induce apoptosis and calpain-mediated proteolysis. This process can be prevented or reduced by hypothermia.	Hours to days to even weeks
Reduced mitochondrial dysfunction and improved energy homeostasis[†]	Mitochondrial dysfunction is a frequent occurrence in the hours to days after a period of ischaemia and may be linked to apoptosis. Hypothermia reduces metabolic demands and may improve mitochondrial function.	Hours to days
Reduction in free radical production[†]	Production of free radicals (for example, superoxide, peroxynitrite, hydrogen peroxide, and hydroxyl radicals) is typical in ischaemia. Mild-moderate (30–35 °C) hypothermia is able to reduce this event.	Hours to days
Mitigation of reperfusion injury[†]	Cascade of reactions following reperfusion, partly mediated by free radicals but with distinctive and various features. These are suppressed by hypothermia.	Hours to days
Reduced permeability of the blood-brain barrier and the vascular wall and reduced oedema formation*	Blood-brain barrier disruptions induced by trauma or ischaemia are moderated by hypothermia. The same effect occurs with vascular permeability and capillary leakage.	Hours to days
Reduced permeability of cellular membranes (including membranes of the cell nucleus)[†]	Decreased leakage of cellular membranes with associated improvements in cell function and cellular homeostasis, including decrease of intracellular acidosis and mitigation of DNA injury.	Hours to days
Improved ion homeostasis	Ischaemia induces accumulation of excitatory neurotransmitters such as glutamate and prolonged excessive influx of Ca^{2+} into the cell. This activates numerous enzyme systems (kinases) and induces a state of hyperexcitability (exitotoxic cascade) that can be moderated by hypothermia.	First minutes to 72 h
Reduced metabolism*	Cellular oxygen and glucose requirements are reduced by 5–8% per °C decrease in temperature.	Hours to days
Depression of the immune response and various potentially harmful pro-inflammatory reactions*	Sustained destructive inflammatory reactions and secretion of pro-inflammatory cytokines after ischaemia can be blocked or mitigated by hypothermia.	First hour to 5 days
Reduction in cerebral thermopooling*	Some areas in the brain have significantly higher temperatures than others. These differences can increase dramatically after injury with temperatures that are up to 2–3 °C higher in injured areas. Hyperthermia can increase the damage to the injured brain cells; this is mitigated by hypothermia.	Minutes to days
Anticoagulant effects*	Microthrombus formation may add to brain injury after CPR. Anticoagulant effects of hypothermia may prevent thrombus formation.	Minutes to days
Suppression of epileptic activity and seizures*	Seizures after ischaemic injury or trauma are common and may add to injury. Hypothermia has been shown to mitigate epileptic activity.	Hours to days

BioMed Central Open Access: Sinclair, HL, & Andrews PJD (2010). Bench-to-bedside review: hypothermia in traumatic brain injury, 2010, **14**, 204.
This table summarises potential beneficial effects of hypothermia, based on experimental and clinical studies.
*Some supporting evidence.
†Animal studies only.
CPR, cardiopulmonary resuscitation.

In patients who are comatose, heavily sedated, or treated with paralytic agents, shivering may be detected by additional monitoring, such as bispectral index (BIS) or electroencephalography (EEG) monitoring. The use of supplemental monitoring has not been extensively studied and evidence-based guidelines are not available.

Hypothermia induction is used for other applications in the critical care unit, including control of severe hyperthermia induced by heatstroke or malignant hyperthermia (MH), a condition induced by a relatively rare triggered response to anesthesic agents. In addition, patients with neurologic conditions will often have markedly elevated temperatures and require cooling methods for temperature reduction. These conditions have diverse pathophysiologies but treatment is focused on safe, rapid cooling. Hoedemaekers *et al.* (2007) examined cooling methods in 50 adult ICU patients randomized to one of the following five methods: (1) conventional cooling with cold intravenous infusions of 30 ml/kg, ice or coldpacks; (2) cooling with water-circulating blankets; (3) air-circulating cooling blankets; (4) gel-coated external cooling device using pads on the back, abdomen, and bilateral thighs; and (5) intravascular cooling using a single lumen central venous catheter inserted into the femoral vein. If the target temperature was not reached within 12 h, ice and cold packs were supplemented. Hoedemaekers *et al.* (2007) found that three cooling methods were equally effective: water-circulating blankets, gel-coated pads, and intravascular cooling. Endovascular cooling was most effective at maintaining the target temperature but was also the most costly method. Conventional cooling was shown to be ineffective, with failure to reach target temperature in 60% of patients randomized to this method.

Hyperthermia

Perspectives on fever have changed over the past decade. In non-life-threatening infections, fever may exert a delimiting effect on the clinical condition, reducing days of infection. However, in severe infections and sepsis, the overwhelming state of systemic inflammation and preexisting state of health make it difficult to predict clinical outcomes associated with fever and its treatment (Hasday, Fairchild, and Shanholtz, 2000; Kiekkas *et al.*, 2010). The impact of fever on ICU mortality in 239 critically ill adult patients without cerebral damage was studied and 44.8% developed fever (Kiekkas *et al.*, 2010). Fever alone was not associated with mortality; however, peak temperature at the higher ranges (39.3 °C and above) resulted in higher ICU mortality than in those with lower peak temperatures. Not surprisingly, patients with higher acuity scores had significantly higher mortality ($p < 0.001$, OR 1.24). In this study, the lower respiratory tract (76.9%), blood (15.4%), and abdomen (7.7%) accounted for the primary sites of infectious causes of fever. Given the associated increased metabolic demand associated with hyperthermia, conclusive evidence favoring antipyretic therapy remains unclear but temperature elevations continue to drive therapy and remain an important assessment parameter. Kiekkas *et al.* (2010) also evaluated the effect of temperature elevation (≥38.3 °C) on other vital parameters, including hourly changes in mean arterial pressure (MAP), heart rate (HR), and arterial oxygen saturation during a 24-h period of intensive care hospitalization. While statistically significant changes in HR and MAP were found in this study, the authors noted that the changes were generally minor and did not represent clinically significant morbidity.

Heatstroke management

Patients admitted for heatstroke present special challenges in care. Bouchama, Dehbi, and Chaves-Carballo (2007) studied the hemodynamic management associated with cooling patients with life-threatening heatstroke, defined as temperatures over 40 °C. Cooling by immersion in iced water was found to be safe and effective in young healthy adults with exertional heatstroke, but posed problems in elderly patients. Ice packs, wet gauze sheets, and use of fans were recommended as reasonable alternatives in elderly patients and consideration given to the use of dantrolene as an adjunct therapy. In addition, Bouchama, Dehbi, and Chaves-Carballo (2007) recommended avoiding antipyretics in heatstroke patients due to the potential of coagulopathy or liver injury but identified the paucity of research in this area.

Malignant hyperthermia

A condition that may develop during the delivery of anesthetics or in the early postoperative period, MH is a critical emergency with elevations of core temperature. Temperature elevations may reach 44 °C (Rosenberg *et al.*,

2007). Triggers include all inhaled anesthetics and succinylcholine, a muscle relaxant. MH is found in all parts of the world and is linked to an autosomal-dominant defect. Larach *et al.* (2010) reported initial MH signs as hypercarbia, sinus tachycardia, and masseter spasm along with elevations in temperature. Generalized musculoskeletal contraction and the development of respiratory and/or metabolic acidosis are common. Dantrolene remains the primary interventional treatment for this condition, is lifesaving, and, with careful fluid management during an acute episode of MH, dantrolene is generally safe (Brandom *et al.*, 2011; Glahn *et al.*, 2010). Published guidelines for recognizing and managing MH crisis including monitoring temperature and treating complications have been advanced by the European Malignant Hyperthermia Group (Glahn *et al.*, 2010). These include measurement of core temperature, routine anesthetic monitoring, IV access, and minimum 24-h monitoring in the ICU. Kim (2012) also reviewed these guidelines, including clinical sign recognition (see Table 2.3).

Table 2.3 Clinical signs associated with malignant hyperthermia. (Adapted from Glagn *et al.* 2010).

Early signs
 Metabolic
 • Inappropriately elevated CO_2 production (raised end-tidal CO_2 on capnography, tachypnoea if breathing spontaneously).
 • Increased O_2 consumption.
 • Mixed metabolic and respiratory acidosis.
 • Profuse sweating.
 • Mottling of skin.
 Cardiovascular
 • Inappropriate tachycardia.
 • Cardiac arrhythmias (especially ectopic ventricular beats and ventricular bigemini).
 • Unstable arterial pressure.
 Muscle
 • Masseter spasm if succinylcholine has been used.
 • Generalized muscle rigidity.
Later signs
 • Hyperkalaemia.
 • Rapid increase in core body temperature.
 • Grossly elevated blood creatine phosphokinase levels.
 • Grossly elevated blood myoglobin levels.
 • Dark-colored urine due to myoglobinuria.
 • Severe cardiac arrhythmias and cardiac arrest.
 • Disseminated intravascular coagulation.

Reproduced by permission of the Korean Society of Anesthesiologists. © Korean Society of Anesthesiologists.

Heart rate monitoring

In general, continuous HR monitoring in the ICU setting is obtained by bedside electrocardiography (ECG). The use of ECG is ubiquitous in the ICU and its application allows for HR, rhythm, and waveform analysis and monitoring. Often, changes in rhythm accompany rate changes and, together, offer a more comprehensive evaluation of the patient's underlying status. In most bedside monitoring systems, respiratory rate and waveforms are also measured and displayed on the oscilloscope using the application of the ECG electrodes. The selection of monitoring leads should be guided by the published standards by Drew and Funk (2006), according to the patient's condition and level of risk for arrhythmia, myocardial ischemia, and/or prolongation of repolarization waveforms (QT interval monitoring) (also see Chapter 4).

The American Association of Critical Care Nurses (2013) has advanced practice alerts guiding alarm management, dysrhythmia monitoring, and ST segment monitoring. For general arrhythmia monitoring, lead V_1 and lead II are recommended for monitoring wide QRS activity and atrial waveforms, respectively. ST segment monitoring guidelines and selection of leads depend on the bedside monitoring system available. Generally, for patients at risk of ST segment changes due to acute coronary syndromes, the more leads that are available for continuous monitoring, the greater is the accuracy of detection of ST segment changes. If the ST fingerprint is known, monitoring the leads that have already shown changes during ischemia is recommended. If these are not available, and with monitoring systems in which only two leads are available for continuous ST segment monitoring, leads III and V_5 are recommended. The practice alerts detail how to select and place leads accurately and how to detect changes at the J point of the QRS. Setting alarms to achieve notification without overactivation may be difficult, especially in patients with intermittent bundle branch block (BBB), pacemakers, or frequent ventricular arrhythmias. Table 2.4 represents the settings currently recommended by evidence. In most cases, clinical guidelines do not specify the timing of monitoring, for example,

Table 2.4 Published class I ECG monitoring guidelines for heart rate and rhythm changes in adults.

Parameter	Recommendation	Source
Heart rate variations		
ST segment changes during early phase of acute coronary syndrome (ACS)	1–2 mm above and below ST baseline at 60 ms from J-point	AACN (2009); Drew et al. (2004)
Post cardiac arrest	ECG monitoring until an implantable cardioverter defibrillator (ICD) is inserted or until correction of cause of arrest is made and resolved	Drew et al. (2004)
Unstable coronary syndromes or newly diagnosed high-risk coronary lesions	Continous monitoring until revascularization; continue at least 24 h if arrhythmias or ST changes occur post intervention	Drew et al. (2004)
Post cardiac surgery	Minimum 24–48 h postop for all patients; for those at risk of atrial fibrillation, monitoring should continue until discharge	Drew et al. (2004)
Post ICD or pacemaker	12–24 h post implantation	Drew et al. (2004)
Patients with Mobitz II block, complete heart block, or new-onset BBB in the setting of acute myocardial infarction (AMI)	Monitor until resolution of block or definitive treatment	Drew et al. (2004)
Acute heart failure or pulmonary edema	Monitor until acute heart failure and/or hemodynamically significant arrhythmias have been resolved for 24 h	Drew et al. (2004)
Intensive care patients	Monitor until weaned from mechanical ventilation and hemodynamically stable	Drew et al. (2004)
Conscious sedation or anesthesia	Continue until patient is awake, alert, and hemodynamically stable	Drew et al. (2004)
QTc interval (normal: <0.46 in women, <0.45 in men)	QTc (corrected for heart rate) should be monitored in all patients on antidysrhythmics, antibiotics, antipsychotics, or other drugs that prolong QT interval; severe bradycardia, hypokalemia, hypomagnesemia, or drug overdose (AACN, 2008, p. 1)	AACN (2008); Drew et al. (2004) (class I monitoring recommendations: patients on proarrhytmic drugs known to cause Torsades de Pointes; new-onset bradycardia, OD from potentially proarrhythmic agent, patients with severe hypokalemia or hypomagnesemia, p. 14)

Adapted from Drew et al. (2004).
Class I recommendations are defined as those in which cardiac monitoring is indicated in most, if not all, participants in this group (p. 2722)

QT interval measurements when continuous monitoring is unavailable. See Chapter 4 for further information on ECG monitoring.

Blood pressure monitoring

BP measurement is very important in monitoring critically ill patients, particularly during shock states and management of changing critical conditions. BP varies in a diurnal pattern, with the highest pressures generally evidenced between 6:00 a.m. and 12:00 a.m. and lowest during sleep (Ogedegbe and Pickering, 2010). While critically ill adults are frequently supine during measurement, variation in measurement can be attributed to arm position relative to torso location and inappropriate cuff sizes selected for patients (especially in obese or very thin individuals; see Table 2.5). Rates of cuff deflation after inflation should be 2–3 mmHg/s (Ogedegbe and Pickering, 2010). An important surveillance issue in BP measurement involves analysis of systems and efficiency and accuracy of measurements in individual patients. Many factors influencing the detection and surveillance of BP will be reviewed.

Table 2.5 Cuff sizes for appropriate BP measurement in adults.

Cuff size	Arm circumference (cm)	Recommended cuff size (cm)
Small adult	22–26	22 length; 12 width
Adult	27–34	30 length; 16 width
Large adult	35–44	36 length; 16 width
Adult thigh	45–52	42 length; 16 width

Adapted from Pickering *et al.* (2005).

Oscillometric blood pressure measurement

The measurement of BP has changed considerably in recent years. The original detection of Korotkoff sounds at the brachial artery using a standard BP cuff, mercury manometer, and stethoscope has gradually been replaced in many critical care and step-down units by automated oscillometric measurement incorporated into bedside monitoring systems. Oscillometric techniques may raise concerns in measurement due to many technical measurement and pulse detection errors that arise in critically ill patients. Tholl, Forstner, and Anlauf (2004) identified issues with oscillometric device accuracy, including calibration, vascular wall elasticity, and size of the artery measured, noting that atherosclerotic vascular changes have a measurement effect on the oscillogram. Ogedegbe and Pickering (2010) identified measurement restrictions that have been evaluated with arm measurement of BP. These include the effects of posture, body positioning, cuff size, and the occurrence of cuff-inflation hypertension. If cuffs are not positioned carefully, oscillometric systems may maintain long inflation cycles, particularly in patients with arrhythmias. As cuff inflation cycles are prolonged, discomfort and bruising may develop, especially when BPs are labile and frequent measurements are conducted.

Aneroid measurement

Portable BP measurement may be conducted intermittently using aneroid sphygmomanometers and many of these systems are wall-mounted although their use has declined over the last decade. These devices have largely replaced mercury manometers due to safety concerns from mercury. Aneroid sphygmomanometers have been generally found to be reliable and accurate although they are sensitive to mechanical damage and should be calibrated annually (Tholl, Forstner, and Anlauf, 2004). With reductions in the use of mercury due to environmental concerns, Tholl, Forstner, and Anlauf (2004) reviewed the issues associated with accuracy using aneroid and oscillometric techniques. These include proper calibration, aneroid susceptibility to inaccuracies following damage, technique of cuff placement and measurement at the level of the heart, arrhythmia influence on oscillometric measurement, and proper deflation rates and rest periods during repeated measurements (Tholl, Forstner, and Anlauf, 2004).

Arterial pressure measurement

The accuracy of noninvasive blood pressure (NIBP) compared with arterial invasive monitoring has been studied in critically ill overweight adults, finding both oscillometric and auscultatory measurements to significantly underestimate BP compared to direct arterial measurement (Araghi, Bander, and Guzman, 2006). One serious inaccuracy of NIBP concerns proper patient arm circumference measurement and appropriate selection of cuff size to obtain an accurate BP. Most unstable patients will have invasive placement of arterial catheters, generally in the radial or femoral artery. In critically ill patients, continuous arterial pressure monitoring allows for rapid evaluation of the effects of therapies and changing clinical condition. However, invasive placement can be affected by many errors, including dislodgement, positional waveforms, requirements of appropriate line management and tubing issues, as well as catheter dynamics. Serious risks accompany the use of intraarterial catheters, including bleeding, infection, and phlebitis. Risks versus benefits of methods of monitoring must be weighed in the selection process. Evaluation of accuracy of methods should be the responsibility of all team members caring for the patient. Mignini, Piacentini, and Dubin (2006) found minimal bias and strong precision in mean BP assessments comparing femoral and radial arterial catheters in critically ill adults, considering the values obtained as clinically interchangeable.

Although comparisons were made during the first 5 min following insertion in this study, the use of radial catheters is common practice in most ICUs given increased risk of infection with femoral line placements. See Chapter 5 for further analysis of arterial pressure monitoring.

Newer noninvasive methods are under investigation for trending BP. Nowak *et al.* (2011) evaluated the use of a finger cuff technology (Nexfin®, Bmeye, The Netherlands) to trend BP and HR in emergency department patients. The Nexfin device uses a small finger cuff with the capacity to display systolic pressure, diastolic pressure, and MAP with estimation of other hemodynamic parameters. Nowak *et al.* (2011) compared the BP and HR variables to those obtained using routine cardiac and NIBP monitoring in 40 adult patients using a convenience sample with data collected every 15 min for 2 h. Both Bland-Altman (mean bias = 0.87) and Pearson correlation (0.83, $p < 0.0001$) suggested acceptable agreement in the derived values. Although further study is under way, newer technologies that provide less invasiveness and may be better tolerated by patients will continually emerge. However, investigation of these devices in patients with arrhythmias such as atrial fibrillation is still needed.

Respiratory monitoring

Most respiratory rate monitoring is conducted through plethysmography sensed by the chest and abdominal movements of the electrodes of the cardiac monitoring system. In many critical care units, respiratory rates are also monitored by ventilator systems designed to track pressure and airflow during each respiratory cycle or by monitoring end-tidal carbon dioxide levels. Generally, patients with advanced respiratory failure who require ventilatory support have multiple methods available for tracking respiratory rate and rhythm (see Chapter 3). These are most important in evaluating trends over time and allowing for the establishment of alarms to alert practitioners to declining or excessive respiratory rates or changing rhythms, such as those associated with Cheyne–Stokes respiration. Table 2.6 demonstrates common abnormal respiratory patterns that are often associated with pulmonary pathologies in the ICU.

Respiratory assessment and monitoring includes active evaluation of patient effort and depth of breathing, use of accessory muscles, expansion and shape of the chest, ability to speak during breathing effort, evidence of nasal flaring, symmetrical chest expansion, and auscultatory findings (Higginson and Jones, 2009). The use of pulse oximetry and capnography enhances respiratory assessment, supplements assessment findings, and guides therapy, often saving costs by allowing for reduction in arterial blood gas sampling during periods of relative stability.

Capnography

Capnography is available in a number of configurations and is widely used during surgery and postanesthesia care. In the ICU, capnography is generally used for intubated, ventilated patients and most bedside monitoring systems have modules for continuous capnogram display. Widespread use of color-changing CO_2 detectors is recommended when a patient is first intubated to ensure that an endotracheal tube is correctly placed. Ccapnography provides waveform displays of the entire ventilatory cycle and continuous numeric display of the partial pressure of end-tidal CO_2 (Pet CO_2). Advantages of continuous capnography include the ability to monitor all phases of inhalation and exhalation, thus allowing for analysis of changes in ventilation, perfusion, and dead space trending (Cheifetz and Myers, 2007). Indications for continuous capnography include monitoring effects of conscious sedation, endotracheal tube displacement, quality of resuscitation efforts, and early findings in patients with pulmonary emboli or low cardiac output conditions (Johnson, Schweitzer, and Ahrens, 2011). Monitoring and surveillance require a strong understanding of the relationship of phases of the ventilatory cycle to the exhalation of CO_2, the clinical condition of the patient, and the ability to troubleshoot alarm conditions. Capnogram waveform analysis is covered in Chapter 3. No randomized trials have shown definitively that continuous monitoring of capnography in intensive care patients alters

Table 2.6 Abnormal respiratory patterns commonly seen in ICU patients.

Assessing Respiratory Patterns

Type	Waveform	Characteristics	Possible Clinical Condition
Eupnea		Normal rate and rhythm for adults and teenagers (12–20 breaths/ min)	Normal pattern while awake
Bradypnea		Decreased rate (<12 breaths/ min); regular rhythm	Normal sleep pattern; opiate or alcohol use; tumor; metabolic disorder
Tachypnea		Rapid rate (>20 breaths/min); hypoventilation or hyperventilation	Fever; restrictive respiratory disorders; pulmonary emboli
Hyperpnea		Depth of respirations greater than normal	Meeting increased metabolic demand (e.g., sepsis, MODS, SIRS, and exercise)
Apnea		Cessation of breathing; may be intermittent	Intermittent with CNS disturbances or drug intoxication; obstructed airway; respiratory arrest if it persists
Kussmaul		Deep, rapid (>20 breaths/ min), sighing, labored	Renal failure, DKA, sepsis, shock
Cheyne-Stokes		Alternating patterns of apnea (10–20 sec) with periods of deep and rapid breathing. Lesions located bilaterally and deep within cerebral hemispheres	Heart failure, opiate or hypnotic overdose, thyrotoxicosis, dissecting aneurysm, subarachnoid hemorrhage, IICP, aortic valve disorders; may be normal in older adults during sleep
Central neurogenic hyperventilation		Rapid (>20 breaths/min), deep, regular. Lesions of midbrain or upper pons thought to be source of pattern	Primary injury (ischemia, infarction, space-occupying lesion); secondary injury (IICP, metabolic disorders, drug overdose)

From Baird and Bethel (2011). © Elsevier.

outcomes although capnography has been a standard of care in intraoperative monitoring for decades (Cheifetz and Myers, 2007).

Shock conditions in critically ill adults

Shock conditions pose critical threats to life and are regularly treated in critical care units worldwide. Over the years, categories of shock have been defined in a number of ways and the evolution of shock management has changed as more effective early assessment and treatments have been studied. At the core of all forms of shock, threats to tissue perfusion and circulatory pathology generally lead to tissue dysoxia (Antonelli *et al.*, 2008). While traditional definitions of shock have focused on hypotension as a major sign, Antonelli and colleagues (2007) published recommendations guiding international shock management with less emphasis on the presence of hypotension and more on fluid responsiveness, markers of regional and microcirculatory changes, and hemodynamic monitoring, including advanced monitoring recommendations for the management of critical care patients in shock states (Antonelli *et al.*, 2007). These include the following:

• The definition for shock is advanced as "a life-threatening, generalized misdistribution of blood flow resulting in failure to deliver and/or utilize adequate amounts of oxygen leading to tissue dysoxia" (p. 577) and not based on the presence of hypotension.

- Measurement of markers of impaired oxygenation should supplement history and physical exam data including markers of inadequate perfusion such as reductions in $ScvO_2$ or SvO_2, increased blood lactate, or increased base deficit (p. 578).
- Resuscitation efforts should target an MAP of 40 mmHg until bleeding is surgically controlled; MAP of 90 mmHg for traumatic brain injury; and for all other shock states, MAP targets are over 65 mmHg (p. 578).
- While preload measures alone should not be used to predict fluid responsiveness in shock states, low levels of static measures (central venous pressure (CVP), right atrial pressure (RAP), pulmonary artery occlusion pressure (PAOP)) should trigger immediate fluid resuscitation efforts in shock states and fluid challenges are recommended to assess fluid responsiveness. Based on literature support, 250 cc of crystalloid or colloid equivalent, or straight leg raise maneuver should target a rise in CVP of at least 2 mmHg, and dynamic measures of fluid responsiveness are not recommended, although it is acknowledged that there may be advantages in selected patient conditions (p. 580).
- Routine measurement of cardiac output is not recommended although ECG or measurement in patients with ventricular failure and persistent shock may be appropriate (p. 581).
- Invasive BP measurement is recommended for refractory shock but use of the pulmonary artery catheter is not endorsed (p. 584).
- Goal-directed therapy for septic shock is supported within 6 h or less and use of supranormal oxygen delivery systems is not recommended.

Further published guidelines for sepsis management and goal-directed therapy will be covered in the following section on septic shock. Important management of shock states requires symptom and response analysis regardless of type of monitoring devices employed. Frequency of vital sign monitoring has generally not been elucidated in the majority of studies or guidelines and must be guided by assessment findings in individual patients and response to treatment.

Cardiogenic shock

Cardiogenic shock is associated with poor peripheral perfusion secondary to primary alterations in heart chamber filling or pumping functions. This may develop as a result of systolic or diastolic dysfunction or a combination of these. Functional or structural changes induced by trauma, pulmonary embolism, pericarditis, cardiac tamponade, or primary pulmonary conditions such as tension pneumothorax may also result in cardiogenic shock and death. Acute myocardial infarction, particularly anterior wall involvement, is a common cause of cardiogenic shock, particularly if papillary muscles or extensive myocardial damage is sustained.

The frequency of cardiogenic shock has significantly declined over the past decade, primarily attributed to improvement in reperfusion interventional cardiology techniques (Babaev et al., 2005). While overall hospital mortality associated with cardiogenic shock significantly declined from 1995 to 2004, rates remained near 50% and application and adherence to the published standards, particularly early interventional strategies, were stressed (Babaev et al., 2005). Published guidelines for management of acute ST elevation and non-ST elevation acute myocardial infarction continue to evolve (Jneid et al., 2013; O'Gara et al., 2013). These are extensively reviewed by national experts associated with the American Heart Association and the American College of Cardiology Foundation and employ evidence-based practice guideline protocols advanced by these organizations. Class I recommendations for treatment of cardiogenic shock include emergency revascularization (percutaneous intervention or coronary artery bypass graft (CABG)) or fibrolytic therapy in patients unable to undergo interventional strategies and class II recommendations including the use of intraaortic balloon pump (IABP) (O'Gara et al., 2013). In a 10-year study of outcomes associated with cardiogenic shock, Babaev et al. (2005) found that nearly 30% of 7356 patients presented with cardiogenic shock while the remaining 70%

developed shock after hospital arrival. Trends associated with improved outcomes were identified with increasing frequency of percutaneous coronary intervention (PCI), while CABG and IABP use remained relatively stable over the study period.

In the most recent updates on interventions for acute ST-segment elevated myocardial infarction (STEMI), the strongest evidence included early recognition of acute myocardial infarction, with a 12-lead measurement and transmittal by emergency medical personnel, expedited hospital intervention (door to balloon times of 90 min or less; door to thrombolytic intervention in areas without rapid access to interventional cardiology procedures of 30 min or less), early pharmacologic interventions to reduce cardiac workload and platelet aggregation, oxygen administration, and pain management (O'Gara et al., 2013). While most hospitals have developed extensive emergency medical system (EMS) and emergency department (ED) protocols that require coordination and intervention across disciplinary units within the hospital, many geographical areas find implementation of published guidelines difficult due to remote access or EMSs that are primarily staffed by volunteers. Collaboration across disciplines is critical to ensure best outcomes for patients at risk of cardiogenic shock and to decrease mortality and morbidity associated with cardiac emergencies.

Anaphylactic shock

Anaphylaxis develops following a hypersensitivity reaction to an antigen, mediated by immunoglobulin E. Medication, foods, insect bites or stings, and radiocontrast dyes are all common antigens that can affect humans (Sheikh, 2013; Soar and Unsworth, 2009). In anaphylactic shock, widespread vasodilation and increased capillary permeability are triggered, with fatality ranging from 1:1000 exposures to food products to 1:100 for medication or insect venom (Kirkbright and Brown, 2012).

Clinical guidelines for the treatment of anaphylaxis have been published (Soar et al., 2008). These include a focus on assessment of airway, breathing, circulation, disability, and exposure (ABCDE), administration of intramuscular adrenalin, and evaluation and protection of patients including long-term management strategies for self-administration of adrenalin (Soar et al., 2008). Figure 2.1 demonstrates the anaphylaxis algorithm in these guidelines. Treatment for anaphylaxis involves administration of adrenalin 1:1000, dosed at 0.01 mg/kg IM with a maximum initial dose of 0.5 mg (Kirkbright and Brown, 2012).

Most patients will receive intravenous (IV) therapy with normal saline. Patients should be kept recumbent to enhance venous return and observed for complications as recurrent symptoms may occur in association with late-phase reactions (Thompson, 2012). Patients with known allergens and prior anaphylaxis should be instructed to carry adrenalin autoinjectors for rapid treatment following future exposure (Soar and Unsworth, 2009). Education is an important aspect of care following anaphylaxis. Despite the widespread use of adrenalin for treatment, no randomized controlled trials have demonstrated its effectiveness; due to its long use and clinical effectiveness in treatment, a Cochrane review noted that ethical issues and the unexpected development of anaphylaxis will continue to restrict the use of controlled trials guiding anaphylactic management (Sheikh et al., 2012). Frequency of monitoring remains understudied but generally minimal monitoring includes ECG, pulse oximetry, and all vital signs until the risk of recurrent anaphylaxis has passed (Soar and Unsworth, 2009). All areas of hospital care should be equipped to treat anaphylaxis.

Hypovolemic shock

Burns, traumatic injuries, and hemorrhagic shock are commonly treated in the ICU but may also develop secondary to operative complications. Over the past decade, more aggressive monitoring and assessment techniques have been identified with the realization that hypotension, skin turgor changes, and capillary refill testing are often nonspecific or late signs in the development of shock conditions (Thompson, 2012). Methods to monitor fluid responsiveness are covered in Chapter 5. Generally, hypovolemic shock states develop in rapidly sequential patterns when hemorrhage and burns occur (see also Chapter 10).

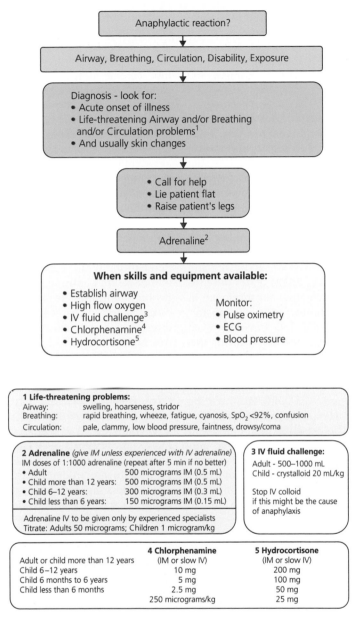

Figure 2.1 Anaphylaxis algorithm. Reprinted with permission from The exact terminology for reprinting states that the credit should read as follows Reprinted with permission from The Royal Australian College of General Practitioners from Kirkbright, SJ, Brown, SGA. Anaphylaxis–Recognition and management. AFP 2012; 41:366–70. © The Royal Australian College of General Practitioners/Australian Family Physician.

It is important to assess preload changes and determine responsiveness to fluid administration, and early detection of the source of the shock is critical to management. Pacagnella *et al.* (2013) conducted a systematic review on indicators for severity of hypovolemic shock and found considerable variation among etiologies. The use of the shock index (SI) was found to be a helpful tool in assessing cardiovascular effects of shock. The SI is calculated as the ratio between the HR and systolic blood pressure (SBP) and allows for a rapid analysis of cardiovascular response to fluid loss. Clear guidelines for complex patient management, including management of patients with concurrent heart failure and trauma, remain difficult and require careful assessment and evaluation.

Sepsis syndromes

Sepsis, as an antecedent of severe sepsis, septic shock, and multisystem organ dysfunction syndrome (MODS), is a complex process that is defined by the presence of systemic inflammatory responses to the presence of an infection and represents the tenth leading cause of death in the United States (CDC, 2010). Data show that sepsis affects more than 1.1 million persons and carries mortality rates as high as 59% (Angus *et al.*, 2001; Legrand *et al.*, 2012; Zuber *et al.*, 2012). Rates of sepsis have increased despite the advancement in treatment options although increasing awareness and published guidelines have improved efforts and raised awareness for reducing this condition. It is imperative to recognize sepsis in its early stages in order to improve outcomes (Dellinger *et al.*, 2013). In accordance, *The Surviving Sepsis Campaign* was instituted by health-care organizations to define sepsis and its sequelae, and to set forth monitoring and therapy guidelines to improve early recognition and treatment for patients at risk for sepsis (Dellinger *et al.*, 2008). These guidelines focused on initial management, identification, and treatment of the infectious source (Dellinger *et al.*, 2008). Initial management recommendations include management strategies for the first 6 h, effective methods of diagnosis, antibiotic treatment, source of the infection, and infection control. Helpful tables summarize hemodynamic support, fluid management, and the use of steroids and other medications. These guidelines have been incorporated into most orientation and educational programs for the preparation of critical care practitioners. Key management strategies include identifying the source of the infection and eliminating it, containing the systemic response, supporting macrocirculatory needs and hemodynamics, and overall support of failing systems. Assessment findings in early sepsis may be seen in Table 2.7.

Monitoring for tissue hypoperfusion is critical. Jones and Puskarich (2011) identifed global variables that reflect tissue hypoperfusion. These include hypotension, tachycardia, low cardiac output, mottled skin, delayed capillary refill, altered mental state, hyperlactemia, and low mixed venous and central oxygen saturation. Giuliano and Kleinpell (2005) surveyed experienced and/or certified critical care nurses and physicians in attendance at two major conferences in 2003 to determine the clinical practice of continuous monitoring for patients with sepsis. Over 600 participants identified invasive BP monitoring, pulse oximetry, cardiac monitoring, and pulmonary artery pressure monitoring as the top continuous monitoring parameters for this patient population. While options for hemodynamic management continue to evolve, sepsis monitoring continues to be complex and the essential role of early intervention and goal-directed therapy has improved outcomes in this highly lethal shock condition. The critical role of a multidisciplinary approach to care is essential to positive outcomes.

While hemodynamic monitoring in sepsis remains controversial, it may augment trends in a patient's condition and tolerance of rapidly changing hemodynamic treatment and management effects. CVP changes remain part of published sepsis guidelines and additional techniques are under investigation to move toward less invasive and more continuous measurement of cardiac output and stroke volume (see Chapter 5).

SIRS, sepsis, and septic shock

Systemic inflammatory response syndrome (SIRS), the prequel to sepsis, is an overwhelming, multisystem response to injury or infection. This response was initially defined by the presence of two or more of four clinical indicators including temperature (>38 °C or <36 °C); HR (>90 beats/min); respiratory changes (>20 breaths/min or $PaCo_2 < 32$ mmHg); and white blood cell elevations (>12 × 10^9/l or <4 × 10^9/l, or >10% bands) (ACCP-SCCM Consensus Conference, 1992; Dellinger *et al.*, 2013). SIRS in the presence of a presumed or documented infection denotes *sepsis* (Table 2.8), while *severe sepsis* indicates the presence of sepsis-induced

Table 2.7 Assessment findings in sepsis.

Clinical indicator	Cause
Cardiovascular	
Increased HR (>100 heats/min)	Sympathetic/autonomic nervous system (SANS) stimulation
Decreased BP (<90 mm Hg systolic, MAP <65 mm Hg)	Vasodilation
CO >7 L/min; CI >4 L/min/ m², CVP <8 mm Hg	Hyperdynamic state secondary to SANS stimulation
Svo_2 >80%	Decreased utilization of oxygen by cells
PAWP usually <6 mm Hg	Venous dilation; decreased preload
SVR < 900 dynes/sec/cm⁻⁵	Vasodilation
Strong, bounding peripheral pulses	Hyperdynamic cardiovascular system (Keeping in mind that patients with preexisting cardiomyopathy will have minimal elevation in cardiac output and drop in SVR)
Respiratory	
Tachypnea (>20 breaths/min) and hyperventilation	Metabolic acidosis which leads to decreases in cerebrospinal fluid pH that stimulate the central respiratory center
Crackles	Interstitial edema occurring with increased vascular permeability
$Paco_2$ <35 mm Hg	Tachypnea and hyperventilation
Dyspnea	Increased respiratory muscle work
Renal	
Decreased urine output (<0.5 ml/kg/hr)	Decreased renal perfusion
Increased specific gravity (1.025–1.035)	Decreased glomerular filtration rate
Cutaneous	
Flushed and warm skin	Vasodilation
Metabolic	
Increasing body temperature (usually >38.3°C [100.9°F])	Increased metabolic activity; release of pyrogens secondary to invading microorganisms; release of interleukin-1 by macrophages
pH < 7.35	Metabolic acidosis occurring with accumulation of lactic acid
Lactic acid >2.5	
↑ Blood sugar or at times profound hypoglycemia	Release of glucagon; insulin resistance
Neurologic	
Changes in LOC	Decreased cerebral perfusion and brain hypoxia
Fluid	
↑ Fluid retention	↑ ADH, ↑ aldosterone

ADH, Antidiuretic hormone; beats/min, beats per minute; *BP*, Blood pressure; *CO*, cardiac output; *CI*, cardiac index; *HR*, heart rate; *LOC*, level of consciousness; *PAWP*, pulmonary artery wedge pressure; *SVR*, systemic vascular resistance.
From Baird and Bethel (2011, p. 925). © Elsevier.

tissue hypoperfusion (altered mental status, shock, oliguria, or elevated lactic acid level) or acute organ dysfunction. *Septic shock* is defined as persistent sepsis-induced hypotension (SBP < 90 mmHg, MAP < 70 mmHg, or SBP drop of >40 mmHg from baseline), despite adequate volume resuscitation (Dellinger *et al.*, 2008). The goal is to implement care bundles within 3 and 6h of symptom presentation to prevent shock development. In the latest international guidelines, recommendations are for serum lactate, blood culture administration prior to antibiotics, and administration of 30 ml/kg crystalloids for hypotension or serum lactate ≥4 mmol/l (Dellinger *et al.*, 2013). Within 6h, recommendations include vasopressor support for hypotension unresponsive to fluid administration, and implementation of central venous pressure monitoring with CV oxygen saturation and reassessment of lactate levels, if initially elevated. Targeted results of resuscitation efforts within 6h are to attain a CVP of 8–12 mmHg, mean arterial pressure ≥65 mmHg, $ScvO_2$ ≥70% or SvO_2 ≥65% and normalization of serum lactate in those with prior elevation (Dellinger *et al.*, 2013, p. 587).

Table 2.8 Risk factors for sepsis.

Age extremes (<1 year and >65 years)

Diabetes
Cancer
Chronic kidney disease
End-stage liver disease
Malnutrition
Alcoholism
Tobacco use
Hypothermia
Mechanical ventilation
Invasive or surgical procedures
Presence of drug-resistant organisms
Prior use of broad-spectrum antibiotics
Major trauma
Major burns
Presence of invasive lines/tubes
• Urinary catheters
• Endotracheal tubes
• Central venous access devices
Immunocompromised
HIV/AIDS
• Neutropenia
• Immunosuppressives
• Chemotherapeutic agents
• Organ transplantation

Adapted from Balk (2000); Esper and Martin (2009); Kleinpell (2003); Legrand et al. (2012); Picard et al. (2006).

Morbidity and mortality due to severe sepsis and septic shock develops from dysfunctional or failed end-organ systems such as the kidneys, lungs, heart, brain, and liver. See also Sepsis in the Immunocompromised Host (Chapter 11).

Monitoring and treatment priorities in sepsis syndromes

Priorities for care of patients admitted to critical care units include the following:

1 Identify patients at high risk for sepsis.
2 Stabilize patients with severe sepsis or septic shock.
3 Administer antimicrobial agents to rapidly eradicate microorganisms following cultures.
4 Treat infectious foci, such as drainage of abscesses/purulent collections or surgical repair of enteric injuries.
5 Monitor acid–base, oxygenation, and hemodynamics in order to optimize oxygen delivery to tissues and organs.

Table 2.9 Sepsis diagnostic criteria.

General

• Hypothermia (core temperature <36 °C)
• Fever (core temperature >38 °C)
• Tachycardia (>90 beats/min)
• Tachypnea (respiratory rate (RR) > 20 breaths/min)
• Confusion or altered mental status
• Hyperglycemia (>120 g/dl in nondiabetics)
• Positive fluid balance (>20 ml/kg over 24 h)

Hematologic/inflammatory
• Leukocytosis (WBC > 12 000)
• Leukopenia (WBC < 4 000)
• Immature neutrophils (bands > 10%)
• Thrombocytopenia (platelets < 100 000/μl)

Hemodynamics
• Hypotension (MAP < 70 mmHg, or SBP < 90 mmHg, or SBP decrease of >40 mmHg from baseline)
• Cardiac index >3.5 l/min/m²
• SvO_2 > 70%
• Stroke volume variation (>15%)

Organ dysfunction
• Acute kidney injury (creatinine rise >0.5 mg/dl or urine output <0.5 ml/kg/h ideal body weight (IBW))
• Arterial hypoxemia (PaO_2/FiO_2 < 300)
• Coagulopathy (international normalized ratio (INR) > 1.5 or partial thromboplastin time (PTT) > 60 s)
• Ileus
• Hyperbilirubinemia (total bilirubin >4 g/dl)
• A-a gradient >20 mmHg

Tissue perfusion
• Lactic acidosis (>1 mmol/l)
• Anion gap >20
• Mottled extremities or decreased capillary refill

Adapted from Cunneen and Cartwright (2004); Levy et al. (2003).

Sepsis diagnosis

The diagnosis of sepsis is based on the assessment of risk factors and clinical signs and symptoms (Table 2.9). An accurate history and physical exam are the first steps in assessing patients for risk factors and signs and symptoms of sepsis. This may be difficult if patients are confused, medicated, or have cognitive impairments that preclude accurate history taking. Use of family, significant others, emergency personnel, and medical records can aid in obtaining a complete history (Nduka and Parrillo, 2011). Signs of early sepsis, such as change in vital signs, restlessness, lethargy, and confusion are often subtle or attributed to other etiologies.

Body temperature

Abnormal body temperature is often the first indicator that a patient is septic. Normal body temperature is 37 °C (+/−1 °C), but this can vary +/−0.5–1 °C based on circadian rhythm and menstrual cycle. Strenuous exercise can increase core temperature by up to 3 °C. Environmental factors such as specialty beds, room temperature, therapeutic interventions (drugs, dialysis, and cardiopulmonary bypass), and endocrine disorders (hypo- or hyperthyroidism) can also alter core temperatures (O'Grady et al., 2008). Hyperthermia in response to infection is defined as a core temperature greater than either 38.3 or 38 °C in neutropenic patients. Almost half of critical care patients have at least one febrile episode and these episodes are more common in medical patients. Hypothermia is defined as a body temperature below 36 °C and may be noted more commonly in surgical patients, the elderly, or in patients with hepatic failure, heart failure, open abdominal wounds, or major burns. Mortality has been associated with both hyper- and hypothermia, but occurs more frequently in hypothermic patients (Laupland et al., 2012; O'Grady et al., 2008).

The presence of hyper- or hypothermia should trigger investigation for cause, especially if signs of SIRS, organ dysfunction, or hypotension are present, but consideration should be given to the accuracy of temperature measurements. The American College of Critical Care Medicine and the Infectious Diseases Society of America have published guidelines ranking pulmonary artery, urinary bladder catheter, and esophageal and rectal probes as more accurate than infrared ear, temporal artery, oral and axillary thermometers (O'Grady et al., 2008).

Cultures

Blood cultures should be obtained when there are clinical signs of infection or sepsis. Approximately 50% of blood cultures are negative in septic patients. Therefore, care should be taken in collecting two sets prior to initiation of antibiotics, transporting the samples to the laboratory, and meticulously preparing the skin with 2% alcoholic chlorhexidine or 1–2% tincture of iodine. A volume of at least 10 ml/ bottle should be drawn, with one being drawn from any vascular access device in place for more than 48 h (Dellinger et al., 2008; O'Grady et al., 2008). Common microorganisms found in cultures guide practitioners in selecting empiric antimicrobial prescriptions.

Intravascular catheters

The risk of bloodstream infections is highest with noncuffed temporary venous hemodialysis catheters, followed by central lines, then peripherally inserted central venous lines and implanted ports (Mermel et al., 2009). It is recommended that short-term catheters be removed and cultured if line sepsis is considered. Cultures of catheter insertion sites are notoriously nonspecific and carry a high frequency of false positive results, leading to unnecessary device removal. Diagnosis of a catheter-related bloodstream infection is based on positive cultures of identical microorganisms from both intracutaneous (5–7 cm of intradermal catheter section) and blood cultures. Central catheters in patients who have fever alone (no signs of SIRS or sepsis) should not routinely be removed (O'Grady et al., 2008).

Other infectious complications in critically ill adults

Pulmonary infections

Hospital-associated pneumonia (HAP) is the second most common nosocomial infection and carries a mortality rate of up to 50%, with the majority of ICU patients having ventilator-associated pneumonia (VAP) (ATS/IDSA, 2005; Dellit et al., 2008; Labeau et al., 2008). VAP carries a mortality rate of 24–76% (Dellit et al., 2008; Kollef et al., 2008). Classic signs and symptoms of pneumonia include fever, cough, leukocytosis, and dyspnea (Andrews, 2012). In ICU patients with endotracheal tubes, fever and increased sputum production (or changes in pulmonary secretion characteristics) are often the first indicators of pneumonia (O'Grady et al., 2008). Sputum sampling for culture and sensitivity can be accomplished via expectoration, tracheal suctioning, or bronchial alveolar lavage (with or without bronchoscopy), with the goal of obtaining a lower respiratory tract sample without oral secretion contamination. Bronchoscopy is particularly helpful in obtaining adequate samples with *Mycobacterium* (acid-fast bacilli), *Pneumocystis jiroveci* (or pneumocystis pneumonia (PCP), *Aspergillus* and other fungi, *Legionella* species, and cytomegalovirus (CMV). Urinary antigen testing for *Streptococcus pneumoniae* and *Legionella* (serogroup 1) is available and provides rapid turnaround times for results. Direct fluorescent antibody staining for influenza A and B should be performed on patients with respiratory symptoms during the fall and into the spring months (Mandell *et al.*, 2007).

A chest radiograph should be obtained to assess for pulmonary infiltrates. Although the anteroposterior (AP portable) method is safer for patients, its reliability may be limited due to patient positioning, disease process, and equipment. If there is difficulty in interpreting the portable film, high-resolution computerized tomography can aid in the diagnosis of complex pleural effusions, cavitations, and posterior and inferior lung disorders (O'Grady *et al.*, 2008). A diagnostic thoracentesis should be performed to obtain cultures in patients with pleural effusions associated with adjacent infiltrates to rule out aerobic or anaerobic empyemas (Mandell *et al.*, 2007).

Urinary tract infections

Bacteriuria due to bladder catheterization is the most common health-care-associated infection in the world. The conventional signs and symptoms of urinary tract infection (UTI) include dysuria, hesitancy, frequency, chills, hematuria, malaise, new onset fever, and flank or pelvic pain but are often absent in ICU patients. Bacteriuria and candiduria as the cause of bacteremia and sepsis occur in less than 15% of patients. Patients with tract obstructions (calculi, tumors), hydronephrosis, renal transplantation, tract manipulation procedures or surgery, neutropenia, and who reside in long-term care facilities have the highest rates of UTI-associated bacteremia. Mortality from bacteremic UTI is cited at approximately 13% (Hooton *et al.*, 2010; O'Grady *et al.*, 2008).

Diagnosis of catheter-associated UTI (CAUTI) is based on the presence of bacteria or fungus, at concentrations over 10^3 colony-forming units (CFU)/ml in patients with signs and symptoms of UTI, and in patients without signs or symptoms or who are wearing a condom catheter, concentrations over 10^5 CFU/ml. The presence of pyuria (WBC $> 10^5$/ml) in a urine sample is indicative of UTI only in community-acquired infections and should not be used in diagnosis. Additionally, cloudy or foul-smelling urine in catheterized patients is not a sensitive indicator of UTI (Hooton *et al.*, 2010; O'Grady *et al.*, 2008). Prevention of CAUTI should be targeted and indwelling catheters removed at the earliest time of stabilization of critically ill septic patients.

In summary, the care of patients with suspected shock syndromes has become increasingly protocolized and systematic. Further outcome studies are warranted to decipher best practices across a range of patient conditions and attributes.

Monitoring during transport

Maintaining the same level of diligent surveillance during transport is often challenging to ICU staff. Day (2010) reviewed the goals of safe transport, including the maintenance of ICU standards of care and monitoring during transport, ensuring patient stability and avoiding complications while achieving the goals of obtaining quality diagnostic study or intervention. In general, if a patient is unstable, transporting should be avoided unless the diagnostic study or intervention is lifesaving. Drew *et al.* (2004) also addressed the imperative of continuous cardiac monitoring during transport equivalent to bedside monitoring in the ECG-monitoring practice standards.

Portable monitoring devices in many models of ICU bedside systems now allow for quick transport readiness. However, transport remains a risky endeavor for patients who are on life-support equipment and often requires the expertise of a cadre of critical care staff for successful monitoring and safety during transport.

Conclusion

Surveillance of vital signs is critical to care management in intensive care settings, particularly during treatment of shock conditions. While vital sign measurement and analysis is part of continual monitoring practices in the ICU, few studies have validated the most effective methods or frequency of monitoring. Given that considerable time is spent by nurses on equipment management, trending, and managing interventions based on vital signs, further research is needed to identify practices that are efficient and enhance good patient outcomes. Rapid treatment and complex management of shock states is critical to good outcomes. While considerable research on conditions such as sepsis and targeted temperature management has emerged in the past decade, further studies are needed, including basic examination of effective BP measurement using variable cuff types, and effectiveness and efficiency studies on all vital measurements. Especially needed are studies that examine measurement techniques that allow optimal discernment of vital changes and measurement systems that provide optimal analysis, enhance safety, and are well tolerated by critically ill patients. The use of technical equipment varies considerably in ICU settings. Nursing surveillance and management of these systems is critical to ensuring accurate data that capably guide therapy and care of critically ill adults.

References

ACCP-SCCM Consensus Conference (1992) Definitions of sepsis and multiple organ failure and guidelines for the use of innovative therapies in sepsis. *Critical Care Medicine*, **20**, 864–874.

American Association of Critical-Care Nurses (AACN) (2008) *AACN Practice Alert. Dysrhythmia Monitoring*, http://www.aacn.org/wd/practice/docs/practicealerts/dysrhythmia-monitoring.pdf?menu=aboutus (accessed July 24, 2014).

American Association of Critical-Care Nurses (AACN) (2009) *AACN Practice Alert. ST Segment Monitoring*, http://www.aacn.org/wd/practice/docs/practicealerts/st-segment-monitoring.pdf?menu=aboutus (accessed July 24, 2014).

American Association of Critical-Care Nurses (AACN) (2013) *Practice Alerts*, http://www.aacn.org/WD/Practice/Content/practicealerts.content?menu=Practice (accessed July 24, 2014).

American Thoracic Society and Infectious Diseases Society of American (ATS/IDSA) (2005) Guidelines for management of adults with hospital-acquired, ventilator-associated, and healthcare-associated pneumonia. *American Journal of Respiratory and Critical Care Medicine*, **181**, 388–419.

Andrews, L.K. (2012) Nursing management: patients with chest and lower respiratory tract disorders, in *Focus on Adult Health Medical-Surgical Nursing* (ed. L.H. Pellico), Wolters Kluwer/Lippincott Williams & Wilkins, Philadelphia, pp. 275–325.

Angus, D.C., Linde-Zwirble, W.T., Lidicker, J. *et al.* (2001) Epidemiology of severe sepsis in the United States: analysis of incidence, outcome, and associated costs of care. *Critical Care Medicine*, **29** (7), 1303–1310.

Antonelli, M., Levy, M., Andrews, P.J.D. *et al.* (2007) Hemodynamic monitoring in shock and implications for management. *Intensive Care Medicine*, **33**, 575–590.

Araghi, A., Bander, J.J., and Guzman, J.A. (2006) Arterial blood pressure monitoring in overweight critically ill patients: invasive or noninvasive? *Critical Care*, **10**, R64.

Australian Resuscitation Council, New Zealand Resuscitation Council (2011) Therapeutic hypothermia after cardiac arrest. ARC and NZRC guideline 2010. *Emergency Medicine Australasia*, **23**, 297–298.

Babaev, A., Frederick, P.D., Pasta, D.J. *et al.* (2005) Trends in management and outcomes of patients with acute myocardial infarction complicated by cardiogenic shock. *Journal of the American Medical Association*, **294**, 448–454.

Baird, M.S. and Bethel, S. (2011) *Manual of Critical Care Nursing*, Elsevier, St. Louis.

Balk, R.A. (2000) Severe sepsis and septic shock. Definitions, epidemiology, and clinical manifestations. *Critical Care Clinics*, **16** (2), 179–192.

Bouchama, A., Dehbi, M., and Chaves-Carballo, E. (2007) Cooling and hemodynamic management in heatstroke: practical recommendations. *Critical Care*, **11**, R54.

Brandom, B.W., Larach, M.G., Chen, M.S., and Young, M.C. (2011) Complications associated with the administration of dantrolene 1987 to 2006: a report from the North American Malignant Hyperthermia Registry of the Malignant Hyperthermia Association of the United States. *Anesthesia and Analgesia*, **112**, 1115–1123.

Centers for Disease Control and Prevention (CDC) (2010) *Ten Leading Causes of Death and Injury*,

http://www.cdc.gov/injury/wisqars/pdf/10LCID_
All_Deaths_By_Age_Group_2010-a.pdf (accessed
July 24, 2014).

Cheifetz, I.M. and Myers, T.R. (2007) Should every
mechanically ventilated patients be monitored
with capnography from intubation to extubation?
Respiratory Care, **52** (4), 423–442.

Cunneen, J. and Cartwright, M. (2004) The puzzle of
sepsis: fitting the pieces of the inflammatory
response with treatment. *AACN Clinical Issues*, **15**,
18–44.

Day, D. (2010) Keeping patients safe during intra-
hospital transport. *Critical Care Nurse*, **30**, 18–32.

Dellinger, R.P., Levy, M.M., Carlet, J.M. *et al.* (2008)
Surviving sepsis campaign: international guidelines for management of severe sepsis and septic
shock: 2008. *Critical Care Medicine*, **36**, 296–327.

Dellinger, R.P., Levy, M.M., Rhodes, A. *et al.* (2013)
Surviving sepsis campaign: international guidelines
for management of severe sepsis and septic shock:
2012. *Critical Care Medicine*, **41** (2), 580–637.

Dellit, T.H., Chan, J.D., Skerrett, S.J., and Nathens,
A.B. (2008) Development of a guideline for the
management of ventilator-associated pneumonia
based on local microbiologic findings and impact
of the guideline on antimicrobial use practices.
Infection Control Hospital Epidemiology, **29** (6),
525–533.

Drew, B.J. and Funk, M. (2006) Practice standards
for ECG monitoring in hospital settings: executive
summary and guide for implementation. *Nursing
Clinics of North American*, **18** (2), 157–168.

Drew, B.J., Califf, R.M., Funk, M. *et al.* (2004)
Practice standards for electrocardiographic monitoring in hospital settings: an American Heart
Association scientific statement from the Councils
on Cardiovascular Nursing, Clinical Cardiology,
and Cardiovascular Disease in the Young: endorsed
by the International Society of Computerized
Electrocardiology and the American Association of
Critical-Care Nurses. *Circulation*, **110**, 2721–2746.

Esper, A.M. and Martin, G.S. (2009) Extending
international sepsis epidemiology: the impact of
organ dysfunction. *Critical Care (London, England)*,
13 (1), 120.

Evans, D., Hodgkinson, B., and Berry, J. (2001) Vital
signs in hospital patients: a systematic review.
International Journal of Nursing Studies, **38**,
643–650.

Frommelt, T., Ott, C., and Hays, V. (2008) Accuracy
of different devices to measure temperature.
MEDSURG Nursing, **17**, 171–176; 182.

Giuliano, K.K. and Kleinpell, R. (2005) The use of
common continuous monitoring parameters. A
quality indicator for critically ill patients with
sepsis. *AACN Clinical Issues*, **16** (2), 140–148.

Glahn, K.P., Ellis, F.R., Halsall, P.J. *et al.* (2010)
Recognizing and managing a malignant hyper-
thermia crisis: guidelines from the European
Malignant Hyperthermia Group. *British Journal of
Anesthesiology*, **105**, 417–420.

Hasday, J.D., Fairchild, K.D., and Shanholtz, C.
(2000) The role of fever in the infected host.
Microbes and Infection, **2**, 1891–1904.

Heart and Stroke Foundation of Canada (2005)
CAEP position statement: therapeutic hypo-
thermia after cardiac arrest. ILCOR Advisory
Statement, October 2002. *CJEM*, **7**, 129.

Henneman, E.A. (2010) Patient safety and technology. *AACN Advanced Critical Care*, **20**, 128–132.

Higginson, R. and Jones, B. (2009) Respiratory
assessment in critically ill patients: airway and
breathing. *British Journal of Nursing*, **18**, 456–461.

Hoedemaekers, C.W., Ezzahti, M., Gerritsen, A., and
van der Hoeven, J.G. (2007) Comparison of cooling
methods to induce and maintain normo- and
hypothermia in intensive care unit patients: a prospective intervention study. *Critical Care*, **11**, R91.

Hooton, T.M., Bradley, S.F., Cardenas, D.D. *et al.*
(2010) Diagnosis, prevention, and treatment of
catheter-associated urinary tract infection in
adults: 2009 international clinical practice guidelines for the Infectious Diseases Society of America.
Clinical Infectious Diseases, **50**, 625–663.

Jneid, H. Alam, M., Virani, S.S., and Bozkurt, B.
(2013) Redefining myocardial infarction: what is
new in the ESC/ACCF/AHA/WHF third universal
definition of myocardial infarction? *Methodist
DeBakey Cardiovascular Journal*, **9**, 169–172.

Johnson, A., Schweitzer, D., and Ahrens, T. (2011)
Time the throw away your stethoscope?
Capnography: evidence-based patient monitoring
technology. *Journal of Radiology Nursing*, **30**, 25–34.

Jones, A.E. and Puskarich, M.A. (2011) Sepsis-
induced tissue hypoperfusion. *Critical Care Nursing
Clinics of North America*, **23**, 115–125.

Kagawa, E., Inoue, I., Kawagoe, T. *et al.* (2010)
Who benefits most from mild therapeutic hypothermia in coronary intervention era? A retrospective and propensity-matched study. *Critical
Care*, **14**, R155.

Kiekkas, P., Velissaris, D., Karanikolas, M. *et al.*
(2010) Peak body temperature predicts mortality
in critically ill patients without cerebral damage.
Heart & Lung, **39**, 208–216.

Kim, D.-C. (2012) Malignant hyperthermia. *Korean
Journal of Anesthesiology*, **63**, 395–401.

Kirkbright, S.J. and Brown, S.G.A. (2012) Anaphylaxis:
recognition and management. *Australian Family
Physician*, **41**, 366–370.

Kleinpell, R.M. (2003) The role of the critical care
nurse in the assessment and management of the

patient with severe sepsis. *Critical Care Nursing Clinics of North America*, **15** (1), 27–34.

Kollef, M.H., Morrow, L.E., Baughman, R.P. *et al.* (2008) Health care-associated pneumonia (HCAP): a critical appraisal to improve identification, management, and outcomes—proceedings of the HCAP Summit. *Clinical Infectious Diseases*, **46** (Suppl 4), S296–S334.

Labeau, S., Vandijck, D., Rello, J. *et al.* (2008) Evidence-based guidelines for the prevention of ventilator-associated pneumonia: results of a knowledge test among European intensive care nurses. *Journal of Hospital Infections*, **70** (2), 180–185.

Larach, M.G., Gronert, G.A., Allen, G.C. *et al.* (2010) Clinical presentation, treatment, and complications of malignant hyperthermia in North America from 1987 to 2006. *Anesthesia and Analgesia*, **110**, 498–507.

Laupland, K.B., Zahar, J., Adrie, C. *et al.* (2012) Determinates of temperature abnormalities and influence on outcome of critical illness. *Critical Care Medicine*, **40**, 145–151.

Legrand, M., Max, A., Peigne, V. *et al.* (2012) Survival in neutropenic patients with severe sepsis or septic shock. *Critical Care Medicine*, **40** (1), 43–49.

Levy, M.M., Fink, M.P., Marshall, J.C. *et al.* (2003) 2001 SCCM/ESICM/ACCP/ATS/SIS international sepsis definitions conference. *Critical Care Medicine*, **31**, 1250–1256.

Mandell, L.A., Wunderink, G., Anzueto, A. *et al.* (2007) Infectious Diseases Society of America/American Thoracic Society consensus guidelines on the management of community-acquired pneumonia in adults. *Clinical Infectious Diseases*, **44**, S27–S72.

Mattox, E. (2012) Medical devices and patient safety. *Critical Care Nurse*, **32**, 60–68.

Menon, V., Slater, I.N., White, H.D. *et al.* (2000) Acute myocardial infarction complicated by systemic hypoperfusion without hypotension: report of the SHOCK trial registry. *American Journal of Medicine*, **108**, 374–380.

Merboth, M.K. and Barnason, S. (2000) Managing pain: the fifth vital sign. *Nursing Clinics of North America*, **35** (2), 375–383.

Mermel, L.A., Allon, M., Bouza, E. *et al.* (2009) Clinical practice guidelines for diagnosis and management of intravenous catheter-related infections: update by the Infectious Diseases Society of America. *Clinical Infectious Diseases*, **49**, 1–45.

Mignini, M.A., Piacentini, E., and Dubin, A. (2006) Peripheral arterial blood pressure monitoring adequately tracks central arterial blood pressure in critically ill patients: an observational study. *Critical Care*, **10**, R43.

Mower, W.R., Sachs, C., Nicklin, E.L. *et al.* (1995) Effect of routine emergency department triage pulse oximetry screening on medical management. *Chest*, **108**, 1297–1302.

Nduka, O.O. and Parrillo, J.E. (2011) The patho-physiology of septic shock. *Nursing Clinics of North America*, **23**, 41–66.

Nolan, J.P., Morley, P.T., Vanden Hoek, T.L., and Hickey, R.W. (2003) Therapeutic hypothermia after cardiac arrest: an advisory statement by the Advanced Life Support Task Force of the International Liaison Committee on Resuscitation. *Circulation*, **108**, 118–121.

Nonose, Y., Sato, Y., Kabayama, H., Arisawa, A., Onodera, M., Imanaka, H., and Nishimura, M. (2012) Accuracy of recordered body temperature of critically ill patients related to measurement site: a prospective observational study. *Anaesthesia & Intensive Care*, **40**, 820–824.

Nowak, R.M., Sen, A., Garcia, A.J. *et al.* (2011) Noninvasive continous or intermittent blood pressure and heart rate patient monitoring in the ED. *American Journal of Emergency Medicine*, **29**, 782–790.

Nunnally, M.E., Jaeschke, R., Bellingan, G.J. *et al.* (2011) Targeted temperature management in critical care: a report and recommendations from five professional societies. *Critical Care Medicine*, **39**, 1113–1125.

O'Gara, P.T., Kushner, F.G., Ascheim, D.D. *et al.* (2013) ACCF/AHA guideline for the management of ST-elevation myocardial infarction: executive summary: a report of the American College of Cardiology Foundation/American Heart Association Task Force on Practice Guidelines. *Circulation*, **127**, 529–555.

Ogedegbe, G. and Picering, T. (2010) Principles and techniques of blood pressure measurement. *Cardiology Clinics*, **28**, 571–586.

O'Grady, N.P., Barie, P.S., Bartlett, J.G. *et al.* (2008) Guidelines for evaluation of new fever in critically ill adult patients: 2008 update from the American College of Critical Care Medicine and the Infectious Diseases Society of America. *Critical Care Medicine*, **36**, 1330–1349.

Pacagnella, R.C., Souza, J.P., Durocher, J. *et al.* (2013) A systematic review of the relationship between blood loss and clinical signs. *PLoS One*, **8** (3), e57594.

Peberdy, M.A., Cretikos, M., Abella, B.S. *et al.* (2007) Recommended guidelines for monitoring, reporting, and conducting research on medical emergency team, outreach, and rapid response systems: an Utstein-style scientific statement: a scientific statement from the International Liaison Committee on Resuscitation (American Heart Association, Australian Resuscitation Council, European Resuscitation Council, Heart and Stroke

Foundation of Canada, InterAmerican Heart Foundation, Resuscitation Council of Southern Africa, and the New Zealand Resuscitation Council); the American Heart Association Emergency Cardiovascular Care Committee; the Council on Cardiopulmonary, Perioperative, and Critical Care; and the Interdisciplinary Working Group on Quality of Care and Outcomes Research. *Circulation*, **116** (21), 2481–2500.

Picard, K.M., O'Donoghue, S.C., Young-Kershaw, D.A., and Russell, K.J. (2006) Development and implementation of a multidisciplinary sepsis protocol. *Critical Care Nurse*, **26** (3), 43–54.

Pickering, T.G., Hall, J.E., Appel, L.J. *et al.* (2005) Recommendations for blood pressure measurement in humans and experimental animals. Part I: blood pressure measurement in humans: a statement for professionals from the subcommittee of professional and public education of the American Heart Association Council on high Blood Pressure Research. *Hypertension*, **45**, 142–161.

Rosenberg, H., Davis, M., James, D. *et al.* (2007) Malignant hyperthermia. *Orphanet Journal of Rare Diseases*, **2** (21). doi: 10.1186/1750-1172-2-21.

Sasson, C., Meier, P., Campbell, J.A. *et al.* (2011) Improving cardiac arrest survival by providing high quality, co-ordinated care: 2010 International Liaison Committee on Resuscitation guidelines. *Future Medicine*, **8**, 721–730.

Schey, B.M., Williams, D.Y., and Bucknall, T. (2010) Skin temperature and core-peripheral temperature gradient as markers of hemodynamic status in critically ill patients: a review. *Heart & Lung*, **29**, 27–40.

Sheikh, A., Simons, F.E.R., Barbour, V., and Worth, A. (2012). Adrenaline atuo-injectors for the treatment of anaphylaxis with and without cardiovascular collapse in the community. *Cochrane Database of Systematic Reviews*, 8. Art No.: CD008935. DOI: 10.1002/14651858.CD008935.pub2.

Sheikh, A. (2013) Emergency management of anaphylaxis: current pharmacotherapy and future directions. *Expert Opinion on Pharmacotherapy*, **14** (7), 827–830.

Sinclair, H.L. and Andrews, P.J.D. (2010) Bench-to-bedside review: hypothermia in traumatic brain injury. *Critical Care*, **14**, 204.

Soar, J. and Unsworth, D.J. (2009) Suspected anaphylaxis requires prompt treatment. *The Practitioner*, **253**, 32–37.

Soar, J., Pumphrey, R., Cant, A. *et al.* (2008) Emergency treatment of anaphylactic reactions—guidelines for healthcare providers. *Resuscitation*, **77** (2), 157–169.

Tholl, U., Forstner, K., and Anlauf, M. (2004) Measuring blood pressure: pitfalls and recommendations. *Nephrology Dialysis Transplant*, **19**, 766–770.

Thompson, C.J. (2012) Cardiovascular problems, in *Advanced Practice Nursing of Adults in Acute Care* (eds J.G. Foster and S.S. Prevost), F.A. Davis, Philadelphia, pp. 239–397.

Zuber, B., Tran, T., Aegerter, P. *et al.* (2012) Impact of case volume on surviival of septic shock in patients with malignancies. *Critical Care Medicine*, **40**, 50–62.

CHAPTER 3

Monitoring for respiratory dysfunction

Alexander P. Johnson[1] and Jennifer Abraham[2]

[1] *Cadence Health, Central DuPage Hospital, Winfield, IL., USA*

[2] *Advocate BroMenn Medical Center, Normal, IL., USA*

Respiratory dysfunction and subsequent failure is a common reason for admittance to the critical care unit. While underlying lung disease may not be the primary cause of respiratory failure, all systems are highly dependent on adequate ventilation. Septic shock, trauma, acidosis, and cardiovascular emergencies can all result in respiratory failure. Underlying comorbidities including obesity can complicate pulmonary support, and should be considered. The clinician's ability to monitor effectively and treat the patient urgently in respiratory failure is critical to the patient's outcome.

This chapter focuses on primary causes of respiratory dysfunction in the critical care unit, strategies for monitoring and treatment, and an overview of ventilatory support. Key elements of monitoring and treatment will be highlighted, as well as supporting evidence and clinical pearls that will hopefully make the content easy to use at the bedside.

Acid-base disturbances & anion gap

A systematic approach to arterial blood gas (ABG) analysis can help accurately and rapidly identify the underlying cause of an acid–base disorder. The four following primary categories of abnormal blood gas changes compartmentalize blood gas interpretation in order to facilitate triage and treatment of critical care patients.

Metabolic acidosis
Disorders causing metabolic acidosis can be categorized into two groups: (1) anion gap metabolic acidosis and (2) non-anion gap acidosis.

This can help clinicians quickly differentiate the underlying cause of the acidosis. An increased anion gap is generally associated with increased acid production or administration, and nonanion gap acidosis is associated with increased bicarbonate loss or loss of bicarbonate precursors. The anion gap is the expected difference between measured serum cations and anions under normal conditions. The normal anion gap is 7–16, and the formula for the gap is as follows:

$$\text{Anion gap} = \left(Na^+ + K^+\right) - \left(Cl^- + HCO_3^-\right)$$

$$\text{Example} \rightarrow AG = \left(142 + 4\right) - \left(106 + 25\right) = 15$$

Be aware that some clinicians omit potassium from the calculation due to its minimal influence on the equation.

Clinical pearls

Many venous chemistry panels list bicarbonate as "CO_2."

Identification of the underlying cause can be further simplified with respect to the fact that three main types of metabolic acidosis are generally seen in intensive care unit (ICU) patients:

1 Renal acidosis
2 Diabetic ketoacidosis
3 Lactic acidosis

The most common of the three causes is lactic acidosis (type-A form). Type-A lactic acidosis is a global indicator of tissue hypoxia and elevated levels should prompt investigation regarding the underlying cause including, but not limited to, bleeding, low cardiac output (e.g., heart failure), or hypovolemia. Common causes of metabolic acidosis are reviewed in Table 3.1 and a diagnostic algorithm for metabolic acidosis is provided in Figure 3.1.

Critical Care Nursing: Monitoring and Treatment for Advanced Nursing Practice, First Edition. Edited by Kathy J. Booker.

© 2015 John Wiley & Sons, Inc. Published 2015 by John Wiley & Sons, Inc.

Table 3.1 Causes of metabolic acidosis.

Anion gap acidosis	Nonanion gap acidosis
Methanol intoxication	GI losses (i.e., diarrhea, fistulas, drains)
Uremia (chronic renal failure)	Renal tubular acidosis (RTA)
Lactic acidosis	Total parenteral nutrition fluids
Ethylene glycol (i.e., antifreeze solution)	Carbonic anhydrase inhibitors
Paraldehyde intoxication	Ammonium chloride ingestion
"Aspirin" (salicylic acid)	
Ketoacidosis	

Anion gap acidosis clinical pearl: The acronym MULEPAK may help practitioners remember the types of anion gap metabolic acidosis. Rule these out, and the nonanion gap types are the likely cause.

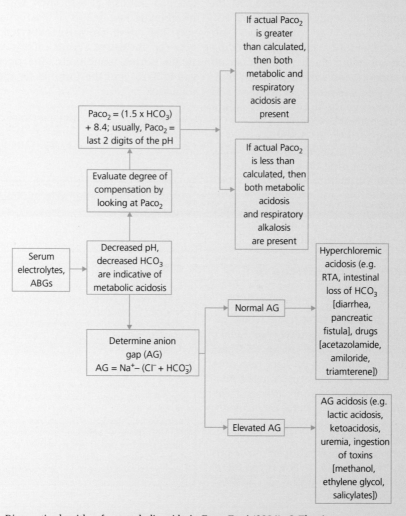

Figure 3.1 Diagnostic algorithm for metabolic acidosis. From Ferri (2004). © Elsevier.

2 Diuretic infusions (e.g., continuous lasix infusion)
3 Excessive administration of $NaHCO_3$

Metabolic alkalosis

Metabolic alkalosis is generally less dangerous than metabolic acidosis. A few common causes of metabolic alkalosis exist:
1 Excessive gastrointestinal (GI) losses (i.e., increased gastric output, vomiting)

See Figure 3.2 for a more detailed diagnostic algorithm for metabolic alkalosis.

Respiratory acidosis

Carbon dioxide (CO_2), a by-product of cellular metabolism, accumulates in the blood due to hypoventilation secondary to a decrease in

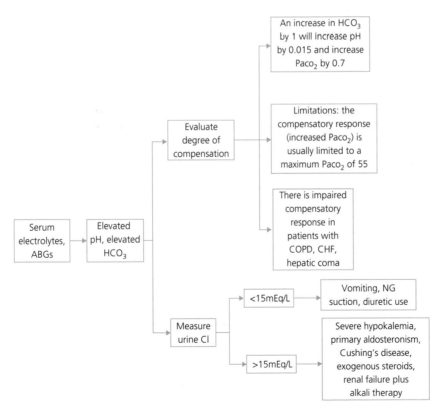

Figure 3.2 Diagnostic algorithm for metabolic alkalosis. From Ferri (2004). © Elsevier.

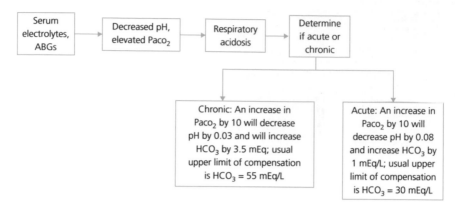

Figure 3.3 Diagnostic algorithm for respiratory acidosis. From Ferri (2004). © Elsevier.

minute ventilation. Initial interventions to treat respiratory acidosis include supporting airway and breathing. This may include airway maneuvers such as a head tilt and chin lift, jaw thrust, or airway devices such as oral and nasopharyngeal airways. Ambu bag-valve mask, bilevel positive airway pressure (BiPAP), or mechanical ventilation may be required to support ventilation, increase minute ventilation, and decrease $PaCO_2$. Reversal of sedative or narcotic agents must also be considered, as well as underlying pathologies such as stroke, seizure, atelectasis, or effects from drug overdose when strategizing how to increase the patient's respiratory rate or depth in order to resolve the acidosis.

Clinical pearls

For every 10 mmHg increase in $PaCO_2$, the pH will decrease by 0.08.

See Figure 3.3 for a more detailed diagnostic algorithm for respiratory acidosis.

Respiratory alkalosis

Respiratory alkalosis generally occurs in association with two main clinical scenarios:

1 **Overventilation due to pain, fear, or other anxiety-provoking stimuli.** Treatment efforts should focus on removing offending stimuli or administering analgesics or anxiolytics as needed. Decreasing mandatory rate and/or tidal volume should be considered in mechanically ventilated patients.

2 **Compensatory mechanisms.** If the respiratory alkalosis exists as a compensatory mechanism for metabolic acidosis, treatment of the underlying cause must be addressed as soon as possible (e.g., diabetic ketoacidosis (DKA). If the patient exhausts the ability to hyperventilate, decompensation or even death may occur.

Clinical pearls

For every 10 mmHg decrease in $PaCO_2$, the pH will increase by 0.08.

See Figure 3.4 for a more detailed diagnostic algorithm for respiratory alkalosis.

Mixed acid–base disorders

When one of the four earlier mentioned acid–base disorders is superimposed upon the other, this is generally referred to as a "mixed" acid–base disorder. Determining whether or not a mixed disorder exists begins with the fact that for every 10 points the CO_2 or HCO_3 increases or decreases, the pH should change proportionately. If not, a mixed disorder is present.

Oxygenation

Estimation of the PaO_2

The predictability of the oxyhemoglobin dissociation curve can allow clinicians to estimate the PaO_2 based on the patient's existing PaO_2 and FiO_2. Provided hemoglobin's affinity for O_2 is normal:

• If the SaO_2 is 99%, then the PaO_2 will be 100 mm.

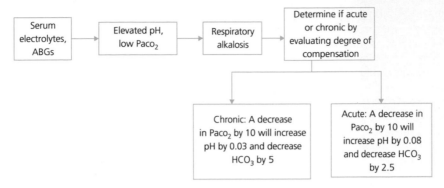

Figure 3.4 Diagnostic algorithm for respiratory alkalosis. From Ferri (2004). © Elsevier.

- If the SaO_2 is 95%, then the PaO_2 will be 80 mm.
- If the SaO_2 is 90%, then the PaO_2 will be 60 mm.
- If the SaO_2 is 85%, then the PaO_2 will be 50 mm.

Clinical Pearls

The "rule of 5s." The FiO_2 multiplied by 5 should be approximately the value that the PaO_2 should be (caution: this estimation is not exact). For example:

$$FiO_2 \times 5 = expected\ PaO_2$$
$$50\% \times 5 = 250\ mmHg$$

A–a Gradient

Calculating the alveolar–arterial oxygen (A–a) gradient provides an indication of how well alveolar oxygen moves into the arterial blood, and whether gas exchange is normal or altered. The A–a gradient differentiates hypoxemic disturbances due to either hypoventilation or low inspired PaO_2 (which have normal A–a gradients) from other causes such as shunting or V/Q mismatch (which have increased A–a gradients). While a decreased A–a gradient is the objective, "normal" values vary with age, FiO_2 concentration, and barometric pressure. Generally, the gradient should be less than 10–15 mmHg on room air. As a general rule, a 3 mmHg increase is expected for every decade of life after the age of 30. An estimation of normal can be gauged by utilization of the following formula:

$$(Age/4)+4$$

Example in a 40 – year – old patient :
$$(40/4)+4=14$$

A–a gradients will be 5–25 mmHg for an $FiO_2 = 21\%$ and should be less than 150 mmHg for an FiO_2 of 100%. Most ABG analyzers calculate the A–a gradient. A more exact estimation can be made using the alveolar gas equation, although this would be cumbersome to calculate at the bedside.

PaO_2/FiO_2 (P/F) ratio

An easier, less complex calculation of pulmonary shunting is the P/F ratio. The ratio is simply the PaO_2 obtained from the ABG divided by the FiO_2 concentration. A normal value is considered anything greater than 250 Torr, and the shunt worsens as the P/F ratio decreases. For example:

$$98/0.21(room\ air) = 466$$
$$PaO_2/FiO_2 = 466\ Torr$$

Values less than 250 are considered abnormal and require investigation regarding the underlying cause. P/F ratios less than 200 are associated with severe shunting such as in adult respiratory distress syndrome (ARDS). The 2008 Surviving Sepsis Campaign International Guidelines for Severe Sepsis and Septic Shock classify pulmonary organ dysfunction as acute lung injury with P/F ratio less than 250 in the absence of pneumonia as the infection source and less than 200 in the presence of pneumonia as the sepsis source (Dellinger *et al.*, 2008).

Acute respiratory failure

A systematic approach to acute respiratory failure facilitates identifying the underlying cause and subsequent treatment. Generally, acute respiratory failure can be classified into three kinds:

1 **Hypercapnic** ($CO_2 > 45$) due to the inability of accessory muscles to provide adequate minute ventilation (e.g., narcotic overdose or inability to compensate for metabolic acidosis any longer).

2 **Hypoxemic** ($PaO_2 < 60$ mmHg) (e.g., severe shunting like pneumonia or ARDS). Passive delivery of O_2 is insufficient to improve oxygenation and patient needs positive end-expiratory pressure (PEEP) or other pressure support delivery.

    PEEP titration can help reduce FiO_2 levels (goal < 60%) and avoid oxygen toxicity. Other causes of hypoxia, such as low cardiac output (circulatory hypoxia) and anemia (anemic hypoxia), should be considered.

3 **Inability to maintain an airway and/or manage secretions** (e.g., altered mental status due to combinations of hypercapnia and hypoxemia).This may occur with profound respiratory muscle weakness due to altered mental status, excessive sedation, or drug overdose states.

Clinical Pearls

Restlessness can be an early sign of hypoxia. Take caution not to sedate the patient or give anxiolytics to the patient with impending respiratory failure.

Clinical Pearls

Do not be afraid to give 100% oxygen to deteriorating patients out of fear that they are CO_2 retainers. In the emergent setting, always give enough oxygen to keep $SaO_2 > 90\%$. Moving forward, downtitrate O_2 as tolerated as the patient is stabilized.

    As a general rule, patients meeting criteria for any of the following parameters may be classified as having acute respiratory failure:
- pH < 7.25
- $PaO_2 < 50$
- $PaCO_2 > 50$
- PaO_2/FiO_2 ratio < 250

Other criteria may include the following:
- Altered mental status
- Tidal volume < 250 ml

Clinical Pearls

Some clinicians affectionately refer to meeting these criteria as being in the "50/50 club."

Capnography

Capnography helps evaluate the adequacy of ventilation and blood flow by measuring end-tidal CO_2 ($PetCO_2$). $PetCO_2$ is the maximum concentration of CO_2 at the end of an exhaled breath. Two common methods of measurement are by using colorimetric devices or by measuring actual CO_2 molecules. CO_2 molecule measurement (called infrared absorption spectrophotometry) provides a waveform (called a capnogram) and is the more useful application for ongoing monitoring in the ICU. This method of ongoing monitoring is reviewed in the following sections.

Monitoring ventilation with PetCO$_2$

Monitoring $PetCO_2$ levels is considered to be a more objective method of assessing ventilation than respiratory rate or the subjective evaluation of respiratory depth (American Academy of Pediatrics, Committee on Drugs, 2002; American Society of Anesthesiologists Task Force on Sedation and Analgesia by non-Anesthesiologists, 2002; Cacho et al., 2010; Greensmith and Aker, 1998; Lightdale et al., 2006; Soto et al., 2004; Vargo et al., 2002). The normal range for $PetCO_2$ can be considered as 35–45 mmHg. Ideally, however, a patient's true $PetCO_2$ baseline should be validated by the $PaCO_2$ on the ABG. $PetCO_2$ and $PaCO_2$ values should trend similarly. Deadspace ventilation accounts for an expected 5 mmHg gradient between the two, with the $PetCO_2$ being lower, provided the patient has healthy lungs. Patients with lung disease such as COPD often have wider $PetCO_2$–$PaCO_2$ gradients. Regardless, $PetCO_2$ levels greater than 50 mmHg or increases of ≥10 mmHg above baseline require pH evaluation via ABG as well as interventions to support the airway and breathing until the patient is considered safe. Applications include monitoring of patients during ventilator weaning, detecting incorrect placement of endotracheal tubes, and

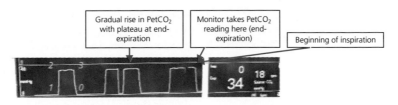

Gradual rise in PetCO$_2$ with plateau at end-expiration

Monitor takes PetCO$_2$ reading here (end-expiration)

Beginning of inspiration

Phase 1 to 2—Signifies the beginning of exhalation. Due to deadspace, gas in this phase contains small amounts of CO$_2$

Phase 2 to 3—Exhalation phase. Air from gas-exchanging portions of the lung (alveolar gas) is detected by the PetCO$_2$ sensor as the wave upslopes.

Phase 3 to 0—Also known as alveolar-emptying phase. Wave suddenly increases and plateaus, with the sharp drop signifying the end of exhalation.

Phase 0 to 1—Inspiratory phase. No PetCO$_2$ detected.

Figure 3.5 Phases of the capnogram.

detecting disconnection from the ventilator. Studies regarding additional uses, such as detecting correct placement of nasogastric tubes, are ongoing.

Figure 3.5 illustrates phases of the capnogram, the PetCO$_2$ waveform displayed on the patient monitor. Monitors also display a respiratory rate (e.g., the number of capnograms per minute). Waveform characteristics reveal information regarding ventilation, for example, hypopnea (small waveform), apnea (no waveform), or obstructive disease such as asthma ("shark-fin" type pattern).

Monitoring blood flow

A normal PetCO$_2$ reading depends upon adequate blood flow to the lungs. Therefore, a decrease (particularly a sudden decrease) in PetCO$_2$ without an associated increase in minute ventilation may suggest a decrease in cardiac output, such as bleeding, heart failure, or increased deadspace (e.g., pulmonary embolus). In these situations, measurement of cardiac output and stroke volume or ABG testing and chest imaging should be considered in order to validate findings.

PetCO$_2$ values have also shown to be prognostic indicators in cardiac arrest. PetCO$_2$ levels less than 10 mmHg after 20 min of cardiopulmonary resuscitation (CPR) have been associated with 0% survival (Ahrens *et al.*, 2001; Levine, Wayne, and Miller, 1997). In addition, increased PetCO$_2$ levels obtained during CPR have been associated with adequacy of chest compressions and return of spontaneous circulation.

Modes of mechanical ventilation

Management protocols for mechanical ventilation have been studied for decades. Critical care teams generally select modes of mechanical ventilation that optimally manage a patient's unique physiologic requirements. Surveillance of patient trends and values requires strong multidisciplinary work, including airway management, sedation protocols, activity coordination, and nutritional support. The modes of mechanical ventilation and airway support systems with monitoring strategies are reviewed later. There is strong support for multidisciplinary management using weaning protocols for liberating patients from mechanical ventilation (Brook *et al.*, 1999; Ely *et al.*, 2001; MacIntyre, 2008; MacIntyre *et al.*, 2001). However, ascertaining readiness for weaning is highly individualized and complex, especially if patients have multiple comorbid conditions or prolonged debilitation.

Continuous positive airway pressure (CPAP) with pressure support

This mode is commonly used during the last phase of weaning trials. No mandatory ventilator breaths are delivered, only patient-triggered spontaneous tidal volumes with the aid of PEEP and pressure support are given to support the patient's spontaneous breathing cycles. This mode facilitates spontaneous breathing and overcomes airway resistance of the endotracheal tube and the ventilator circuit. This is generally accomplished with a pressure support between 5 and 10 cm H_2O.

Synchronized intermittent mandatory ventilation (SIMV)

Machine-delivered tidal volumes are delivered at a set volume and minimum mandatory rate entered by the clinician. Breaths can be patient- or ventilator-triggered. However, in between mandatory tidal volume ventilator breaths, the patient can pull spontaneous tidal volumes as well with the assistance of PEEP and pressure support.

Assist/control ventilation (AC)

Machine-delivered tidal volumes are delivered at a set volume and minimum mandatory rate set by the clinician. These breaths can be patient- or ventilator-triggered. The main difference between AC and SIMV is that in AC, *ALL* ventilator breaths are delivered at the mandatory, preset tidal volume. Therefore, the work of breathing in AC is less as opposed to SIMV. Graphics illustrating the differences between CPAP with pressure support, SIMV, and AC are displayed in Figure 3.6.

Pressure control ventilation

A minimum mandatory rate is set by the clinician; however, tidal volumes are patient-specific. Rather than tidal volumes predetermined by set volume, they are determined according to mean airway pressure. The ventilator will deliver the tidal volume until a preset pressure is achieved and then stop the inspiratory flow. Advantages of pressure control include the minimization of volutrauma and barotrauma associated with AC ventilation.

Airway pressure release ventilation (APRV)

This mode is characterized by higher baseline airway pressures, which may be viewed as a nearly continuous alveolar recruitment maneuver. Airway pressure then periodically drops to zero, aiding in carbon dioxide elimination and theoretically stimulating the diaphragm in order to eventually facilitate the weaning process. This mode allows unrestricted spontaneous breathing throughout the respiratory cycle.

Pressure-regulated volume control (PRVC)

This mode is an AC/pressure control hybrid. Volumes will be delivered at a preset amount as

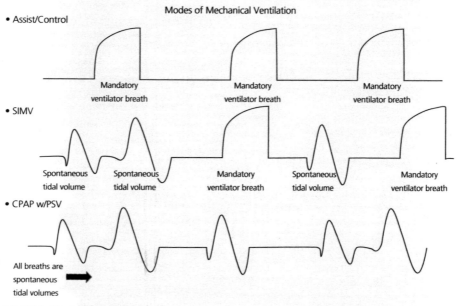

Figure 3.6 CPAP, PS, and AC patterns.

in AC, to a preset pressure limit as in pressure control, or whichever occurs first during a particular breath.

Inverse ratio ventilation

The normal physiologic inhalation time/exhalation time (I/E) ratio is 1:3. The use of inverse ratio ventilation involves increased inspiratory times delivered by the ventilator and expiratory times are decreased to achieve I/E ratios of less than 1:3 to as much as 1:1. This mode is part of a strategy to improve PaO_2 and SaO_2 levels by prolonging the inhalation phase. Patients must be paralyzed and sedated to tolerate this process due to comfort concerns created by such an unnatural inhalation–exhalation pattern. Caution must be taken to avoid hyperinflation.

Oscillatory ventilation

This mode is associated with respiratory rates of 150–300 breaths per minute (i.e., Hertz, or "cycles" per minute) and tidal volumes of approximately 50 ml (determined by the "amplitude" setting). A set airway pressure is determined by the clinician. This mode is often used in severe ARDS in order to avoid the risk of volutrauma and barotrauma that may be associated with AC or pressure control modes. Patients ventilated according to this mode should be paralyzed and sedated via continuous infusion.

Overview of protective lung ventilation in ARDS

The ARDS Network is a collaborative designed to facilitate knowledge transfer and protocolization regarding evidence-based care for patients with ARDS. The National Heart, Lung, and Blood Institute as well as the National Institutes of Health collaborate within the ARDS Network to determine best practice for ARDS management (NHLBI ARDS Network, 2014).

Inclusion criteria include the acute onset of ARDS

1 $PaO_2/FiO_2 \leq 300$
2 Bilateral (patchy, diffuse, or homogeneous) infiltrates consistent with pulmonary edema
3 No clinical evidence of left atrial hypertension

Guidelines for ventilator setup and adjustment
1 Calculate predicted body weight (PBW):

$$\text{Males} = 50 + 2.3 [\text{height (inches)} - 60]$$
$$\text{Females} = 45.5 + 2.3 [\text{height (inches)} - 60].$$

2 Select AC mode.
3 Set initial TV to 8 ml/kg PBW.
4 Reduce TV by 1 ml/kg at intervals ≤ 2 h until TV = 6 ml/kg PBW.
5 Set initial rate to approximate baseline minute ventilation (not > 35 bpm).
6 Adjust TV and RR to achieve pH and plateau pressure goals given later.
7 Set inspiratory flow rate above patient demand (usually > 80 l/min).

ARDSNet protocol goals

1 Oxygenation goal: PaO_2 55–80 mmHg or SpO_2 88–95% (NHLBI ARDS Network, 2008)
   (i) Use incremental FiO_2/PEEP combinations to achieve goal. Higher PEEP levels will decrease FiO_2 and may be preferred in patients with high FiO_2 who can tolerate higher PEEP (stable BP, no barotrauma).
2 Plateau pressure goal: ≤ 30 cm H_2O
3 Low tidal volume strategy to avoid volutrauma and barotrauma
4 pH goal: 7.30–7.45
   (i) "Permissive hypercapnia"—a strategy designed to avoid overventilating the patient and that allows the pH to be maintained modestly at less than 7.35 to avoid barotrauma.
   (ii) "clinical pearl"—patients will generally tolerate permissive hypercapnia (pH ~ 7.2, oxygen saturation < 90% to 85–90%).
5 I/E ratio goal: 1:1.0–1:3.0

Monitoring for complications during mechanical ventilation

High peak airway pressures on mechanical ventilation

High peak airway pressures (>30–40 cm H_2O) require immediate attention as potential causes may range from minor to life-threatening.

Causes essentially range from least severe to most severe and may include the following:

- Coughing. Consider suctioning, sedating, or administering a bronchodilator.
- Bronchospasm: Bronchodilator may be needed.
- Patient–ventilator asynchrony: Patient may need sedation or ventilator settings to be adjusted.
- Excessive set tidal volumes being administered.
- Right mainstem intubation (right mainstem bronchus is at a more obtuse angle than the left).
- Mucous plugging.
- Pneumothorax.
- Endotracheal tube occlusion.

High peak airway pressures may be resolved with medication (e.g., sedation, analgesia), suctioning, or adjusting ventilator settings. However, airway pressure alarms associated with acute changes in tidal volume, minute ventilation, vital signs, or decreased SaO_2 should immediately be evaluated by disconnecting the patient from the ventilator and ambu bagging with 100% O_2.

Response to bagging—monitoring and treatment

If bagging the patient is *NOT* difficult, the patient can be placed back on the ventilator. The patient should be reevaluated for the need for sedation, a change in ventilator settings, or bronchospasm, and treated accordingly.

If bagging the patient *IS* difficult, the airway must be evaluated for obstruction or another cause of diminished air movement. Determination of the underlying cause can be facilitated by the advancement of a coudé suction catheter through the endotracheal tube.

If the suction catheter *CANNOT* be passed through the endotracheal tube, assess for biting. Increasing the sedation and bite blocks may enable resolution of these obstructions. Thick mucous plugs or clots blocking the airway may be loosened with aggressive bagging and lavaging with saline. Emergent bronchoscopy may be considered; however, patients who continue to deteriorate may need to be extubated so that a new endotracheal tube can be placed. If the suction catheter *CAN* be passed, consider bronchospasm, pneumothorax, right mainstem intubation, or obstruction in the tracheobronchial tree lower than the endotracheal tube itself.

Auto-PEEP effect

Mechanically ventilated patients require adequate expiratory time to avoid barotrauma and hyperinflation injury. Inadequate airflows, excessive tidal volumes, narrow endotracheal tubes, water clogging ventilator circuits, and high respiratory rates limit expiratory time and place the patient at risk for an "air-trapping" condition termed auto-PEEP (see Fig. 3.7). Auto-PEEP can be determined by performing an expiratory hold maneuver on the ventilator. Risks of auto-PEEP include reduction of venous return, hypotension, increased work of breathing, and patient–ventilator triggering difficulty.

Auto-PEEP can be corrected by adding extrinsic (set) PEEP, lowering tidal volumes, sedating in some cases, and prolonging exhalation times (or decreasing inhalation time) of the ventilator I/E ratio.

Weaning from mechanical ventilation

The majority (~70%) of patients on ventilators can be weaned successfully in a single weaning period (Luetz *et al.*, 2012). MacIntyre and colleagues (2001) published an evidence-based review and guidelines for ventilator weaning, including criteria to be utilized during spontaneous breathing trials and weaning protocols. Evidence-based guidelines have also been published specifically for nonphysician providers (Ely *et al.*, 2001). Table 3.2 is based on those criteria. Several randomized trials have shown that weaning protocols driven by registered nurses (RNs) and respiratory therapists (RTs) improved efficiency of weaning as opposed to physician-directed weaning (Blackwood *et al.*, 2010; Ely *et al.*, 2001). Although these guidelines may appear seemingly dated, they have been described as having stood the "test of time" (MacIntyre, 2008) and updates have not been published. However, to date no data have shown which specific weaning strategy is best (e.g., CPAP and pressure support ventilation (PSV) versus T-piece), much like no specific weaning protocol has been shown to be better than another.

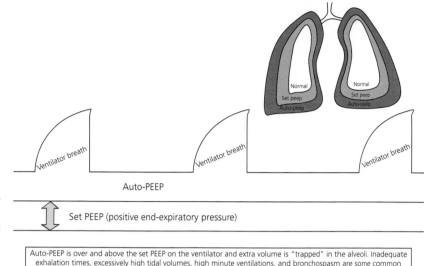

Auto-PEEP

+

0

Set PEEP (positive end-expiratory pressure)

Auto-PEEP is over and above the set PEEP on the ventilator and extra volume is "trapped" in the alveoli. Inadequate exhalation times, excessively high tidal volumes, high minute ventilations, and bronchospasm are some common causes, enabling ventilator breaths to become "stacked."

Figure 3.7 Auto-PEEP effect.

Table 3.2 Parameters for liberating (weaning) from mechanical ventilation.

Weaning parameter	Reference range
Respiratory rate	<30 breaths/min
Spontaneous tidal volume	325–400 ml (4–6 ml/kg)
Minute ventilation (V_E)	<10–15 l/min
Negative inspiratory force (NIF)	−20 to −30 cm H_2O
pH	≥7.25
SaO_2	≥90%
PaO_2	≥60 mmHg
FiO_2	Requiring <0.40–0.50
PaO_2/FiO_2 ratio	>150–200
PEEP	Requiring <5–8 cm H_2O
Rapid shallow breathing index (respiratory rate/ tidal volume)	<100 breaths/min/l
Hemodynamic stability	As evidenced by minimal or low-dose vasopressor therapy and absence of active myocardial ischemia
Secretions	Minimal secretions, adequate cough effort
Heart rate	≤140
Blood pressure	Stable with no (or minimal) vasopressors
Mental status	For example, arousable, Glasgow Coma Scale (GCS)≥ 13, and/or no continuous sedative infusions
Evidence of some reversal of the underlying cause of the respiratory failure	

Regardless of the specific weaning strategy used, the ultimate goal is to wean to extubation as soon as the patient can safely tolerate it. This is because mechanical ventilation itself is not without risk. Complications are common, including ventilator-associated pneumonia, deep vein thrombosis, paralytic ileus, deconditioning, skin breakdown, and vocal cord paralysis. A daily weaning readiness evaluation should be performed for possible spontaneous breathing trial based on criteria such as those listed in Table 3.2, provided the underlying cause of respiratory failure is improved or resolved.

Research also clarifies that daily interruption of continuously infusing sedatives leads to decreased ventilator days when compared to controls, and that intermittently given sedation leads to shorter vent days compared with continuous infusion of sedation (Brook *et al.*, 1999; Grap *et al.*, 2012; Kress *et al.*, 2000; Luetz *et al.*, 2012; Roberts, Haroon, and Hall, 2012).

Some patients will exhibit respiratory failure shortly after extubation despite excellent objective evaluation of readiness and appropriate precautions. These patients may be more appropriate for tracheostomy. Although an optimal rate of reintubation is not known, 5–15% has been published as a "healthy" 24-h failure rate (e.g., reintubation rate) for non-neurologically impaired ICU patients (Ely *et al*,

Clinical Pearls

For difficult-to-wean patients (48–72 h after resolution of the underlying cause of respiratory failure), consider applying the WEANS NOW checklist or the Burns Wean Assessment Program (BWAP) protocol to help ensure that all barriers to wean ability are being addressed (Burns *et al.*, 2010). In prior testing, a score of 50 on the BWAP was predictive of successful weaning. Burns *et al.* (2010) retrospectively analyzed over 1800 patients on whom the BWAP had been prospectively applied and found that 88% of weaning attempts were successful (Burns *et al.*, 2010). The BWAP is designed to assess 12 items as general assessment indicators, including metabolic factors, sleep, and general body endurance, and 14 items that assess respiratory assessment parameters (Burns *et al.*, 2010). For the WEANS NOW checklist, see Table 3.3.

Table 3.3 *WEANS NOW* checklist to assess failure to wean 48–72 h after resolution of underlying condition causing respiratory failure.

Weaning parameters	Readiness to wean (see Table 3.2)
Endotracheal tube	Ideal to use largest ET tube possible
	Consider use of PSV+ during SBT to overcome intrinsic resistance of ET tube
Aterial blood gases	Prevent or treat metabolic alkalosis
	Maintain PaO_2 at 60–65 mmHg to avoid blunting of respiratory drive
	For CO_2-retaining patients, keep $PaCO_2$ at or above their baseline
Nutrition	Provide nutritional support as needed
	Avoid electrolyte imbalances
	Avoid excessive caloric intake (may increase CO_2 production)
Secretions	Clear regularly
	Avoid dehydration if possible
Neuromuscular factors	Avoid agents that may exacerbate neuromuscular weakness in at-risk patients (neuromuscular blockers, aminoglycosides, clindamycin)
	Avoid unnecessary corticosteroids
Obstruction of airways	Bronchodilator use as appropriate
	Rule out possibility of foreign bodies in airway
Wakefulness	Avoid oversedation
	Wean in morning or when patient is most awake

Modified from Green *et al.* (2004).
ET, endotracheal; PSV, pressure support ventilation; SBT, spontaneous breathing trial.

2001). Higher than 15% may be reflective of weaning that is perhaps too aggressive and less than 5% may not be aggressive enough.

Clinical pearls

Ventilator weaning for acute-on-chronic respiratory failure (e.g., COPD exacerbation) may be facilitated by the use of noninvasive positive pressure ventilation (NIPPV).

Postextubation stridor: Monitoring and treatment

Postextubation stridor is an emergent condition and is documented to occur in up to 16% of patients (usually occurring in <15 min after extubation) (Critical Care Alert, 2012). This obstruction is usually related to laryngeal edema and treatment is aimed at initiating local vasoconstriction and reducing airway edema.

First-line treatment includes airway precautions and nebulized (racemic) epinephrine. The literature also suggests that humidified O_2, the cuff leak test, parenteral steroids, laryngeal ultrasound, and inhalation of an oxygen/helium mixture may help avoid or alleviate postextubation stridor, although randomized controlled trials would be needed to definitively confirm the efficacy of these treatments (Cheng *et al.*, 2011; Ding, Wang, and Wu, 2006; Jaber *et al.*, 2009; Markovitz, Randolph, and Khemani, 2009; Wittekamp *et al.*, 2009).

Patients with vocal cord paralysis after longer-term intubation display a lower pitched, "looser," upper airway sound and typically do not appear in as much distress, although these sounds may sometimes be confused with stridor. However, these patients must be evaluated for swallowing dysfunction to gauge the risk of aspiration.

Noninvasive positive pressure ventilation

NIPPV may be used in select patients as a strategy to avoid placement of an advanced airway (but should not be used to delay imminent intubation). NIPPV provides close to full mechanical ventilatory support with the settings of a conventional ventilator (can be pressure-cycled or volume-cycled modes) used via a tight-fitting mask (can be a mouth or nasal mask). A mouth mask may be preferred over a nasal mask due to the increased airway resistance of the nasal passages and the likelihood of positive pressure loss through the mouth, which may also be perceived as uncomfortable for the patient. Monitoring and adjusting the mask to attain a good seal and fit is key in order to maintain comfort and minimize air leak, positive pressure loss, eye drying, and skin breakdown.

Hypercapnic respiratory failure tends to respond well to NIPPV. The literature has shown improved outcomes with regard to COPD exacerbations, cardiogenic pulmonary edema, and hypoxemic respiratory failure in immunocompromised hosts with pulmonary infiltrates (Esteban *et al.*, 2008; Keenan *et al.*, 2011; Kollef *et al.*, 2008). However, in general, hypoxemic respiratory failure doesn't respond as well to NIPPV. The American Association of Respiratory Care has criteria for which to consider NIPPV in patients with COPD exacerbation (see Table 3.4).

Contraindications to NIPPV primarily include instability or inability to maintain an airway such as the following:

- Cardiac or respiratory arrest, or unstable cardiac rhythm
- Hemodyamic instability
- Nonrespiratory organ failure
- Facial surgery, trauma, or deformity

Table 3.4 American Association of Respiratory Care criteria for noninvasive positive pressure ventilation for exacerbation of COPD.

Must meet two or more of the following and have *no* contraindications
1 Respiratory distress with moderate-to-severe dyspnea
2 Arterial pH < 7.35 with $PaCO_2 > 45$
3 Respiratory rate ≥ 25 breaths/min

- Severe encephalopathy or inability to protect airway
- Upper airway obstruction
- Severe upper GI bleeding, risk for aspiration, or inability to clear secretions

Patients who fail NIPPV require endotracheal intubation and mechanical ventilation, pending the patient's code status. Signs of failure of NIPPV therapy include the following:

- Worsening gas exchange (should see improvement on ABG within 1 h)
- Worsening tachypnea, dyspnea, or asynchrony with mechanical breaths
- Hemodynamic instability
- Mental status changes

Even if the patient responds to NIPPV therapy, close ongoing monitoring is critical in order to evaluate for potential decline in status. Clinicians must continue to watch for changes in mental status, respiratory rate, accessory muscle use, tidal volumes, ventilator synchrony, and comfort. When in doubt of potential deterioration, obtain an ABG and do not be misled by a seemingly normal SaO_2, because desaturation is often a late sign of patient changes.

Tension pneumothorax

Tension pneumothorax is a cause of obstructive shock and is a medical emergency. In the intensive care setting, pnueumothorax more commonly occurs as a complication of mechanical ventilation, central line placement, or status post thoracentesis. A tension pneumothorax in patients with these problems results when air enters the pleural space via a tear in the lung or tracheobronchial tree and is not allowed to escape during expiration, creating a one-way valve effect. Intrathoracic pressure then builds which compresses the heart and great vessels and decreases venous return. Signs and symptoms include tachypnea, dyspnea, hypoxia, tachycardia, hypotension, restlessness, agitation, absent breath sounds and hyperresonance on the affected side and tracheal deviation toward the contralateral side.

Emergent treatment—needle thoracostomy

Urgent decompression must be done by inserting a large bore needle (16 gauge is good, 14 gauge is better) in the second intercostal space, midclavicular line. Conventional chest tube placement should immediately follow.

> **Clinical Pearls**
>
> Cutting off the finger and fingertip of a rubber glove and securing it over the end of the angiocath will create a rudimentary one-way valve until the chest tube can be placed (glove will collapse over the end of the angiocath during inspiration). A three-way stopcock can also serve as a valve, but will have to be turned periodically to allow air to escape.

Chest radiograph interpretation

The chest radiograph may be the most frequently performed imaging study in the critical care unit. A significant amount of information may be obtained from the radiograph; however, a systematic approach to interpretation is recommended in order to avoid clinical concerns going unrecognized.

Radiologic criteria for evaluation may be broken down into five areas:

1 Heart size and configuration—a cardiothoracic ratio of 0.60 is the upper limit of normal, greater than 0.60 may suggest cardiomegaly.
2 Pulmonary vascularity—normal lung fields have a light, white, "lacey" appearance. Heavier interstitial lung markings or generalized haziness over the lung fields may suggest pulmonary edema.
3 Aeration of the lungs—overall expansion, radiolucency, and density of the right and left lungs should be equal.
4 Lung infiltrates—observe for the presence or absence of pulmonary infiltrates (areas of increased densities). Types of densities and their distribution may lead to a diagnosis.
5 Mediastinal shift—the trachea, heart, and great vessels shift toward the side with the decreased lung volume or away from the hemithorax with increased lung volume.

It is important to remember that even though the lungs may be the primary focus for obtaining the film, all areas of the radiograph warrant evaluation including the air-filled spaces, soft tissue, and all bony structures. Other aspects to evaluate include (i) liver size (may vary with the progression of right-sided heart failure), (ii) abdominal gas pattern, (iii) catheter tube and position, (iv) bony structure (evaluate for fractures, dislocation, hypodensities, and bony anomolies), and (v) it is also important to know the age of the patient and progression of any previous radiologic findings. Figure 3.8 shows an illustration of normal landmarks.

Pathologies commonly encountered in the ICU that may be identified on the chest radiograph include the following:

- ARDS—Generalized, bilateral pulmonary infiltrates ("ground glass" appearance, progressing to complete white-out) known as noncardiogenic pulmonary edema. In order to differentiate from heart failure, normal brain natriuretic peptide (BNP) and/or pulmonary artery wedge pressure less than 18 mmHg help confirm ARDS.
- Pleural effusion—Characteristics include blunting of costophrenic angle in an upright patient, suggesting fluid accumulation.
- Pneumothorax—A portion of the lung border appears to be shifting toward the mediastinum, leaving a fully dark, delineated area between the lung border and preexisting lung field. Pneumothorax can occur anywhere along the lung border, but is most common in the apices.
- "White out" areas—May be due to blood (hemothorax), severe atelectasis, or mucous plugging.
- Describing infiltrates—Infiltrates should be described according to their distribution. For example, symmetrical versus asymmetrical, diffuse versus nondiffuse, alveolar (ill-defined margins), or interstitial (stringy appearance).

> **Clinical Pearls**
>
> Be aware that the pulmonary vasculature may be obscured on supine chest x-rays, because blood is no longer flowing dependently to the lower lobes.

Sleep-disordered breathing in the critical care unit

Normal sleep can affect respiratory physiology in several ways, including decreased hypoxic ventilatory drive, decreased hypercapnic ventilatory drive, increased airway resistance, and increased arousal threshold to increased airway

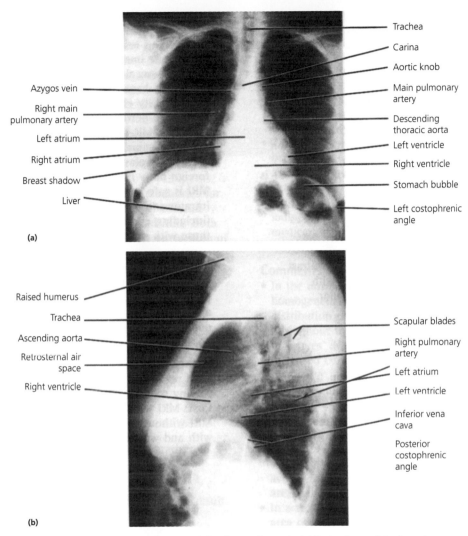

Figure 3.8 Common landmarks and structures of the chest radiograph. (a) Projection and the lateral. (b) Projection. From Ferri (2004). © Elsevier.

resistance. The addition of comorbidities (e.g., COPD) can exacerbate this otherwise normal physiology. Sleep issues abound in critical care units (Hardin, 2009). Sleep disorders that impact patients in the ICU include obstructive sleep apnea (OSA), central sleep apnea (CSA), and obesity hypoventilation syndrome (OHS). However, sometimes the primary pathology occurs as repeated upper airway collapse during sleep (Dhand, 2010). The obesity epidemic and increased recognition of how sleep disorders exacerbate/cause heart disease have contributed to the growing field of sleep medicine, and should increase practitioners' surveillance of and monitoring for these disorders (Dhand, 2010). While few monitoring guidelines have been published, perioperative management of patients with obstructive sleep apnea–hypopnea syndrome (OSAHS) has been advanced by the American Society of Anesthesiologists Task Force on Perioperative Management of Patients with Obstructive Sleep Apnea (2006). These include avoidance of systemic opiods when possible, supportive use of postextubation oxygenation, CPAP and NIPPV application as soon as feasible after surgery, avoidance of supine positioning of patients with OSA, and continuous pulse oximetry until room air SaO_2 remains greater than 90% during sleep.

Obstructive sleep apnea

OSA is characterized by excess soft tissue in the upper airway that limits airflow and results in obstruction, which has been associated with postoperative complications, increased ICU admissions, onset of inpatient delirium, and greater length of hospital stay (Chung et al., 2008). Hypopneas (resulting in reductions of tidal volume by 50% with breaths and generally accompanied by at least a 4% decline in oxygen saturation) and apneas (no tidal volume) cause repeated disruptions in progression through the sleep cycle and microarousals (Bradley and Floras, 2009). Sleep disruptions in the ICU setting are significant, particularly in mechanically ventilated patients and have been studied extensively over the past several decades (Cabello et al., 2008; Freedman et al., 2001; Frighetto et al., 2004). Sleep quality is also significantly affected by sedatives in ICU patients (Frighetto et al., 2004). Although difficult to use in the ICU, polysomnography studies have shown significant disruptions of sleep architecture in ICU patients (Cabello et al., 2008; Parthasarathy and Tobin, 2002) and nurse observations and actigraphy have not been validated as alternatives in the ICU (Beecroft et al., 2008). Sleep disturbances have been linked to higher rates of stress hormones, inflammatory mediators, and cardiac arrhythmias (Bijwadia et al., 2009; Ryan et al., 2008).

Alonso-Fernandez et al. (2005) also found an increased frequency of ST-segment depression indicative of myocardial ischemia in patients with OSAHS compared with controls. In addition, OSAHS patients had more arrhythmias and elevated daytime urinary epinephrine levels. Redeker (2008) reviewed the many challenges to research sleep measurement in the critical care setting, including physiologic monitoring and scoring of sleep variables, impact of multiorgan dysfunction and interventional treatments, and challenges in accurate detection of behavioral, perceptual, and temporal variations in sleep patterns.

Obstructions during the sleep cycle result in paradoxical respiratory effort and apneas that lead to increased arousals and desaturations. OSA can be classified by severity according to the apnea–hypopnea index. Patients exhibit daytime sleepiness because of increased stress hormones and nighttime catecholamine surges. Long-term effects have been linked to hypertension, heart failure, and stroke (Epstein et al., 2009).

OSA impacts the course of hospitalization in the ICU because it is a risk factor for respiratory failure and is largely undiagnosed. It is estimated that nearly 80% of men and 93% of women with moderate to severe OSA are undiagnosed (Chung et al., 2008). Endotracehal intubation of these patients is challenging due to a crowded oropharynx and may require the assistance of a video scope or bronchoscopy.

Central sleep apnea

CSA is more commonly associated with heart failure. It differs from OSAHS in mechanism and presentation, is generally diagnosed by polysomnography, and is associated with apnea in the absence of rib cage or abdominal movements. Grimm et al. (2009) found that CSA is common in patients with implantable cardioverter defibrillators (ICDs), detected in 57 of 129 (44%) patients with first ICD implant. While OSAHS was also diagnosed in 25% of patients, CSA patients were found to have more severe cardiomyopathy (57% versus 26% of patients with OSA). Serizawa et al. (2008) also studied 71 patients with polysomnography within 1 week after ICD and found sleep-disordered breathing diagnosis in 47 of 71 (66%). Sleep-disordered breathing predicted life-threatening arrhythmias that occurred most often during sleep.

Ryan and colleagues (2008) found that the timing of ventricular ectopy differed during sleep-disordered breathing, with the majority of ventricular arrhythmias occurring during the apneic/hypopneic phases in patients with OSAHS and during hyperventilatory stages in patients with CSA. Although a number of mechanisms may account for these alterations, the definitive cause remains unknown.

Obesity hypoventilation syndrome

OHS is a consequence of morbid obesity. The hallmark sign of OHS is "awake hypercapnia ($PaCO_2 > 45\,mmHg$) in the obese patient ($BMI > 30\,kg/m^2$) after other causes that could account for awake hypoventilation, such as lung or neuromuscular disease, have been excluded" (Piper and Grunstein, 2011, p. 292). Nowbar *et al.* (2004) identified the prevalence of OHS in approximately 50% of patients weighing over $50\,kg/m^2$ and the growing proportion of obesity in the United States predicts rising frequency of this disorder. The majority of patients with this condition have complex interactions of altered central respiratory drive, upper airway obstruction and resultant increased work of breathing, and hormonal influences (Piper and Grunstein, 2011). Treatment with CPAP and reductions in CO_2 are generally effective. Expiratory positive airway pressure (EPAP) may be added if continued problems with oxygen saturation or hypercapnia are not resolved with CPAP. Long-term management with tracheostomy or bariatric surgery may also be indicated although further outcome studies are needed.

While OHS is characterized by daytime hypercapnia, actual definitions vary in the literature. Signs and symptoms of OSA and OHS can be systematically identified with screening strategies such as the "STOP-BANG" questionnaire (Abrishami, Khajehdehi, and Chung, 2010; Chung *et al.*, 2008). Questionnaires can be valuable tools for quick prediction of sleep disorders as they can be applied and scored easily as part of routine daily practice. The "STOP-BANG" is considered to be a questionnaire with strong positive predictive value based on the high-quality methodology of its validation studies (Abrishami, Khajehdehi, and Chung, 2010; Chung *et al.*, 2008). Questions from this tool include the following:

1 Do you snore loudly? (louder than talking or loud enough to be heard through closed doors?
2 How loud do you snore? (can it be heard in another room?) How often do you snore?
3 Has your snoring ever bothered anyone?
4 Do you often feel tired, fatigued, or sleepy during the daytime?
5 How often do you feel tired or fatigued after you sleep?
6 During your waking time, do you feel tired, fatigued, or not up to par?
7 Has anyone noticed that you quit breathing during your sleep?
8 Do you have or are you being treated for high blood pressure?
9 Have you ever nodded off or fallen asleep while driving a vehicle? If so, how often? (Chung *et al.*, 2008, p. 816)

Heightened awareness of the clinical manifestations of sleep-disordered breathing in critically ill adults is necessary for accurate monitoring and anticipation of risk.

The STOP-BANG questionnaire is a standardized patient screening using yes/no questions that risk-stratifies patients for OSA based on the number of "yes" responses observed. Answering "yes" to less than three questions indicates that a low risk of OSA exists. Obtaining positive answers to three or more questions indicates a high risk of OSA. Questionnaires such as this can be implemented using protocols for appropriate patient placement (floor versus step-down versus ICU) to prevent adverse outcomes (Dhand, 2010). Patients with a $pH < 7.30$, altered mentation, or intolerant of positive pressure ventilation should be admitted to the ICU (Lee and Mokhlesi, 2008). Medication management of these patients should include limiting the administration of sedating medication that may exacerbate potential airway compromise. Patients at high risk should also be considered for further assessment by a sleep specialist, use of airway precautions, and CPAP or BiPAP therapy as appropriate while in the ICU and while screened for perioperative risk factors. In fact, more recent data suggest that long-term positive pressure ventilation for OHS is associated with mortality benefit (Priou *et al.*, 2010).

CPAP and BiPAP therapy

A first-line approach for treating obstructive sleep disorders in the ICU is often CPAP or BiPAP therapy. CPAP is essentially a positive pressure delivery system that applies PEEP via a tight-fitting facemask or nasal appliance (i.e., "nasal pillows") in order to maintain an open airway during sleep. PEEP delivered in this

Table 3.5 Treatment options for sleep-disordered breathing in the critical care unit (*assuming data from prior sleep study is not available*).

Sleep disorder	Treatment
OSAHS without associated hypercapnia	CPAP with close monitoring that includes continuous pulse oximetry and telemetry
Hypercapnia related to OSAHS alone	CPAP at a pressure that resolves obstructive events to correct hypercapnia (with continuous monitoring as above)
Hypercapnia that involves sleep-related hypoventilation	BiPap generally required (with continuous monitoring as above)

BiPAP, CPAP plus end-expiratory airway pressure; CPAP, continuous positive airway pressure; OSAHS, obstructive sleep apnea–hypopnea syndrome.

setting may also be referred to as EPAP. CPAP is generally not considered a therapy designed to correct hypercapnia, unless the hypercapnia is due solely to uncomplicated OSA.

BiPAP provides an increased amount of ventilatory support over CPAP and is the preferred method between the two to treat more complex hypercapnia. The increased ventilatory support in BiPAP is due to the combination of inspiratory positive airway pressure (IPAP) and EPAP it provides. IPAP lessens work of breathing by delivering flow during inspiration to a predetermined airway pressure. The IPAP minus the EPAP (i.e., the "delta") correlates with tidal volumes and the degree of ventilation (Lee and Mokhlesi, 2008). BiPAP modes may consist of time-cycled, machine-triggered breaths, spontaneous, or a combination.

Without data from a sleep study to diagnose the sleep disorder and titrate CPAP or BiPAP settings, little evidence exists to guide initial settings to start BiPAP and CPAP therapy. Typical initial settings may be an EPAP of 5–7 cm H_2O for CPAP and an IPAP/EPAP of 10–12 cm H_2O over 5 cm H_2O for BiPAP. CPAP and BiPAP initiated empirically should be followed with continuous cardiac and pulse oximetry monitoring, and ABGs as optimal settings are being determined. Failure to titrate pressure settings high enough to overcome airway obstruction could result in apneas, desaturations, or even death. One can reasonably assume that patients with severe OSA or OHS will require higher pressures. However, pressures titrated too high may result in patient discomfort, gastric distension, mask leak, eye dryness, and skin irritation. More

specific pressure titration guidelines can be found on the American Academy of Sleep Medicine web site (Morgenthaler *et al.*, 2008).

Patients already diagnosed with OSA or OHS prior to admission should be instructed to have their home CPAP device brought to the hospital (to use while sleeping during the day as well as at night). One may consider tracheostomy in OSA patients refractory to CPAP and BiPAP but this is generally a last resort (Dhand, 2010). Airflow through a tracheostomy allows the patient to completely bypass the upper airway soft tissue that causes the obstruction. Table 3.5 displays a general guide to empirically initiating CPAP or BiPAP according to the sleep disorder.

Cardiovascular aspects to monitor include an increase in myocardial oxygen demand during sleep-disordered breathing. Systemic blood pressure can surge up to as high as 250/150 mmHg during post-apnea arousal (Naughton, 2008). This state of elevated afterload is implicated in OSA-associated chronic heart failure.

Approach to cardiogenic dyspnea in acute heart failure

The advent of the serum BNP measurement has significantly aided clinicians to differentiate cardiogenic versus noncardiogenic forms of pulmonary edema (Hunt *et al.*, 2009). BNP is released in response to increased preload and stretch of ventricular tissue. BNP levels less than 250 mg/ml may indicate acute lung injury and help rule out heart failure as a cause of dyspnea. Serum levels of BNP > 250 mg/ml are suggestive of decompensated heart failure, reduced ejection fraction (Hunt *et al.*, 2009), and may serve as a prognostic indicator in heart failure risk stratification. Although laboratory references may suggest that normal values are less than 100 mg/ml, recent studies suggest a higher threshold may be required (i.e., around 250 mg/ml) in order to discriminate heart failure dyspnea from other causes in the ICU (Principi *et al.*, 2009; Rana *et al.*, 2006). Bhardwaj and Januzzi (2009) illustrate a more detailed diagnostic and monitoring algorithm for acute heart failure utilizing BNP.

The higher the levels of BNP, the more severe is the heart failure. In fact, increases in BNP≥75 pg/ml at 24 h after ICU admission carry a threefold increased likelihood that the patient will require intubation (Vander Werf *et al.*, 2010).

However, serial values closer than 48–72 h apart during an individual hospitalization are not recommended because BNP levels to do not decrease consistently after treatment. Decreased renal clearance, a common occurrence in critically ill patients, may also influence values to remain elevated, thus limiting the BNP's diagnostic value (Rana *et al.*, 2006). BNP has been found to be superior to clinical judgment for diagnosing acute decompensated heart failure and, in one trial, was able to improve diagnostic accuracy from 74 to 81% (Bhardwaj and Januzzi, 2009), and because of this, BNP testing has been associated with improvments of length of stay in hospital (Hunt *et al.*, 2009; Lam *et al.*, 2010). If diagnosed, treatment for acute heart failure may include the following:

- Oxygen
- BiPAP (decreases work of breathing, lowering myocardial oxygen demand, and decreases preload by increasing intrathoracic pressure and pressure to the inferior vena cava, thus lowering venous return)
- Morphine IVP (decreases afterload, preload, and perceived shortness of breath)
- Lasix (decreases preload)
- Nitroglycerin (if hypertensive, to decrease preload and afterload)

Clincians must also be aware of noncardiac causes of BNP elevation, such as acute pulmonary embolism, pulmonary hypertension, septic shock, hyperthyroidism, renal insufficiency, and advanced liver disease (Bhardwaj and Januzzi, 2009; Hunt *et al.*, 2009).

Clinical Pearls

When patients with a history of heart failure are thought to have hypovolemic shock (systolic blood pressure (SBP)<90 mmHg), aggressive fluid resuscitation to perfuse end organs must be strongly considered while measures to support airway and breathing are simultaneously undertaken.

Conclusions

Pulmonary management of critically ill adults is a mainstay of monitoring and treatment in critically ill patients. While considerable research has been conducted in mechanically ventilated patients, significant difficulties arise in researching patient conditions that are widely heterogeneous. Monitoring protocols for early detection and safety have been reviewed in this chapter but further research is needed to establish evidence-based guidelines for optimal care and outcomes.

References

Abrishami, A., Khajehdehi, A., and Chung, F. (2010) A systematic review of screening questionnaires for obstructive sleep apnea. *Journal of Canadian Anesthesiology*, **57**, 423–438.

Ahrens, T., Schallom, L., Bettorf, K. *et al.* (2001) End-tidal carbon dioxide measurements as a prognostic indicator of outcome in cardiac arrest. *American Journal of Critical Care*, **10** (6), 391–398.

Alonso-Fernandez, A., Garcia-Rio, F., Racionero, M.A. *et al.* (2005) Cardiac rhythm disturbances and ST-segment depression episodes in pateitns with obstructive sleep apnea-hypopnea syndrome and its mechanisms. *Chest*, **127**, 15–22.

American Academy of Pediatrics, Committee on Drugs (2002) Guidelines for monitoring and management of pediatric patients during and after sedation for diagnostic and therapeutic procedures: addendum. *Pediatrics*, **110**, 836–838.

American Society of Anesthesiologists Task Force on Perioperative Management of Patients with Obstructive Sleep Apnea (2006) Practice guidelines for the perioperative management of patients with obstructive sleep apnea. *Anesthesiology*, **104**, 1081–1093.

American Society of Anesthesiologists Task Force on Sedation and Analgesia by Non-Anesthesiologists (2002) Practice guidelines for sedation and analgesia by non-anesthesiologists. *Anesthesiology*, **96**, 1004–1017.

Beecroft, J.M., Ward, M., Younes, M. *et al.* (2008) Sleep monitoring in the intensive care unit: comparison of nurse assessment, actigraphy and polysomnography. *Intensive Care Medicine*, **34**, 2076–2083.

Bhardwaj, A. and Januzzi, J. (2009) Natriuretic peptide-guided management of acutely destabilized heart failure. *Critical Pathways in Cardiology*, **8** (4), 146–150.

Bijwadia, J.S. and Ejaz, M.S. (2009) Sleep and critical care. *Current Opinion in Critical Care*, **15**, 25–29.

Blackwood, B., Alderdice, F., Burns, K.E.A. *et al.* (2010) Protocolized versus non-protocolized weaning for reducing the duration of mechanical ventilation in critically ill adult patients. *Cochrane Database of Systematic Reviews* (**5**), CD006904. doi: 10.1002/14651858.CD006904.pub2.

Bradley, T.D. and Floras, J.S. (2009) Obstructive sleep apnoea and its cardiovascular consequences. *Lancet*, **373**, 82–93.

Brook, A., Ahrens, T., Schaiff, R. *et al.* (1999) Effect of a nursing-implemented sedation protocol on the duration of mechanical ventilation. *Critical Care Medicine*, **27**, 2609–2615.

Burns, S., Fisher, C., Tribble, S.S.E. *et al.* (2010) Multifactor clinical score and outcome of mechanical ventilation weaning trials: Burns Wean Assessment Program. *American Journal of Critical Care*, **19**, 431–440.

Cabello, B., Thille, A.W., Drouot, X. *et al.* (2008) Sleep quality in mechanicallly ventilated patients: comparison of three ventilatory modes. *Critical Care Medicine*, **36**, 1749–1755.

Cacho, G., Pérez-Calle, J., Barbado, A. *et al.* (2010) Capnography is superior to pulse oximetry for the detection of respiratory depression during colonoscopy. *Revista española de enfermedades digestivas: organo oficial de la Sociedad Española de Patología Digestiva*, **102** (2), 86–89.

Cheng, K.C., Chen, C.M., Tan, C.K. *et al.* (2011) Methylprednisone reduces the rates of postextubation stridor and reintubation associated with attenuated cytokine responses in critically ill patients. *Minerva Anestesiologica*, **77** (5), 503–509.

Chung, F., Yegneswaran, B., Liao, P. *et al.* (2008) STOP questionnaire: a tool to screen patients for obstructive sleep apnea. *Anesthesiology*, **108**, 812–821.

Critical Care Alert (2012) The cuff-leak test for predicting post-extubation stridor: are we focusing on the wrong question? The cuff-leak test for predicting post-extubation stridor: are we focusing on the wrong question? *Critical Care Alert*, http://search.proquest.com/docview/1221175822?accountid=28051 (accessed July 26, 2014).

Dellinger, R.P., Levy, M.M., Carlet, J.M. *et al.* (2008) Surviving Sepsis Campaign: international guidelines for management of severe sepsis and septic shock: 2008. *Critical Care Medicine*, **36**, 296–327.

Dhand, R. (2010) Sleep disorders: diagnosis and treatment. *Respiratory Care*, **55** (10), 1389–1396.

Ding, L., Wang, H., and Wu, D. (2006) Laryngeal ultrasound: a useful method in predicting post-extubation stridor. A pilot study. *European Respiratory Journal*, **27** (2), 384–389.

Ely, E.W., Meade, M.O., Haponik, E.F. *et al.* (2001) Mechanical ventilator weaning protocols driven by nonphysician health-care professionals: evidence-based clinical practice guidelines. *Chest*, **120**, 454–463.

Epstein, L.J., Kristo, D., Strollo Jr, P.J. *et al.* (2009) Clinical guideline for the evaluation, management, and long-term care of obstructive sleep apnea in adults. *Journal of Clinical Sleep Medicine*, **5** (3), 263–276.

Esteban, A., Ferguson, N.D., Meade, M.O. *et al.* (2008) Evolution of mechanical ventilation in response to clinical research. *American Journal of Respiratory and Critical Care Medicine*, **177**, 170–177.

Ferri, F. (2004) *Ferri's Best Test: A Practical Guide to Clinical Laboratory Medicine and Diagnostic Imaging*, Elsevier-Mosby, Philadelphia.

Freedman, N.S., Gazendam, J., Levan, L. *et al.* (2001) Abnormal sleep/wake cycles and the effect of environmental noise on sleep disruption in the intensive care unit. *American Journal of Respiratory and Critical Care Medicine*, **163** (2), 451–457.

Frighetto, L., Marra, C., Bandali, S. *et al.* (2004) An assessment of quality of sleep and the use of drugs with sedating properties in hospitalized adult patients. *Health and Quality of Life Outcomes*, **2**, 1–10.

Grap, M.J., Munro, C.L., Wetzel, P.A. *et al.* (2012) Sedation in adults receiving mechanical ventilation: physiological and comfort outcomes. *American Journal of Critical Care*, **21**, e53–e64.

Green, G.B., Harris, I.S., Lin, G.A. *et al.* (2004) *The Washington Manual of Medical Therapeutics*, 31st edn, Lippincott Williams & Wilkins, Philadelphia, p. 192.

Greensmith, J. and Aker, J. (1998) Ventilatory management in the postanesthesia care unit. *Journal of Perianesthesia Nursing*, **12**, 370–381.

Grimm, W., Sharkova, J., Heitmann, J. *et al.* (2009) Sleep-disordered breathing in recipients of implantable defibrillators. *PACE*, **32**, S8–S11.

Hardin, K.A. (2009) Sleep in the ICU. *Chest*, **136**, 284–294.

Hunt, S.A., Abraham, W.T., Chin, M.H. *et al.* (2009) 2009 focused update incorporated into the ACC/AHA 2005 guidelines for the diagnosis and management of heart failure in adults: a report of the American College of Cardiology Foundation/American Heart Association task force on practice guidelines developed in collaboration with the international society for heart and lung transplantation. *Journal of the American College of Cardiology*, **53** (15), e1–e90.

Jaber, S., Jung, B., Chanques, G. *et al.* (2009) Effects of steroids on reintubation and post-extubation stridor in adults: meta-analysis of randomized controlled trials. *Critical Care*, **13** (2), R49–R59.

Keenan, S.P., Sinuff, T., Burns, K.E.A. *et al.* (2011) Clinical practice guidelines for the use of noninvasive positive-pressure ventilation and noninvasive continuous positive airway pressure in the acute care setting. *Canadian Medical Association Journal*, **183**, E195–E214.

Kollef, M., Bedient, T., Isakow, W., and Witt, C. (2008) *The Washington Manual of Critical Care*, Lippincott, Williams & Wilkins, Philadelphia.

Kress, J.P., Pohlman, A.S., O'Connor, M.F., and Hall, J.B. (2000) Daily interruption of sedative infusions in critically ill patients undergoing mechanical ventilation. *The New England Journal of Medicine*, **342**, 1471–1477.

Lam, L.L., Cameron, P.A., Schneider, H.G. *et al.* (2010) Meta-analysis: effect of B-type natriuretic peptide testing on clinical outcomes in patients with acute dyspnea in the emergency setting. *Annals of Internal Medicine*, **153** (11), 728–735.

Lee, W.Y. and Mokhlesi, B. (2008) Diagnosis and management of obesity hypoventilation syndrome in the ICU. *Critical Care Clinics*, **24**, 533–549.

Levine, R.L., Wayne, M.A., and Miller, C.C. (1997) End-tidal carbon dioxide and outcome of out of hospital cardiac arrest. *New England Journal of Medicine*, **337**, 301–306.

Lightdale, J.R., Goldmann, D.A., Feldman, H.A. *et al.* (2006) Microstream capnography improves patient monitoring during moderate sedation: a randomized, controlled trial. *Pediatrics*, **117** (6), e1170–e1178.

Luetz, A., Goldmann, A., Weber-Carstens, S., and Spies, C. (2012) Weaning from mechanical ventilation and sedation. *Current Opinion in Anesthesiology*, **25**, 164–169.

MacIntyre, N.R. (2008) Ventilator discontinuation process: evidence and guidelines. *Critical Care Medicine*, **36** (1), 329–330.

MacIntyre, N.R., Cook, D.J., Ely Jr, E.W. *et al.* (2001) Evidence-based guidelines for weaning and discontinuing ventilatory support: a collective task force facilitated by the American College of Chest Physicians; the American Association for Respiratory Care; and the American College of Critical Care Medicine. *Chest*, **120**, 375S–396S.

Markovitz, B., Randolph, A., and Khemani, R. (2009) Corticosteroids for the prevention and treatment of post-extubation stridor in neonates, children, and adults. *Cochrane Database of Systematic Reviews* (**2**), CD001000. doi: 10.1002/14651858.CD001000.pub2.

Morgenthaler, T.I., Aurora, R.N., Brown, T. *et al.* (2008.) Practice parameters for the use of autotitrating continuous positive airway pressure devices for titrating pressures and treating adult patients with obstructive sleep apnea syndrome: an update for 2007 An American Academy of Sleep Medicine report. *Sleep*, **31** (1), 141–147.

National Heart Lung and Blood Institute (NHLBI) ARDS Network (2008) *NIH NHLBI ARDS Clinical Network Mechanical Ventilation Protocol Summary*, www.ardsnet.org/node/77791 (Accessed September 27, 2014).

National Heart Lung and Blood Institute (NHLBI) ARDS Network (2014), http://www.ardsnet.org/ (accessed August 7, 2014).

Naughton, M. (2008) Common sleep problems in ICU: heart failure and sleep-disordered breathing syndromes. *Critical Care Clinics*, **24**, 565–587.

Nowbar, S., Burkart, K.M., Gonzales, R. *et al.* (2004) Obesity-associated hypoventilation in hospitalized patients: prevalence, effects, and outcome. *The American Journal of Medicine*, **116** (1), 1–7.

Parthasarathy, S. and Tobin, M.J. (2002) Effect of ventilator mode on sleep quality in critically ill patients. *American Journal of Respiratory and Critical Care Medicine*, **166**, 1423–1429.

Piper, A.J. and Grunstein, R.R. (2011) Obesity hypoventilation syndrome. Mechanisms and management. *American Journal of Respiratory Critical Care Medicine*, **183**, 292–298.

Principi, T., Falzetti, G., Elisei, D. *et al.* (2009) Behavior of B-type natriuretic peptide during mechanical ventilation and spontaneous breathing after extubation. *Minerva Anestesiologica*, **75** (4), 179–183.

Priou, P., Hamel, J.F., Person, C. *et al.* (2010) Long-term outcome of noninvasive positive pressure ventilation for obesity hypoventilation syndrome. *Chest*, **138** (1), 84–90.

Rana, R., Vlahakis, N.E., Daniels, C.W. *et al.* (2006) B-type natriuretic peptide in the assessment of acute lung injury and cardiogenic pulmonary edema. *Critical Care Medicine*, **34** (7), 1941–1946.

Redeker, N.S. (2008) Challenges and opportunities associated with studying sleep in critically ill adults. *AACN Advanced Critical Care*, **19**, 178–185.

Roberts, D.J., Haroon, B., and Hall, R.I. (2012) Sedation for critically ill or injured adults in the intensive care unit. A shifting paradigm. Drugs, **72**, 1881–1916.

Ryan, D.M., Juvet, S., Leung, R., and Bradley, T.D. (2008) Timing of nocturnal ventricular ectopy in heart failure patients with sleep apnea. *Chest*, **133**, 934–940.

Serizawa, N., Yumino, D., Kajimoto, K. *et al.* (2008) Impact of sleep-disordered breathing on life-threatening ventricular arrhythmia in heart failure patients with implantable cardioverter-defibrillator. *American Journal of Cardiology*, **102**, 1064–1068.

Soto, R., Fu, E., Vila Jr, H., and Miguel, R. (2004) Capnography accurately detects apnea during monitored anesthesia care. *Anesthesia & Analgesia*, **99**, 379–382.

Vander Werf, B.D., Watt, J., Joseph, B. *et al.* (2010) Can plasma B-type natriuretic peptide levels predict need for mechanical ventilation after injury? *American Journal of Surgery*, **200** (6), 845–850.

Vargo, J.J., Zuccaro Jr, G., Dumot, J.A. *et al.* (2002) Automated graphic assessment of respiratory activity is superior to pulse oximetry and visual assessment for the detection of early respiratory depression during therapeutic upper endoscopy. *Gastrointestinal Endoscopy*, **55**, 826–831.

Wittekamp, B.H., van Mook, W.N., Tjan, D.H. *et al.* (2009) Clinical review: post-extubation laryngeal edema and extubation failure in critically ill adult patients. *Critical Care (London, England)*, **13** (6), 233.

CHAPTER 4

Electrocardiographic monitoring for cardiovascular dysfunction

Catherine Winkler

Fairfield University, Fairfield, CT., USA

Cardiovascular disease is the leading cause of mortality and morbidity in the United States accounting for approximately 33.6% of deaths annually (Xu *et al.*, 2010). Although death rates from cardiovascular disease (CVD) have declined in recent years, the overall burden of the disease remains very high. Heart disease is more common among people aged 65 and older; however, the onset of heart disease in younger individuals is gradually becoming more prevalent. More than 150 000 Americans who died because of CVD in 2007 were less than 65 years old (Xu *et al.*, 2010). In addition, more than 61.8 million people currently live with CVD, which can be a major cause of disability producing more than 2.1 million hospitalizations each year (Center for Disease Control and Monitoring, 2010). The cost of expenditure on heart disease in 2010 was $316.4 billion (Xu *et al.*, 2010). Heart disease expenditure estimates include hospitalizations, procedures, physician visits, medications, and lost productivity. Accordingly, cardiovascular admissions continue to predominate in the intensive care unit (ICU) and in the step-down units where advanced practice registered nurses (APRNs) will encounter electrocardiographic (ECG) monitoring as an important component of clinical care.

Physiologic guidelines

The control of risk factors for CVD such as hypertension, hyperlipidemia, smoking, diabetes, obesity, and lack of physical activity remain a central issue for many Americans. Data from the National Health and Nutrition Examination Survey Center for Disease Control and Monitoring, 2010 indicate that 30.5% of US adults (≥20 years of age) have hypertension and that 15% of US adults have elevated cholesterol levels (≥240 mg/dl). Furthermore, despite 40 years of smoking cessation recommendations, in 2009, among Americans (≥18 years of age), 23.1% of men and 18.3% of women continued to be cigarette smokers (Lloyd-Jones *et al.*, 2010). Regrettably, Americans diagnosed with diabetes mellitus represent 8.0% of the adult population and this number is rising, along with an astonishing estimated prevalence of obesity in US adults (≥20 years of age) of 68% in 2008 (NHANES, 2008). These factors along with 36% of Americans who report that they do not engage in any physical activity (Lloyd-Jones *et al.*, 2010) present a challenge for nurse practitioners who are engaged in population health initiatives. Frequently, patients with heart disease have more than two of these risk factors and other comorbidities such as kidney disease and respiratory illnesses. These associated conditions further complicate treatment and present a conundrum to hospitals and all health-care providers who are struggling to provide preventive care as well as treat diseases in a cost-effective manner.

Many hospitals meet the challenge of triaging acute cardiovascular hospitalizations through the development of alternative care settings. Settings such as chest pain centers, observation units, post-anesthesia recovery, or intermediate care units together with the

Critical Care Nursing: Monitoring and Treatment for Advanced Nursing Practice, First Edition. Edited by Kathy J. Booker.
© 2015 John Wiley & Sons, Inc. Published 2015 by John Wiley & Sons, Inc.

traditional inpatient units, telemetry, step-down, and intensive care try to deliver the right care to the right patient at the right time in the right locale. The delivery of cost-effective, high-quality care to patients with heart disease is conducted by ensuring that core measures are met in the inpatient setting, that the patient experience is constructive with education and medication reconciliation provided, and that outcomes are optimized. Likewise, one of the ways that high-quality efficient care can be achieved is through "targeted" ECG monitoring that is determined by the surveillance needs of the patient. Surveillance in this context involves a review of the practice standards for ECG monitoring (Drew *et al.*, 2004) and other related evidence-based literature, following criteria as determined by the practice setting with established ECG monitoring levels, and defining the monitoring goals based on the patient's clinical needs. ECG monitoring can range from simple heart rate and basic rhythm interpretation to complex cardiac arrhythmias, myocardial ischemia, and prolonged QT-interval surveillance (Drew *et al.*, 2004).

Goals of monitoring

Targeted or patient-centric ECG monitoring is best applied when an immediate assessment of the patient is made to determine the level of optimal monitoring. Based on the diagnosis on admission and changes in the patient's clinical condition during hospitalization, ongoing medical decisions are predicated on the interventions and specific goals of care. The rating system devised by the American College of Cardiology Emergency Cardiac Care Committee (Jaffe *et al.*, 1991) includes three categories: class I cardiac monitoring is indicated for all patients within the group (post cardiac arrest, acute coronary syndrome, etc.); class II monitoring may be beneficial for some patients but not essential for all (syncope, post myocardial infarction [MI], etc.); and class III monitoring in which monitoring has no therapeutic benefits (permanent rate-controlled atrial fibrillation [AF]). After a decision is made regarding the category of

ECG monitoring and the level of intensity that is required for a patient, the specific inpatient setting is selected as well as a plan for the monitoring timeframe. ECG monitoring is one of the most important tools to diagnose cardiac disease and alterations associated with changing health status. Therefore, important clinical decisions such as the medication therapy, device adjustments (e.g., pacemaker and implantable cardioverter defibrillator [ICD]), further diagnostic testing, cardiac consultation, unit transfers, and length of stay are made every day using ECG monitoring data. The American Heart Association (AHA) practice standards (Drew *et al.*, 2004) provide direction for ECG monitoring that will assist APRNs in deciding which patients are best served by ECG monitoring during an episode of care. Equally important to realize is the power of misdiagnosis of the ECG monitoring data that can result in adverse patient outcomes from undertreatment to selection of the wrong therapy. Recognizing artifacts and other pitfalls resulting from patient movement, outside electrical interference, and misplaced electrodes and leads will ultimately result in improved patient outcomes (Baranchuk *et al.*, 2009). Registered nurses must establish the proper location and the correct preparation for electrode placement for proper ECG monitoring and ongoing comparison of rhythm strips over time.

APRNs and expert staff nurses are central in deciding on the goals of monitoring for an individual patient as they are in the best position to detect clinical problems early to mitigate them to optimize patient outcomes. A patient is monitored for a variety of reasons: to detect changes in a patient's clinical condition, to diagnose a problem, to assess a response to an intervention, to prevent an undesirable event, and for surveillance before and after surgery. Through an understanding of the patient's underlying health-care issues and the pathology, the nurse can select the leads that will supply the best and most clinically significant information.

To provide optimum care and establish appropriate ECG monitoring, it is important to review the cardiac diseases that are clinically managed using this technology.

Table 4.1 Biomarkers used for diagnosis of acute MI.

Test	Estimated peak (h)	Sensitivity and specificity	Description
Troponin Subunits Tn1, TnT	12	↑↑↑ sensitivity and specificity	Troponin is released with the degradation of actin and myosin filaments. Released in 2–4h/ persists for up to 7 days
Creatine kinase or CK-MB	10–24	↑↑ relatively specific when skeletal muscle damage is absent	CK-MB facilitates movement of high-energy phosphates into and out of mitochondria. It is in many types of tissues even in the skeletal muscle. Short duration; it cannot be used for late diagnosis of acute MI but can be used to suggest infarct extension if levels rise again. Normal within 2–3 days

CK-MB, creatine kinase–myocardial band; h, hours; MI, myocardial infarction.

Indications for ECG monitoring include the following conditions: post successful cardiopulmonary resuscitation; acute coronary syndrome (ACS); cardiac arrhythmias; heart failure; electrolyte abnormalities; critical illnesses; and drug overdose (if there is a potential pro-arrhythmic complication) (Drew *et al.*, 2004; Jevon, 2010). All of these clinical diagnoses need ECG monitoring to exam and assess for cardiac dysfunction. Nurse practitioners are in a position to assist in setting the standards for ECG monitoring in their facility through their recommendations and leadership.

Post cardiopulmonary resuscitation

The purpose of ECG monitoring in the early days of coronary care units was the immediate recognition of cardiac arrest. However, it was quickly realized that nurses needed not only to identify and respond to cardiac arrest but also to detect life-threatening arrhythmias to decrease mortality in patients who had an acute MI (Webner, 2011). From this time forward with the technological improvements in ECG surveillance, it was understood that cardiac arrhythmias could result in hemodynamic instability and sudden cardiac death (Webner, 2011). Education of staff involved in arrhythmia detection of emergent arrhythmias such as asystole and ventricular tachycardia include bradycardias, heart blocks, and both wide and narrow complex tachycardias. Beyond early recognition and response to cardiac arrest, nurses are now charged with post-cardiopulmonary resuscitation support, which requires continuous assessment of physiological parameters through hemodynamic monitoring, recognition of typical complications (MI, adult respiratory distress syndrome, deep vein thrombosis, pulmonary emboli), and timely interventions. Patients resuscitated from cardiac arrest should be a top priority for monitoring until the reversible cause such as hyperkalemia is corrected or until an ICD is implanted. Acute coronary syndrome is a common cause of cardiac arrest; subsequently, the clinician needs to evaluate the patient's 12-lead ECG and cardiac biomarkers (see Table 4.1). As a result of a high incidence of ischemia, aggressive treatment of ST-elevation MI needs to begin immediately along with emergent percutaneous coronary intervention (PCI) in the context of concurrent ongoing life support.

Monitoring elements

It is important to identify the essential post-resuscitation clinical problems of the patient before deciding on monitoring needs. Patients who continue to be hemodynamically unstable will require monitoring for arrhythmia detection and ongoing ischemia. Depending on the cause of the cardiac arrest and the medications that the patient had been taking, even QT-interval prolongation may be an ongoing concern that will require surveillance. Clinicians need to recognize ECG changes indicative of impending torsades de pointes and implement interventions to prevent this and subsequent cardiac arrest (Sommargren and Drew, 2007).

Evidence-based treatment guidelines

The guidelines published by the American College of Cardiology [ACC] (Jaffe *et al.*, 1991) and practice standards (Drew and Funk, 2004) recommend monitoring the patient until hemodynamically stable and the clinical problem is corrected. The primary reasons for bedside cardiac monitoring include arrhythmia detection, ST-segment monitoring, and QT-interval monitoring as identified by Drew and colleagues (2004), and they may all apply to the patient who is recovering from cardiac arrest. The best lead for monitoring arrhythmias is V_1; the next best is V_6. Use of V_1 allows the practitioner to more easily view P waves, differentiate left and right bundle branch blocks, and distinguish ventricular from supraventricular rhythms with aberrant conduction (Kumar, 2008). Monitoring for ST-segment changes will allow for rapid intervention and leads III and V_3 are recommended by the American Association of Critical Care Nurses (AACN) if the involved coronary arteries are unknown (Bourgault, 2009). If the patient has a prior history of ischemia, then it is best to monitor the patient in a more directed way in the leads that reflect the vessels involved in the ischemic event (see Table 4.2). Prolongation of the QT-interval can also occur because of a genetic predisposition or through acquired abnormalities such as renal failure and acute pancreatitis. In the acute care setting, often the etiology for QT-interval prolongation is related to medications such as some antibiotics, antipsychotics, and antiarrhythmics (Sommargren and Drew, 2007). Patients in this situation would need to be monitored for QT-interval prolongation until the medication is discontinued or dosage established with no lengthening of the QTc. The QTc is considered prolonged when it is greater than 0.47 s in males and greater than 0.48 s in females. If the QTc is greater than 0.50 s in anyone, it can be associated with higher risk for torsades de pointes (Moss, 1999).

Table 4.2 Monitoring recommendations, vessels, and selected leads.

Type of monitoring	Coronary vessel involved	Lead selection
Arrhythmia monitoring Primary lead	LAD	V_1—intraventricular septum
Arrhythmia monitoring Secondary lead	Left circumflex	V_6—lateral wall
Ischemia monitoring	LAD	V_3—anterior wall V_1, V_2, V_4
Ischemia monitoring	RCA	III—inferior wall II, aVF
Ischemia monitoring	Left circumflex	V_5 and V_6—lateral wall I, aVL—sometimes no change V_1, V_2, or V_3 for reciprocal changes posterior wall
If ischemic footprint unknown	LAD and RCA	V_3 and III—anterior and inferior leads
Demand ischemia	Left circumflex	V_5—lateral wall
QT-interval monitoring	N/A	Monitor in the lead with best-defined T wave

LAD, left anterior descending; RCA, right coronary artery.

Clinical Pearls—Patient Management and Treatment

Survival rates at discharge for patients who experience in-hospital cardiac arrest are only 27% among children and 18% among adults (Lloyd-Jones et al., 2010). The National Registry for Cardiopulmonary Resuscitation in 2007 identified that for the events reported, 93% were monitored or witnessed and that ventricular fibrillation or pulseless ventricular tachycardia was listed as the first recorded rhythm (Lloyd-Jones et al., 2010). Continuous cardiac monitoring for recurrent arrhythmias, ST-segment monitoring for ongoing ischemia, and tracking the QT-interval in patients with known clinical risk factors are important elements for hemodynamic optimization and multidisciplinary goal-directed therapy protocols to improve survival (Gaieski et al., 2009).

Acute coronary syndromes

In 2006, when primary and secondary discharge diagnoses were considered together, there were 1 365 000 unique hospitalizations for ACS, of which 765 000 were male and 600 000 were female (National Hospital Discharge

Survey, 2008). Patients in the early phases of ACS such as ST-elevation/non-ST-elevation MI, unstable angina, or rule-out MI should be monitored for a minimum of 24 h for an uncomplicated MI or for at least 24 h after complications (e.g., ongoing chest pain) have resolved (Drew *et al.*, 2004). For patients who are experiencing ACS or a rule-out MI diagnosis, monitoring will involve a greater intensity based on the admission diagnosis. Levels of monitoring intensity are established based on best practice recommendations, which are generated from AHA published standards (2004) and Jaffe and colleagues (1991). Those patients who have an acute MI can be at risk for reperfusion arrhythmias with the incidence of 7.5% after an infarct (Al-Khatib *et al.*, 2002). Furthermore, patients with elevated troponin levels compared to those patients with normal levels are more likely to develop arrhythmias after PCI (Bonnemeier *et al.*, 2003). These patients should be monitored for 12–24 h because of the possibility of an abrupt closure. Early revascularization does not guarantee optimal myocardial perfusion in patients undergoing primary angioplasty. In some patients, perfusion remains impaired and therefore identifying worsening ST-segment elevation post PCI is critically important (Aude and Mehta, 2006). In general, stenting the artery has provided patients with less frequent reocclusions post procedure. Patients receiving thrombolytic therapy for an acute MI should be monitored for at least 12–24 h if event-free to assure that the culprit artery remains patent. Lastly, patients with a potential for vasospasm (Prinzmetal angina, cocaine) should be monitored for ST-segment changes until after therapy is initiated or till they are event-free for 12–24 h. Patients who do not have an arrhythmia may have ECG monitoring discontinued unless they have enduring ST-segment changes and QT-interval deviations that require continuous monitoring. Sometimes there are practical limitations to using ST-segment monitoring such as when a patient is physically restless. Under these circumstances, ST-segment monitoring may not be possible because of fluctuating changes in the baseline ECG pattern. There are several methods to improve ST-segment monitoring to include early identification of body position changes on the monitor and recorded strips to serve as a reference. Nurses should also adjust the alarm parameters for the individual patient once the baseline is established, and carefully prepare the electrode site placing the leads in the proper location. Establishing a reference point for the ST-segment, adjusting the alarm range, and securing the electrodes will all help to minimize false alarms while still providing cardiac monitoring for those patients who are restless.

Monitoring for ST-segment changes is important for those at risk for myocardial ischemia including patients who have unstable angina, chest pain, or post-op patients with a history of heart disease as well as those in critical care who may have a primary diagnosis other than cardiac but are at risk for demand ischemia. It is imperative to differentiate ischemia from infarction. Ischemia is caused by a reduction in blood supply, resulting in less oxygen delivered to a region of the heart. ECG changes during an ischemic event are represented by contiguous T wave inversions and/or ST-segment depression. ST-segments that are 1 mm or more below baseline following the J-point or where the QRS complex meets the T wave are considered to be ischemic. Infarction develops when there is prolonged ischemia leading to myocardial necrosis. Infarction can be diagnosed by ST segments that will elevate ≥1 mm in limb leads and ≥2 mm in chest leads representing the earliest signs of an evolving MI. Prompt intervention may prevent myocardial injury and infarction. As referenced in the practice standards, biphasic T waves in leads V_2 and V_3 could represent Wellen's sign (Drew *et al.*, 2004). It is a critical finding because it is associated with significant stenosis of the left anterior descending coronary artery and may be indicative of an MI.

Monitoring ST-segments can be challenging; therefore, a baseline must be established with the patient in a supine position. If the patient moves or changes positions, it can cause ST-segment variations and false alarms as referenced earlier. The key to minimizing false alarms is to set alarm parameters accurately and monitor for trends in the ST segment. If one does not know the pattern of changes in ST segments because prior ischemic changes were not noted and the coronary arteries involved are unknown, then it is best to select leads III and V_3 per AACN recommendations (Bourgault, 2009). However, lead V_5 is the best for monitoring demand ischemia. The problem with monitoring in just one lead is that as much as 50% of the ST-segment depression events may be missed in a single lead configuration; therefore, multiple-lead monitoring provides the greatest coverage for ischemic changes (Booker et al., 2003) and should be used whenever possible. Booker and colleagues (2003) report that demand ischemia may be transient in noncontiguous leads without the patient experiencing symptoms. Patients with these conditions, as well as the availability of fibrinolytic therapy and PCI, have contributed to the change in focus for continuous cardiac monitoring from just arrhythmia detection to ischemia monitoring as well. Oversight of ST-segment changes is important not only to assess and treat patients with known heart disease but also to protect patients who either experience silent or unreported ischemia (Drew and Krucoff, 1999) and for those who are at risk for reocclusion of target vessels after PCI.

Monitoring elements

Arrhythmia monitoring is compulsory because ischemia and infarction may cause lethal arrhythmias. In addition to arrhythmia monitoring, patients with ACS need surveillance because ST-segment elevation is an independent predictor of mortality, even after controlling for multiple clinical factors (Langer et al., 1998). These patients have top priority because of ongoing ischemia that may result in an acute MI or an extension of an MI. As referenced earlier, the toughest decision with patients who have ACS is the selection of the best lead to monitor for ST-segment pattern changes. The inherent risk is that the wrong choice will result in missing an evolving event. It is important to note that a left bundle branch block or pacemaker-dependent rhythms present challenges to the diagnosis of acute ischemia because of alterations in the QRS complex and T wave that obscure typical ischemic changes. To aid in a definitive diagnosis of acute MI, it is best, when possible, to contrast the new pattern with an old ECG. This will help to determine if a preexisting left bundle branch block had presented before the

acute event. With a new-onset left bundle branch block, the recommendations are to determine if the new bundle with ST-segment elevation of 1 mm or more is concordant with the QRS complex; if the ST-segment depression of 1 mm or more is present in lead V_1, V_2, or V_3; and if ST-segment elevation of 5 mm or more is discordant from the QRS complex in the right-sided leads (Wackers, 1987). Lastly, pericarditis, which is an acute inflammation of the pericardium, can cause both PR depressions and ST-segment elevations during the patient's initial presentation to the hospital. Through this acute phase of pericarditis, the ST-elevations are usually diffuse throughout the precordial and limb leads in a nonanatomic distribution (Wang, Asinger, and Marriott, 2003), differentiating it from an acute MI presentation. Once treated, all ECG changes will return to baseline.

Evidence-based treatment guidelines

Research supports continuous ST-segment monitoring to enable the practitioner to monitor all potential ischemic zones (Drew and Krucoff, 1999; Johnson, 2008; Leeper, 2007). The 2004 Practice Standards for Electrocardiographic Monitoring in Hospital Settings provides the "best practice" for continuous ECG monitoring based on expert opinion (Drew et al., 2004). The consensus guidelines outline ECG indicators (in the absence of left ventricular hypertrophy and left bundle branch block) as new ST-segment elevations at the J-point in two contiguous leads with the cutoff of more than 2 mm in men and 1.5 mm in women in leads V_1 and V_2 and/or more than 1 mm in the other leads. The guidelines also describe acute myocardial ischemia as ST-segment depression of greater than 0.5 mm in two contiguous leads and/or T wave inversion greater than 1 mm in two contiguous leads with a prominent R wave (Sandau and Smith, 2009). Over 20 years ago, Krucoff and colleagues (1988) initially described ST-segment monitoring as helpful to identify recurrent myocardial ischemia after MI or PCI. In a randomized controlled trial of 424 patients presenting to the emergency department with chest pain, researchers used ST-segment monitoring as one component of their protocol during the patient's stay in the chest pain center.

They found that it was influential as a cost-effective alternative to hospital admission for those patients with an intermediate risk of unstable angina (Farkouh *et al.*, 1998). In another study, Gibler and associates (2005) found that half of the patients with acute coronary syndrome who demonstrated ST-segment depression on the initial 12-lead ECG went on to have an MI within hours. However, even with these early studies as well as ongoing evidenced-based experience, ST-segment monitoring outside the catheterization lab has been slow in translating into practice.

Selection of the appropriate lead is the key to accurate bedside monitoring. Each lead reflects the electrical activity in a specific region of the heart and the corresponding vessel that supplies it (Table 4.2). Changes that occur in one or more leads will help the practitioner identify the vessel(s) and region of the heart that are likely affected by ischemia or infarction. Patients with a right coronary artery occlusion, which supplies the inferior wall of the left ventricle, should be monitored in leads II, III, and aVF. It is important to keep in mind that lead II will display the least significant change. Anterior wall infarctions are usually associated with occlusions of the left anterior descending branch of the left coronary artery, for which, subsequently, the best leads are V_3 and V_4. For the intraventricular septum, leads V_1 and V_2 are well matched for detecting ischemic changes in the septal region. The lateral wall infarctions are usually associated with occlusion of the left circumflex artery and in one-third of cases there are no visible changes. When ischemic changes do occur in a patient, they are visualized in leads I, aVL, V_5, and V_6. Reciprocal depression ST-segment changes will occur in leads V_1, V_2, and V_3 when there is a posterior infarction or posterior leads may be applied (Fig. 4.1).

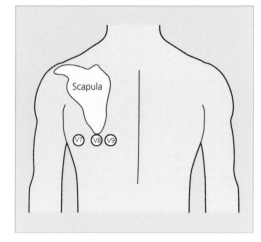

Figure 4.1 Posterior V7–V9 placement. From Morris and Brady (2002). © BMJ.

Clinical Pearls—Patient Management and Treatment

It is also important to note that ST-segment monitoring may need to be specifically ordered if it is not automatically turned on when a patient is attached to the system. Although most cardiac monitors have computerized ischemia monitoring, often the nurse must activate it in order to have it monitor for ST-segment changes. Unlike computerized arrhythmia monitoring, which is automated, ST-segment ischemia monitoring must often be manually turned on (Drew *et al.*, 2004). Unfortunately, computerized ischemia monitoring is still underused in the acute care setting (Funk *et al.*, 2010). It is not clear why both ST-segment and QT-interval prolongation are undermonitored but according to Funk and colleagues (2010), it may be related to lack of knowledge on the part of nurses and/or the absence of physician support for the practice. Anecdotally, some physicians believe that the incidence of reocclusions post procedure is so low because of stent use that ST-segment monitoring is not as important as it might have been in the earlier days of PCI. Funk and colleagues (2009) observe that for over 50 years continuous ECG monitoring has been primarily focused on arrhythmia detection. In fact, some hospitals with old ECG-monitoring equipment only have arrhythmia monitoring. However, ST-segment does have a place in clinical care and ST-segment monitoring should be applied to provide surveillance not only to those with acute MI but also to patients who experience demand ischemia or have silent ischemia without symptoms.

ST-segment alarms should be set for 1 mm above and below baseline when monitoring in V_1 or V_6. Alarm limits can be set tighter with the limb leads using parameters set at 0.5 mm above and below the baseline (Webner, 2011). In contrast, for post-coronary artery bypass graft (CABG) patients, leads may need to be set with a wider range to accommodate the associated ST-segment changes that may occur due to perioperative inflammation. The recommendation is to monitor the ST-segments 1.5 mm above and below the patient's baseline during the postsurgical phase of recovery. If continuous 12-lead monitoring is unavailable in the acute phase of illness, a 6-lead telemetry system should be used to monitor V_1 for arrhythmias and the second V lead for detection of ischemia. It is important to note that, for patients who have intermittent ventricular pacing with ST/T wave abnormalities, a left bundle branch block, or an intermittent right bundle branch block, continuous ST-segment monitoring is not recommended because these rhythm patterns will trigger false alarms (Drew *et al.*, 2004). A special consideration is the identification of the patient who has a right ventricular infarct. This can occur in the context of an inferior wall MI and it is imperative that it is recognized because nitrates are contraindicated, whereas they are typically used in the management of most other types of MI (Calder, 2008). In addition to ST elevations in II, III, and aVF to definitively diagnose a right ventricular infarct, it is essential to move chest leads V_3 through V_6 from the usual left side of the chest to the right. If a right ventricular infarct is present, ST elevations will appear in the right-sided V_4 (Garvey *et al.*, 2006) and may also be present in additional RV leads. Another circumstance is when a posterior infarction is suspected because of ST depressions in V_1, V_2, and V_3 with large R waves. A posterior ECG can be obtained by repositioning leads V_4 through V_6 (Fig. 4.2). The V_4 lead is placed on the left posterior axillary line, V_5 at the border of the left scapula, and V_6 near the vertebrae, to note any ST elevations (Garvey *et al.*, 2006).

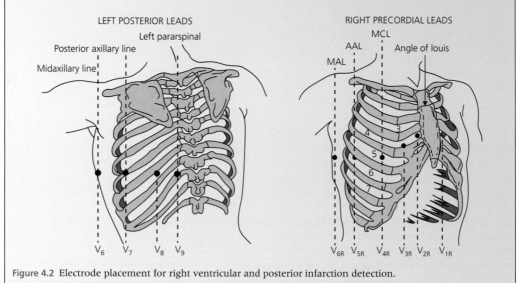

Figure 4.2 Electrode placement for right ventricular and posterior infarction detection.

Cardiac arrhythmias

Published literature such as the practice standards for ECG monitoring (Drew *et al.*, 2004) and the practice alert on dysrhythmia monitoring (Bourgault, 2009) require a patient to be monitored when there is a significant risk for life-threatening arrhythmias, specifically ventricular tachycardia, ventricular fibrillation, and asystole. Drew and colleagues (2004) recognize that nurses have the lead responsibility in attaching the ECG monitor and screening true from false alarms, documenting the onset and termination of tachyarrhythmias, and recording rhythm strips from the atrial epicardial pacemaker in patients who have had cardiac surgery. As discussed under the headings of post cardiac arrest and acute coronary syndrome, patients who have been resuscitated and/or have unstable coronary syndromes and newly diagnosed high-risk coronary lesions are at high risk

for arrhythmias. Interventions such as early revascularization, beta-blockers, nitrates, angiotensin-converting enzyme inhibitors, and other antiplatelet and antithrombotic agents have decreased the incidence and time course of problematic arrhythmias (Drew *et al.*, 2004). Similarly, ECG monitoring data from 278 patients with acute coronary syndrome who participated in a larger prospective study evaluating myocardial ischemia were found to have fewer life-threatening arrhythmias, but experienced frequent benign premature ventricular contractions (PVCs) and nonsustained ventricular tachycardia (Winkler et al., 2013). Frequent PVCs and other serious ventricular ectopy may be a marker for more severe heart disease; however, they are not independent predictors of adverse outcomes. ECG monitoring needs to be established for only those individuals who are at risk for significant arrhythmias as outlined in the practice standards rather than for those who have benign or chronic arrhythmias. Patients who have undergone angioplasty, experience a complication in the catheterization lab, or have an inconclusive outcome should also be monitored for 24 h or longer if arrhythmias have occurred. When the intra-aortic balloon pump is used to support cardiac function, arrhythmia recognition and tracking may be difficult because of changes in the overall ECG pattern. Generally, tracking arrhythmias is central to patient care to sort out and review only those arrhythmias that contribute to a decrease in effectiveness of the heart.

Patients who have undergone cardiac surgery should be monitored for 48–72 h or longer, possibly until discharge, if they are at high risk for developing AF according to the practice standards (Drew *et al.*, 2004). The risk factors for post-op AF include advanced age, past history of AF, valve disease, and in those with a preoperative hold of beta-blockers. Patients who undergo structural heart procedures such as valvuloplasty, transcatheter aortic valve replacement, and atrial septal closure devices as well as those who have the mini-maze procedure should also be monitored for arrhythmias for 12–24 h and longer as warranted based on the clinical course.

Another category of patients who need ECG monitoring are those who have a temporary or new device such as an ICD or pacemaker implanted during their course of hospitalization. For example, a patient with a temporary pacemaker or transcutaneous pacing pads has a short-term set of connections where lead or pad dislodgement is possible. Oversensing or loss of capture could easily occur necessitating an immediate intervention. This is especially important if the patient is device-dependent. Similarly, patients with AV block who are, or could easily become, hemodynamically unstable need ECG monitoring until the block either resolves or definitive treatment (ICD or pacemaker) is implemented.

Wolf–Parkinson White syndrome is associated with sudden cardiac death. Usually during AF, there is fast anterograde conduction over the accessory pathway and so patients need to be carefully monitored until they can be treated, often with an ablation. Torsades de pointes is a life-threatening arrhythmia that is associated

with long QT syndrome and PVCs that might trigger this arrhythmia, which could degenerate into ventricular fibrillation. Therefore, intensive ECG monitoring is clinically indicated until the patient can be stabilized. Any other life-threatening arrhythmias, especially in those patients with heart disease where hemodynamic instability is likely, should be monitored until the cause is determined and treated.

Monitoring elements

The expected practice is to select the best monitoring lead for the patient based on the type of arrhythmia that the patient has or is suspected to develop during their inpatient stay. Lead V_1 is the best to distinguish ventricular tachycardia from supraventricular tachycardia with aberrant conduction, recognize atrial activity, and differentiate between left and right bundle branch blocks with lead V_6 as a second choice (Johnson, 2008).

Evidence-based treatment guidelines

The practice standards for ECG monitoring in the hospital setting (Drew *et al.*, 2004) outline the three classes of arrhythmia monitoring. Class I indications have been listed for post cardiac arrest, acute coronary syndrome, after cardiac surgery, nonurgent PCI with complications, device implants, temporary pacemaker, and transcutaneous pacing, and those with AV block, Wolf–Parkinson White, and long QT syndrome. In addition, patients who are on the intraaortic balloon pump, with acute heart failure/pulmonary edema, with any hemodynamically unstable arrhythmia, in the ICU, or undergoing conscious sedation should be monitored for arrhythmias. Those patients who are post acute MI, with chest pain syndromes, have undergone uncomplicated, nonurgent PCI, and who require adjustments of medications to control the rate of tachyarrhythmias, all fall into class II monitoring, where this may benefit only some patients. Additionally, patients who are also classified as group II for ECG monitoring include those who undergo pacemaker lead replacement but are not pacemaker-dependent, uncomplicated ablation of an arrhythmia, routine diagnostic cardiac catheterization, subacute heart failure, syncope evaluation, and lastly, those who are terminally ill but have an arrhythmia that is uncomfortable with symptoms of palpitations and shortness of breath that require arrhythmia management (Drew *et al.*, 2004). There are patients who, although they may be very ill, fit into class III where they do not require ECG monitoring because they are at very low risk for an occurrence. Patients who undergo uncomplicated surgical procedures, hemodialysis, and patients with stable arrhythmias such as rate-controlled AF or the occasional PVCs in the absence of a moderating condition such as electrolyte abnormality or myocardial ischemia are all in class III (see Table 4.3).

Table 4.3 ECG monitoring arrhythmia classifications.

Class I	Class II	Class III
Highest risk	**Moderate risk**	**Low risk/ECG monitoring not required**
Post cardiac arrest	Post acute myocardial infarction	Postoperative uncomplicated surgical procedures
Acute coronary syndrome	Chest pain syndromes	Hemodialysis
Postoperative cardiac surgery	Uncomplicated, nonurgent PCI	Stable arrhythmias such as rate-controlled atrial fibrillation
Nonurgent PCI with complications	Tachyarrhythmias requiring medication adjustments	Occasional PVCs in the absence of a moderating condition such as electrolyte abnormality or myocardial ischemia
Device implants	Pacemaker lead placement and not pacemaker-dependent	
Temporary pacemaker and transcutaneous pacing	Uncomplicated ablation of arrhythmias	
AV block	Routine, diagnostic catheterization	
Wolf–Parkinson White	Subacute heart failure	
Long QT syndrome	Syncope	
Intra-aortic balloon pump	Terminally ill with arrhythmia, which causes palpitations or SOB and requires management	
Acute heart failure/pulmonary edema		
Hemodynamically unstable arrhythmia		
In intensive care		
Undergoing conscious sedation		

AV, atrial-ventricular; ECG, electrocardiographic; PCI, percutaneous coronary intervention.

Clinical Pearls—Patient Management and Treatment

Patients who have the potential for a prolonged QTc measurement not only have top priority for QT-interval monitoring but also for arrhythmia monitoring. Patients who have been started on a QT-prolonging medication have a primary diagnosis of an overdose from a potentially proarrhythmic medication, a heart rate of less than 40 beats/min or a pause of over 2 seconds severe hypokalemia, or hypomagnesemia are also candidates for monitoring. They should be observed until the underlying disorder is corrected, the offending drug is discontinued, or the potentially proarrhythmic dosage is established with no prolonged QTc. There is no definitive threshold with QT prolongation. However, a QTc beyond 0.50 ms is considered precariously extended, increasing the risk for torsades de pointes, a rare polymorphic ventricular tachycardia (Rodin, 2008). An interesting finding in a study by Pickham and colleagues (2010) is that women received a greater proportion of QT-prolonging drugs, had more frequent electrolyte disturbances, and experienced a greater risk for QT interval prolongation and, consequently, torsades de pointes than men. Since QTc prolongation develops over hours, constant measurement is not necessary. However, when possible, a baseline QTc measurement should be followed and recalculated every 8–12 h. It is also best to measure the QTc in the same lead by calculating the length of the QT-interval in seconds and then correcting it for heart rate. Some ECG monitors have electronic calipers available; otherwise, a manual calculation of the QTc is required. The most common QT-interval calculation formula in use was introduced by Bazett (1920) and many monitoring systems have this formula automatically embedded in monitoring software. The six antiarrhythmic drugs that are especially likely to cause QT prolongation include disopyramide, dofetilide, ibutilide, procainamide, quinidine, and sotalol (Drew *et al.*, 2004).

Acute heart failure

Arrhythmias such as AF that have an associated rapid ventricular rate can either cause or result from acute decompensated heart failure. Patients with acute heart failure or pulmonary edema should have arrhythmia monitoring until the signs/symptoms of acute heart failure have resolved and no hemodynamically significant arrhythmias occur for 24 h (Drew and Funk, 2006). Patients with stable heart failure admitted for rate control through medication titration should be monitored on telemetry to determine drug efficacy. Those with severe heart failure who require inotropic drugs that have pro-arrhythmic properties (e.g., dobutamine, milrinone) or are having infusion rate adjustments also need ECG monitoring. Additionally, patients with heart failure with a recent history of revascularization should be monitored in V_1 for arrhythmia detection and another V lead for ischemia monitoring. Those with subacute or mild heart failure can benefit from ECG monitoring although in a prospective analysis of the utility of telemetry monitoring in 711 patients, medical decisions for this patient population were guided by cardiac monitoring only 17% of the time (Opasich *et al.*, 2000). Even though telemetry monitoring in this study played a weaker role than expected, the authors speculated that perhaps cardiac monitoring provided patients and physicians with reassurance of the success of the therapeutic approach and in some instances might have had an effect on avoiding inappropriate interventions. Kumar (2008) also observed that criteria were established using admission diagnosis with monitoring recommended for 24–72 h for patients with heart or respiratory failure who experienced syncope. Patients who have acute heart failure requiring admission to the ICU should be monitored until hemodynamically stable. In non-ICU patients, monitoring should continue for a period of 24–72 h for heart failure patients who also experience syncope or other comorbidities, which make them more vulnerable for arrhythmias. Conditions such as post-op revascularization, ongoing ischemia, or rhythm disturbances are examples that warrant continuation of ECG monitoring.

Monitoring elements

Continuous ECG monitoring for patients with acute heart failure is justified to watch for new-onset arrhythmias in lead V_1 and when medication or device (ICD, pacemaker) therapy is being adjusted (Drew *et al.*, 2004) since sinus tachycardia is often a normal physiological response to acute decompensated heart failure. Drugs such as inotropic agents and vasodilators used to treat heart failure can also exacerbate sinus tachycardia and may be arrhythmogenic. Although there are many cardiac and noncardiac causes of AF, it is very common in patients who have heart failure. Consequently, the incidence of AF increases with the progression of clinical heart failure (Naccarelli *et al.*, 2003). In the absence of randomized clinical trials, it is still prudent to monitor patients in the subacute phase of heart failure while medications, device therapy, or both are being manipulated.

Clinical Pearls—Patient Management and Treatment

The most common reasons for readmissions are when the ICD has fired in a patient who experiences ventricular arrhythmias (61%) and progressive heart failure (13%) (Kapoor, 2002). Therefore, it is reasonable to monitor the patient while an ICD is interrogated or through the time frame needed to correct the underlying cause of the defibrillator firing and after having alleviated heart failure symptoms.

Electrolyte abnormalities

Electrolyte abnormalities of potassium, calcium, and magnesium have been associated with life-threatening arrhythmias. Conditions in which there is a depletion of electrolytes after cardiac surgery, or lowered electrolyte values occurring due to a variceal bleed treated with vasopressin, or after receiving massive blood transfusion may potentiate the incidence of tachyarrhythmias in these very ill patients. Inadequate levels of potassium, calcium, and magnesium can prolong the QT-interval, which can increase the risk of ventricular arrhythmias and cardiac arrest. Hyperkalemia is sometimes seen in patients with renal insufficiency or in patients who take angiotensin-converting enzyme inhibitors. Elevated potassium levels may increase myocardial excitability and impair the conduction system (Kahloon *et al.*, 2005). Low potassium levels may also cause arrhythmias, especially in patients with underlying heart disease and those with digoxin toxicity (Hoes *et al.*, 1994). Hypomagnesemia and hypocalcemia, especially in the setting of other risk factors, can lead to prolongation of the QT-interval. Electrolytes need to be carefully monitored and treated as needed in all patients, especially those with underlying disease.

Monitoring elements

Patients need to be monitored for as long as they are symptomatic with either arrhythmias or QT-interval prolongation. Once they are hemodynamically stable and the underlying condition is treated, ECG monitoring may be discontinued.

Evidence-based treatment guidelines

There are no specific evidence-based guidelines other than the AHA practice standards that list electrolytes as a high potential risk factor for the generation of arrhythmias or prolongation of the QT-interval (Drew *et al.*, 2004).

Clinical Pearls—Patient Management and Treatment

Patients who are experiencing electrolyte abnormalities should be monitored while their levels are corrected through an intervention although there is no recommended threshold for monitoring patients in the absence of ECG deviations. ECG abnormalities typically occur when the potassium level exceeds 6.5 mmol/l, but normal ECGs (particularly in renal failure patients) have been reported in patients with potassium levels above 9.0 mmol/l (Szerlip, Weiss, and Singer, 1986).

Critical illnesses

Continuous ECG monitoring is a recommendation for patients who are critically ill under a class I category for cardiac monitoring. Patients admitted to the ICU with major trauma, respiratory failure, sepsis, shock, pulmonary embolus, a major noncardiac surgery (especially in elders with a history of coronary artery disease or who have cardiac risk factors), renal failure with electrolyte abnormalities as referenced earlier or drug overdose as listed later, and other serious illnesses should be monitored with the length of time determined by the specific clinical condition (Drew *et al.*, 2004). In addition, patients whose respiratory failure is linked to hypoxemia, hypercapnea, or uncompensated respiratory acidosis should be considered for ECG monitoring secondary to the risk of arrhythmias as well as patients who have suffered an ischemic or hemorrhagic stroke (Kumar, 2008). Patients who are ill enough to be admitted to the ICU may require all three types of cardiac monitoring: arrhythmia, ST-segment, and QT-interval, depending on the etiology of their condition. Class II cardiac monitoring is suggested for patients with acute neurological events like subarachnoid hemorrhage who are prone to QT prolongation even though according to Sommargren and colleagues (2002) these patients usually do not develop torsades de pointes.

Monitoring elements

Careful consideration should be given to the subset of patients with critical illnesses who, although do not meet the AHA practice standards for ECG monitoring (Drew *et al.*, 2004) in some instances, may warrant surveillance based on the severity of their illness and the goals of their care.

Evidence-based treatment guidelines

The AHA guidelines do not include some noncardiac conditions where there may be good evidence to provide ECG monitoring. One area of consideration for cardiac monitoring is for those patients who require massive blood transfusions defined as replacing the person's entire blood volume within 24 h (Chen and Hollander, 2007). Hypocalcemia and hypomagnesemia (both from citrate toxicity) could develop in patients who require massive amounts of blood. In one study by Wilson and colleagues (1992), patients with hypocalcemia experienced mortality rates of 71% compared to those with normal calcium levels whose morality rate was 41%. Even though hypomagnesemia alone is unlikely to cause arrhythmias, it is thought to potentiate the effect of coexisting hypocalcemia (Meikle and Milne, 2000). Patients who have gastrointestinal hemorrhage after endoscopy may benefit from ECG monitoring because life-threatening arrhythmias have been reported in the literature (Eden, Teirstein, and Weiner, 1983; Faigel, Mets, and Kochman, 1995; Mauro et al., 1988). Torsades de pointes could occur in patients who have had neuroleptic medication during the procedure and QT prolongation has occurred with intravenous vasopressin, especially when patients have other electrolyte abnormalities (Faigel, Mets, and Kochman, 1995).

Clinical Pearls—Patient Management and Treatment

Expert staff and APRNs are positioned to use ECG monitoring based on the patient's underlying pathophysiology. Hospitalized patients who are often older adults with comorbidities should be assessed hourly with the clinical indications for ECG monitoring applied when indicated.

Drug overdose

Patients with an overdose or drug toxicity without an arrhythmia should be monitored for 24–48 h, and longer if there is an arrhythmia or a high potential for one to develop. As referenced under the arrhythmia section, certain drugs, particularly those that have a risk for prolonged QT-interval and, subsequently, torsades de pointes, require heightened surveillance of the patient for possible problems. Concurrently, if the patient has other risk factors including older age, history of heart disease, low ejection fraction, or acquired or genetic predisposition to QT prolongation, these conditions may predispose the patient to an untoward outcome. A drug overdose of known arrhythmogenics such as digitalis, tricyclic antidepressants, phenothiazines, and narcotics as well as polypharmacy use exponentially increases the likelihood of an adverse event (see also Chapter 13).

Monitoring elements

It is important to be aware of the side effects and interactions of all medications to avoid a poor outcome. Optimal management is possible when medications can be fully reconciled by the APRN or nurse while educating the patient.

Evidenced-based guidelines

There are no specific guidelines for ECG monitoring of patients with drug overdose other than the recommendations put forth by the AHA in the practice standards for ECG monitoring (Drew et al., 2004).

Clinical Pearls—Management and Training

Drug overdose can be purposeful or accidental due to the high number of medications that patients take and the complexities of their illness. Polypharmacy or taking more than five medications along with coexisting risk factors and illnesses in the context of complex drug regimens contributes to noncompliance as well as adverse drug reactions. It is estimated that patients who are prescribed 10 or more medications have over a 90% chance of experiencing one or more clinically significant adverse events (Nolan and O'Malley, 1988). Twenty years later this problem continues because patients are prescribed many medications that interact adversely and/or the side effects often go unrecognized. APRNs and registered nurses are instrumental in medication reconciliation and education to preempt potential adverse outcomes.

Unnecessary arrhythmia monitoring and underutilization of ischemia and QT-interval monitoring

Almost as important as understanding when a patient requires ECG monitoring is recognizing when they do not. Unnecessary monitoring increases health-care costs, diverts nursing and medical staff from other important work, and may give patients an incorrect message about the status of their cardiac health. It is vital, especially in today's health-care environment, to apply the ECG-monitoring practice standards (Drew et al., 2004). Based on expert opinion, these standards assist in delineating resources for specific conditions and assure that they are not overutilized and instead are applied efficiently to care that is appropriate.

Sometimes physicians use monitored beds for patients who might only require frequent observation and nursing care. When systematic, rigorous standards for inpatient telemetry admissions are not applied, monitored beds quickly become inaccessible and patients are forced to remain in emergency settings or for prolonged stays in post-anesthesia areas. These decisions contribute to overcrowding or ICU delayed transfers, potentially increasing length of stay.

Conversely, Funk and colleagues (2010) found that undermonitoring for ischemia and QTc prolongation occurred frequently in hospitalized patients. In the analysis of baseline data from their randomized clinical trial (PULSE), the authors found that, of the patients with an indication for ischemia monitoring, only 35% of patients were being monitored, but 26% with no indication were monitored for ST-segment changes. Likewise, only 21% of patients with an indication for QTc monitoring had a QTc documented while 18% with no indication for QTc had it documented. Undoubtedly, as technology advances, ECG monitoring and human oversight of the patient remains indispensable, the criteria of evolving clinical models of care must be frequently reexamined through cost-effectiveness research with the aim to deliver the right type and dose of cardiac monitoring.

References

Al-Khatib, S.M., Granger, C.B., Huang, Y. et al. (2002) Sustained ventricular arrhythmias among patients with acute coronary syndromes with no ST-segment elevation: incidence, predictors, and outcomes. *Circulation*, **106**, 309–312.

Aude, Y.W. and Mehta, J.L. (2006) Do we need continuous ECG monitoring in patients transferred for primary angioplasty? *European Heart Journal*, **27**, 249–250.

Baranchuk, A., Shaw, C., Alanazi, H. et al. (2009) Electrocardiography pitfalls and artifacts: the 10 commandments. *Critical Care Nurses*, **29**, 67–73.

Bazett, H.C. (1920) An analysis of the time-relations of electrocardiograms. *Heart*, **7**, 353–370.

Bonnemeier, H., Wiegand, U.K., Giannitsis, E. et al. (2003) Temporal repolarization in homogeneity and reperfusion arrhythmias in patients undergoing successful primary percutaneous coronary interventions for acute ST-segment elevation myocardial infarction: impact of admitting troponin T. *American Heart Journal*, **145**, 484–492.

Booker, K.J., Holm, K., Drew, B.J. et al. (2003) Frequency and outcomes of transient myocardial ischemia in critically adults admitted for noncardiac conditions. *American Journal of Critical Care Nurses*, **12**, 508–517.

Bourgault, A. (2009) *A Practice Alert: Dysrhythmia Monitoring*, http://classic.aacn.org/AACN/aacnnews.nsf/GetArticle/ArticleThree218 (accessed July 22, 2014).

Calder, S. (2008) Clinical pearls and pitfalls of electrocardiogram interpretation in acute myocardial infarction. *Journal of Emergency Nursing*, **34**, 324–329.

Center for Disease Control and Monitoring (2010) *Summary Health Statistics for U.S. Adults: National Health Interview Survey, 2009*, http://www.cdc.gov/nchs/data/series/sr_10/sr10_249.pdf (accessed July 22, 2014).

Chen, E.H. and Hollander, J.E. (2007) When do patients need admission to a telemetry bed? *The Journal of Emergency Medicine*, **33**, 53–60.

Drew, B.J. (2004) Better cardiac monitoring boosts patient outcomes. *ED Management*, **16**, 42–43.

Drew, B.J. and Funk, M. (2006) Practice standards for ECG monitoring in hospital settings: executive summary and guide for implementation. *Critical Care Nursing Clinics of North America*, **18**, 157–168.

Drew, B.J. and Krucoff, M.W. (1999) Multi-lead ST segment monitoring in patients with acute coronary syndromes: a consensus statement for healthcare professionals. ST Segment Monitoring Practice Guideline International Working Group. *American Journal of Critical Care*, **6**, 372–388.

Drew, B.J., Califf, R.M., Funk, M. et al. (2004) Practice standards for electrocardiographic monitoring in hospital settings: An American Heart Association scientific statement from the Councils on Cardiovascular Nursing, Clinical Cardiology and Cardiovascular Disease in the Young: Endorsed by the International Society of Computerized Electrocardiology and the American Association of Critical Care Nurses. *Circulation*, **110**, 2721–2746.

Eden, E., Teirstein, A., and Weiner, I. (1983) Ventricular arrhythmia induced by vasopressin: torsades de pointes related to vasopressin-induced bradycardia. *Mt. Sinai Journal of Medicine*, **50**, 49–51.

Faigel, D.O., Mets, D.C., and Kochman, M.L. (1995) Torsades de pointes complicating the treatment of bleeding esophageal varices: association with neuroleptics, vasopressin and electrolyte imbalance. *American Journal of Gastroenterology*, **90**, 822–824.

Farkouh, M.E., Smars, P.A., Reeder, G.S. *et al.* (1998) A clinical trial of a chest pain observation unit for patients with unstable angina. *New England Journal of Medicine*, **339**, 1882–1888.

Funk, M., May, J., Stephens, K. *et al.* (2009) Substandard quality of ECG monitoring in current clinical practice: preliminary results of the practical use of the latest standards for electrocardiography (PULSE) trial. *Circulation*, **120**, S414.

Funk, M., Winkler, C.G., May, J.L. *et al.* (2010) Unnecessary arrhythmia monitoring and underutilization of ischemia and QT interval monitoring in current clinical practice: baseline results of the practical use of the latest standards for electrocardiography. *Journal of Electrocardiology*, **43**, 542–547.

Gaieski, D.F., Fuchs, B., Carr, B.G. *et al.* (2009) Practical implementation of therapeutic hypothermia after cardiac arrest. *Hospital Practice*, **37**, 71–83.

Garvey, J.L., Monk, L., Granger, C.B. *et al.* (2006) Rates of cardiac catheterization cancelation for ST-segment elevation myocardial infarction after activation by emergency medical services or physicians. *Emergency Medicine Clinics North America*, **24**, 209–225.

Gibler, W., Cannon, C., Blomkalns, A.L. *et al.* (2005) Practical implementation of the guidelines for unstable angina/non–ST-segment elevation myocardial infarction in the emergency department. *Circulation*, **111**, 2699–2710.

Hoes, A.W., Grobbee, D.E., Peet, T.M., and Lubsen, J. (1994) Do non-potassium-sparing diuretics increase the risk of sudden cardiac death in hypertensive patients? Recent evidence. *Drugs*, **47**, 711–733.

Jaffe, A.S., Atkins, J.M., Field, J.M. *et al.* (1991) Recommended guidelines for in-hospital cardiac monitoring of adults for the detection of arrhythmia. *American College of Cardiology*, **18**(6), 1431–1433.

Jevon, P. (2010) An introduction to electrocardiographic monitoring. *British Association of Critical Care Nurses*, **15**, 34–37.

Johnson, K. (2008) Practice alert: ST-segment monitoring. *AACN*, 1–4, http://www.aacn.org/WD/Practice/Docs/ST_Segment_Monitoring_04-2008.pdf (accessed July 22, 2014).

Kahloon, M.U., Aslam, A.K., Aslam, A.F. *et al.* (2005) Hyperkalemia induced failure of atrial and ventricular pacemaker capture. *International Journal of Cardiology*, **105**, 224–226.

Kapoor, W. (2002) Current evaluation and management of syncope. *Circulation*, **106**, 1606–1609.

Krucoff, M., Parente, A., Bottner, R. *et al.* (1988) Stability of multilead ST-segment "fingerprint" over time after percutaneous transluminal angioplasty and its usefulness in detecting reocclusion. *American Journal of Cardiology*, **61**, 1232–1237.

Kumar, D.W. (2008) Cardiac monitoring: new trends and capabilities. *Cardiac Insider*, **2–4**.

Langer, A., Krucoff, M.W., Klootwijk, P. *et al.* (1998) Prognostic significance of ST segment shift early after resolution of ST elevation in patients with myocardial infarction treated with thrombolytic therapy: the GUSTO-I ST segment monitoring substudy. *Journal of American College of Cardiology*, **31**, 783–789.

Leeper, B. (2007) Saving lives with continuous ST-segment monitoring. *American Nurse Today*, **12–14**.

Lloyd-Jones, D.J., Adams, R.J., Brown, T.M. *et al.* (2010) Heart disease and stroke statistics-2010 update. A report from the American Heart Association. *Circulation*, **121**, e46–e250.

Mauro, V.F., Bingle, J.F., Ginn, S.M., and Jafri, F.M. (1988) Torsades de pointes in a patient receiving intravenous vasopressin. *Critical Care Medicine*, **16**, 200–201.

Meikle, A. and Milne, B. (2000) Management of prolonged QT interval during a massive transfusion: calcium, magnesium or both? *Canadian Journal of Anaesthesia*, **47**, 792–795.

Morris, F. and Brady, W.J. (2002) ABC of clinical electrocardiography: acute myocardial infarction—Part I. *British Medical Journal*, **324**, 831–834.

Moss, A.J. (1999) The QT interval and torsade de pointes. *Drug Safety*, **21**, 5–10.

Naccarelli, G.V., Hynes, B.J., Wolbrette, D.L. *et al.* (2003) Atrial fibrillation in heart failure: prognostic significance and management. *Journal of Cardiovascular Electrophysiology*, **14**, S281–S286.

Nolan, L. and O'Malley, K. (1988) Prescribing for the elderly. Part I: sensitivity of the elderly to adverse drug reactions. *Journal of American Geriatric Society*, **36**, 142–149.

Opasich, C., Capomolla, S., Riccardi, P.G. *et al.* (2000) Does in-patient ECG monitoring have an impact on medical care in chronic heart failure patients? *European Journal of Heart Failure*, **2**, 281–285.

Pickham, D., Helfenbein, E., Shinn, J.A. *et al.* (2010) How many patients need QT interval monitoring in critical care units? Preliminary report of the QT in practice study. *Journal of Electrocardiology*, **43**, 572–576.

Rodin, D.M. (2008) Cellular basis of drug induced torsades de pointes. *British Journal of Pharmacology*, **154**, 152–157.

Sandau, K.E. and Smith, M. (2009) Continuous ST-segment monitoring: protocol for practice. *Critical Care Nurse*, **4**, 39–51.

Sommargren, C.E. and Drew, B.J. (2007) Preventing torsades de pointes by careful cardiac monitoring in hospital settings. *AACN Advanced Critical Care*, **18** (3), 285–293.

Sommargren, C.E., Zaroff, J.G., Banki, N., and Drew, B.J. (2002) Electrocardiographic repolarization abnormalities in subarachnoid hemorrhage. *Journal of Electrocardiology*, **35** (Suppl.), 257–262.

Szerlip, H.M., Weiss, J., and Singer, I. (1986) Profound hyperkalemia without electrocardiographic manifestations. *American Journal of Kidney Disease*, **6**, 461–465.

Wackers, F.J. (1987) The diagnosis of myocardial infarction in the presence of left bundle branch block. *Cardiology Clinic*, **5**, 393–401.

Wang, K., Asinger, R.W., and Marriott, H.J. (2003) ST-Segment elevation in conditions other than acute myocardial infarction. *New England Journal of Medicine*, **349**, 2128–2135.

Webner, C. (2011) Applying evidence at the bedside. *Dimensions of Critical Care Nursing*, **30**, 8–18.

Wilson, R.F., Binkley, L.E., Sabo Jr, F.M. *et al.* (1992) Electrolyte and acid base changes with massive blood transfusions. *The American Surgeon*, **58**, 535–544.

Winkler, C., Funk, M., Schindler, D.M., *et al.* (2013). Arrhythmias in patients with acute coronary syndrome in the first 24 hours of hospitalization. *Heart & Lung*, **42**, 422–427.

Xu, J., Kochanek, K.D., Murphy, S., and Tejada-Vera, B. (2010) Deaths: final data for 2007. National Center for Health Statistics. *National Vital Statistic Report*, **58**, 1–135.

CHAPTER 5

Hemodynamic monitoring in critical care

Kathy J. Booker

School of Nursing, Millikin University, Decatur, IL., USA

Hemodynamic monitoring overview

Rapid assessment techniques develop with experience and are critical in the surveillance of all patients admitted to intensive care unit (ICU) settings. Combining continuous electro-cardiographic data with hemodynamic assessments provides minute-to-minute assessment data that must be analyzed carefully. In this chapter, monitoring systems that inform care providers about the impact of the hemodynamic status of critically ill adults will be reviewed.

Mathews (2007) broadly defined hemody-namics as the forces involved with blood circulation. Functional hemodynamic moni-toring has been defined as "that aspect of the measure of cardiovascular variables, either alone or in response to a physiologic pertur-bation, that defines a pathophysiological state, drives therapy or identifies cardiovascular insufficiency more accurately and often earlier than possible by analysis of static hemodynamic variables" (Hadian and Pinsky, 2007, p. 318). The evolution of hemodynamic monitoring from static variables to those capable of trend-ing continuous fluctuations in stroke volume (SV) and cardiac output (CO) has changed the landscape of hemodynamic monitoring over the past decade. The application of less invasive techniques to more accurately predict volume responsiveness offers considerable advantages although systems still remain fallible, especially in patients with spontaneous breathing or cardiac rhythm irregularities.

Understanding hemodynamic monitoring requires both a foundation in pressure-detection systems used extensively over the last four decades and newer technologies based on fluid responsiveness and SV indices, still under inves-tigation. Increasingly, research is focused on patient outcomes of hemodynamic monitoring systems. Over the past decade, direct arterial pressure waveform analysis and other hemo-dynamic variables have been studied using monitoring devices that are less invasive than pulmonary artery catheters (PACs). Stroke volume variation (SVV) and CO calculated from arterial pressure systems have emerged as accu-rate methods for trending hemodynamic status although research has been equivocal and newer systems are not applicable in all critically ill patients (Bendjelid and Romand, 2003; Berkenstadt *et al.*, 2001; Cannesson *et al.*, 2011; Liu *et al.*, 2010; Marik *et al.*, 2009; Wiesenack *et al.*, 2003). Liu *et al.* (2010) found SVV, moni-tored by peripheral arterial lines, to be accurate indicators of cardiac preload and CO. Marik *et al.* (2009) conducted a systematic review on arterial waveform variables and fluid responsiveness in mechanically ventilated patients, concluding that arterial pressure–derived estimates of volume responsiveness yielded higher accuracy when compared with static measures. Although arterial-derived variables to assess fluid respon-siveness have been found to be reliable in a number of studies, many factors influence reli-able measurement and most studies have been done with patients on controlled mechanical ventilation to control for cardiac conditions affected by changing intrathoracic pressure (Marik *et al.*, 2009). As new technology has emerged, parameters that can be monitored or calculated have changed considerably. Terms and normal values associated with hemody-namic monitoring are reviewed in Table 5.1.

Table 5.1 Terms associated with hemodynamic monitoring.

Term	Definition	Normal values
Arterial pressure (AP)	The pressure exerted on the walls of blood vessels by circulating blood ejected into the arterial circulation	115/75
Arterial oxygen saturation	The saturation of oxygen on the hemoglobin molecule; represents the majority of delivered oxygen to tissues	95–98%
Arteriovenous oxygen content difference $(C[a-v]O_2)$	The difference between arterial and venous O_2 content, reflecting oxygen supply and demand: $CaO_2 \times CvO_2$	4–6 ml/vol%
Cardiac index (CI)	Cardiac output divided by body surface area	2.5–3.5 l/min/m²
Cardiac output (CO)	Amount of blood ejected from the ventricles per minute	4–6 l/min
Central venous pressure (CVP)	Pressure measured in the thoracic vena cava representing cardiac filling pressure or preload of the RV	2–6 mmHg
Left ventricular stroke work index (LVSWI)	$SVI (MAP - PAOP) \times 0.0136$	40–75 g/m²/beat
Mixed central venous saturation $(ScvO_2)$	Venous admixture of venous blood returned to the RA; approximates SvO_2 but does not include the venous return from the coronary circulation	60–80%
Mixed venous oxygen saturation (SvO_2)	Venous admixture oxygenation status once all venous blood has been returned to the RV $(CO \times CaO_2 \times 10) - VO_2$	60–80%
Oxygen consumption	Body usage of available oxygen delivered to tissues, calculated by $CO \times 10 \times C(a-VO_2)$	200–250 ml/min
Oxygen delivery (DO_2)	Arterial delivery of oxygen to tissues factoring arterial oxygen content and CO: $CaO_2 \times CO \times 10$	800–1000 ml/min
Passive leg raising (PLR)	A test used to estimate fluid responsiveness, conducted by raising the legs passively, subsequently causing an estimated 300–500 ml venous return to the heart, mimicking fluid administration. Used to assess improvements in vital signs and tissue oxygenation induced by additional preload	Fluid responsiveness to PLR is measured by change in CO/CI or stroke volume > 10–15%
Pulmonary artery pressure (PAP)	Pressure exerted by blood flow in the pulmonary artery	20–30/8–15 mmHg
Pulmonary artery occlusive pressure (PAOP)	Pressure measured when a balloon-tipped PAC is inflated and floats into an occlusive branch of the pulmonary artery; reflects forward pressure from left atrium and LV assuming no mitral valve dysfunction	6–12 mmHg
Pulse pressure (PP)	Systolic blood pressure – diastolic blood pressure, reflective of arterial wall stiffness	<40 mmHg
Pulse pressure variation (PPV)	A calculated measure of pulse variation using arterial or pulse oximetry pulse variation to estimate fluid responsiveness expressed as a percentage improvement. Calculated as a percentage: $$PPV = 100 \times \frac{(PP_{max} - PP_{min})}{[(PP_{max} + PP_{min})/2]}$$	PPV > 13–15% has been associated with fluid responsiveness in mechanically ventilated critically ill patients (Napoli, 2012)
Right atrial pressure (RAP)	Pressure measured within the right atrium of the heart	4–6 mmHg
Right ventricular stroke work index	$SVI (PAM - RAP) \times 0.0136$	4–8 g/m²/beat
Stroke volume (SV)	Volume of blood ejected from ventricles with each cardiac contraction	50–70 ml/beat indexed to patient's size (stroke volume index [SVI]): SV/body surface area

Table 5.1 (*Continued*)

Term	Definition	Normal values
Stroke volume variation (SVV)	A measure taken from the arterial pressure curve in newer noninvasive hemodynamic systems; affected by intrathoracic pressure changes and cardiac arrhythmias; research supported only in mechanically ventilated patients. Possibly less affected by vasomotor tone (Napoli, 2012). Calculated by arterial pressure systems and displayed as a percentage: $$SVV = \frac{SV_{max} - SV_{min}}{SV_{mean}}$$	SVV varies based on patient populations: 9.5% predictive in neurosurgery patients; 10–13% in other surgical populations. These percentages are indicators of predicted positive response to fluid administration (preload responsiveness)
Venous oxygen content (CvO$_2$)	Venous oxygen content following tissue level extraction: Hgb × 1.34 × SvO$_2$	15.5 ml/vol%

Adapted from Baird and Bethel (2011); Cannesson *et al.* (2011); Napoli (2012).

Table 5.2 Principles of hemodynamic monitoring.

1 No hemodynamic monitoring technique can improve outcomes by itself.
2 Monitoring requirements may vary over time and can depend on local equipment availability and training.
3 There are no optimal hemodynamic values that are applicable to all patients.
4 We need to combine and integrate variables.
5 Measurements of SvO$_2$ can be helpful.
6 A high cardiac output and a high SvO$_2$ are not always best.
7 Cardiac output is estimated, not measured.
8 Monitoring hemodynamic changes over short periods of time is important.
9 Continuous measurement of all hemodynamic variables is preferable.
10 Non-invasiveness is not the only issue.

Adapted from Vincent *et al.* (2011). © BioMed Central, Ltd.

The multitude of developing hemodynamic systems has created confusion, particularly due to variation in systems, limited study findings on diverse critical care patient conditions, and variable outcome end points (Vincent *et al.*, 2011). See Table 5.2 for key elements of hemodynamic monitoring systems advanced by Vincent *et al.* (2011). Various hemodynamic monitoring systems will be reviewed within this chapter.

Hemodynamic monitoring systems

Pulmonary artery catheter monitoring

PACs have been used since the 1970s following the development of the PAC by Drs. Swan and Ganz (Rajaram *et al.*, 2013). Following widespread adoption of this catheter as a monitoring tool for critically ill patients, clinicians and researchers began to question its use, noting less-than-optimal outcomes and potential deleterious complications in patients (Harvey *et al.*, 2005; Manoach, Weingart, and Charchaflieh, 2012). Despite a long history of PAC use in critical care units, evidence has demonstrated limited application due to risks associated with placement, potential complications, weak clinical outcomes, and considerable user error (Harvey *et al.*, 2010; Isakow and Schuster, 2007; Manoach, Weingart, and Charchaflieh, 2012; NHLBI ARDS, 2006).

PACs are inserted through a central vein (generally the subclavian or internal jugular) and advanced through the right atrium, right ventricle, and into the pulmonary artery (PA; see Fig. 5.1). The PAC ports allow for multiple blood sampling, monitoring of right heart and PA pressures, and are equipped with an inflatable balloon at the distal tip to allow for brief PA occlusion to obtain intermittent pressures reflective of left ventricular end-diastolic pressure (LVEDP). Theoretically, with normal mitral valve function, the pulmonary artery occlusive pressure (PAOP) aligns with LVEDP at end expiration and, often, PA diastolic pressures are similar to LVEDP. Problems with distal tip positioning, mitral valve insufficiency or stenosis, ventricular compliance, and technical issues may all affect the accurate measurement of PAOP. In addition, pressure does not equate to volume and allows for only estimations of volume status.

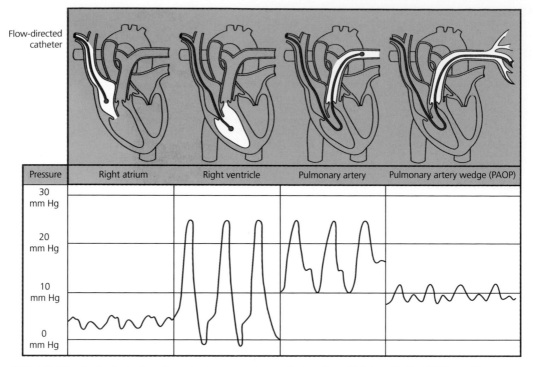

Figure 5.1 Waveforms during insertion of pulmonary artery catheters. From Baird and Bethel (2011, p. 90).
© Elsevier.

Intermittant or continuous cardiac output (CCO) monitoring is possible using a PAC.

Specially developed PACs also allow for continuous monitoring of mixed venous oxygenation (SvO$_2$). Table 5.3 reviews factors affecting SvO$_2$.While CCO values and SvO$_2$ provide significant information on overall hemodynamic status and systemic oxygenation, newer methods add significantly to decisions regarding fluid volume responsiveness. Preload, afterload, and contractility measures are often computed from values obtained by PACs in an effort to optimize hemodynamic status. Standard PAC monitoring may be used more frequently in patients with severe known cardiac disease or conditions in which trending continuous SvO$_2$ is helpful.

Nursing management and care of patients with PACs is considerable. Following insertion, ports may be used for administration of multiple intravenous fluids, blood products, and blood sampling. When not in use, ports must be maintained with flush protocols to prevent clotting at blood/port interfaces and

management of sterility at the insertion site requires considerable attention to prevent central line infections. PACs are inserted through a separate introducer catheter, which must also be managed. When proximal ports are used for central venous pressure (CVP) monitoring and the distal port used for PA pressure monitoring, pressurized sterile systems must be maintained and monitored frequently during the shift. Derived values from a PAC are generally obtained every 4 h and continuous or intermittent CO measures are also trended. While monitoring frequency is guided by orders or standing protocols, outcome studies have not clearly linked monitoring to improved outcomes (Rajaram *et al.*, 2013).

Central venous pressure monitoring and management

The use of central venous catheters (CVCs) to support hemodynamic management is common in the ICU. Central lines serve a number of purposes including multiple infusion ports for

Table 5.3 Factors affecting SvO_2.

Svo_2 is a sensitive indicator of oxygen supply/demand balance, If Svo_2 decreases to less than 50%, the patient should be rapidly assessed for the cause of an increased oxygen demand, or decrease in supply. Anemia, hypoxemia, and decreased CO may result in markedly reduced oxygen delivery. In the presence of the high metabolic demands imposed by critical illness, a reduction in O_2 delivery or further increase in O_2 demand can produce profound instability in the patient. Changes in Svo_2 often precede overt changes reflective of physiologic instability.

Factor	Effect on Svo_2	Clinical Examples
Arterial Oxygen Saturation		
↑ Sao_2	↑ Svo_2	Supplemental oxygen
↓ Sao_2	↓Svo_2	Reduced oxygen supply (e.g., ARDS, ET suctioning, removal of supplemental oxygen, pulmonary disease, asthma, respiratory failure, obstructive sleep apnea)
Cardiac Output		
↑CO	↑Svo_2	Administration of inotropes to increase contractility
↓CO	↓Svo_2	Dysrhythmias, increased SVR, MI, hypovolemia, ↑HR, or ↓HR
Hemoglobin		
↓Hgb	↓Svo_2	Hemorrhage, hemolysis, severe anemia in patients with cardiovascular disease
Oxygen Consumption		
↑Vo_2	↓Svo_2	States in which metabolic demand exceeds oxygen supply (e.g., shivering, seizures, hyperthermia, hyperdynamic states)
↓Vo_2	↑Svo_2	States in which there is failure of peripheral tissue to extract or use oxygen: Significant peripheral arteriovenous shunting: cirrhosis, renal failure Redistribution of blood away from beds where oxygen extraction occurs: sepsis, acute pancreatitis, major burns Blockage of oxygen uptake or utilization: cyanide poisoning (including nitroprusside toxicity), carbon monoxide poisoning
Mechanical Problems	↑Svo_2	Wedged PA catheter creates falsely elevated Svo_2

ARDS, acute respiratory distress syndrome; *CO*, cardiac output; *ET*, endotracheal; *Hgb*, hemoglobin; *MI*, myocardial infarction; *PA*, pulmonary artery; *SVR*, systemic vascular resistance.
Baird & Bethel (2011). *Manual of Critical Care Nursing*. Elsevier.

incompatible solutions, delivery of fluids at higher flow rates than peripheral catheters, monitoring and trending CVP, use for short-term dialysis, and the ability to trend central venous blood for oxygenation and laboratory analysis. While monitoring CVP as a measure of preload is generally inaccurate due to the wide range of physiological conditions that influence values, many other indications for CVCs in critically ill patients continue (Marik, Baram, and Vahid, 2008). Factors that may influence changes in compliance or volume in the central veins include changes in CO, peripheral venous constriction, position changes, arterial dilation, blood or fluid loss through trauma, hyperthermia, hypothermia, conditions that engage the Valsalva maneuver, muscle contraction, and exertion. While still a central component of sepsis guidelines, CVP

monitoring is generally not used to guide therapy, especially with the emergence of other hemodynamic techniques offering greater hemodynamic precision. However, the role of CVCs in newer systems for SVV will be explored later in this chapter.

Central venous pressure trending limitations

Marik, Baram, and Vahid (2008) conducted a classic systematic review and identified the inaccuracies of the CVP as an indicator of intravascular volume, noting that CVP values were no better than chance in estimating fluid responsiveness. Other studies have identified collapse of the superior vena cava during positive pressure ventilation when CVP is less than 10mmHg (Jellinek *et al.*, 2000; Viellard-Baron *et al.*, 2003), technically invalidating its predictive value.

Osman *et al.* (2007) found that cardiac filling pressures were not helpful in predicting fluid responsiveness in patients with sepsis. Neither CVP nor PAOP predicted fluid responsiveness even when low stroke volume index (SVI) values were known. Use of CVP trending is more valuable than individual assessments and may be used along with other hemodynamic parameters to supplement assessment rather than independently used as a driver for therapeutic intervention.

Arterial line monitoring and management

Arterial lines are frequently inserted in critically ill adults to monitor continuous blood pressure and allow frequent arterial sampling for trending arterial blood gas analysis, especially in patients on mechanical ventilation. Increasingly, arterial lines are also used for functional hemodynamic monitoring. As a vascular access device, arterial line systems require special pressurized tubing and monitoring systems that include a transducer and continuous waveform analysis for safe application and trending. Guidelines for management and monitoring of arterial lines have been published (Kunde, 2012). High-level (I and II) supportive recommendations for management identify that arterial catheters do not require routine changing although these catheters should not be overlooked when assessing for infectious sources; flush systems do not require heparin for thrombi prevention; and general safety of arterial lines is established, noting less than 1% major complications (Kunde, 2012). Actual frequency of monitoring and documentation are not addressed in this guideline although the recommendation of checking all connections at the beginning of each shift is emphasized. In critically ill patients, the use of arterial pressure systems requires heightened surveillance due to the very rapid blood loss and risk for exsanguination associated with dislodgement or tubing disconnection. Alarms should be enabled at all times to alert nursing staff to changes in arterial pressure and waveforms displayed continuously to aid in the surveillance of this technology.

Newer techniques for SVV measurement and management use arterial waveform analysis to calculate SV. Combined with CVP-derived measures of central venous oxygenation, adequacy of hemodynamic states may be trended. Bridges (2008) reviewed functional hemodynamic studies that have contributed to critical care practice using arterial-based systems, highlighting the paucity of outcome studies and identifying the numerous limitations in the accuracy of systems, including respiratory variation in spontaneously breathing patients, dynamic responsiveness of systems, calibration issues, and uncertainty in cutoff points for management decisions based on SVV and systolic pressure variation (SPV). These variables will be further explored.

Hemodynamic monitoring guidelines and outcomes

Hemodynamic monitoring must be linked to treatments that improve patient outcomes (Garcia and Pinsky, 2011; Napoli, 2012; Pinsky, 2007; Pinksy and Payen, 2005). All monitoring systems reviewed earlier may place patients at additional infectious and functional risk, a common critique of traditional PA monitoring systems. Harvey *et al.* (2005) observed that approximately 10% of over 500 critically ill patients randomized to PAC use developed complications, including hematoma at the insertion site, arterial punctures, arrhythmias requiring treatment, and pnemothoraces. No differences in mortality or length of stay were observed in the PAC versus non-PAC groups. Similar complications and frequency were noted in a comparison study of trauma patients in which PAC versus transthoracic ultrasonography outcomes were compared (Tchorz *et al.*, 2012). In the National Heart, Lung, and Blood Institute clinical trials network for adult respiratory distress syndrome (ARDS) (2006), comparisons of CVC-guided treatments versus PACs in 1000 patients detected fewer complications in the CVC group with no improvement in patient outcomes with the use of PACs (NHLBI ARDS, 2006). The recommendations from this network include abandonment of the use of PACs for patients with acute lung injury monitoring.

The goal in all hemodynamic monitoring is to allow for trend analysis and evaluation of interventional techniques to prevent and treat tissue hypoperfusion. Prevention of deterioration and measureable hemodynamic improvement in critically ill patients are key goals of critical care management in the ICU. While newer techniques often involve placement of arterial catheters and central venous lines, these are considered less invasive forms of hemodynamic monitoring compared with the use of PACs. Many newer techniques based on SV responsiveness also have limitations in that ventricular function is not directly trended (Marik *et al.*, 2009) and due to inaccurate arterial waveform analysis in patients with arrhythmias such as atrial fibrillation. Indeed, in the monitoring guidelines for patients in shock, Antonelli *et al.* (2007) observed that CO monitoring lacks a gold standard and is not recommended as a routine measurement in patients with shock. See Chapter 2 for further synopsis of these guidelines in patients with shock conditions. Nursing surveillance is required for hemodynamic monitoring and patient safety, management of hemodynamic variables, and appropriate functioning of systems to ensure data accuracy.

Functional indicators of hemodynamic monitoring

Types of functional monitoring that have been validated through research include volume challenge, passive leg raising, changes in CVP during spontaneous breathing, and changes in left ventricular output during positive pressure ventilation (Pinksy and Payen, 2005). The cornerstone of newer hemodynamic techniques is the ability to assess fluid responsiveness, identified "as an increase of 10–15% in stroke volume (SV), cardiac output (CO), or cardiac index (CI) in response to volume expansion" (Napoli, 2012, p. 2). Early goal-directed therapy (EGDT) is foundational to the preservation of hemodynamic stability at early stages of clinical deterioration, particularly in sepsis (Antonelli *et al.*, 2007; Rivers *et al.*, 2012). A review of outcome studies over a decade following the introduction of EGDT and sepsis bundles, in over 18 000 adult patients, concluded that EGDT significantly reduced mortality and progressive organ failure, health-care costs, and inflammatory response (Rivers *et al.*, 2012). Nursing is key to implementation of EGDT protocols and most emergency and critical care units have adopted sepsis initiatives (see Chapter 2).

Perioperative optimization

Perioperative hemodynamic optimization has been studied extensively. The use of blood pressure as a guide for hemodynamic status is misleading due to the many factors affecting blood flow and pressure. Generally, complex and interactive factors affect vascular flow and tissue oxygenation, altered significantly during surgery, perioperative recovery, and in many critical conditions requiring ICU stays.

Interventions to ensure adequate tissue oxygen delivery (DO_2) intraoperatively using goal-directed fluid therapy have been effective (Kirov, Kuzkov, and Moinar, 2010). Blood pressure and heart rate often mask hypovolemia in perioperative and critically ill patients. Compensatory mechanisms to sustain CO involve increased heart rate, vasoconstriction, and increased peripheral oxygen extraction. Blood pressure reductions are considered a late sign, accompanied by poor organ perfusion and reduced urinary output. Prevention of this cascade is always the goal.

Transesophageal monitoring

Esophageal Doppler techniques estimate SV and CO more directly through Doppler technology. Transesophageal Doppler (TED) techniques evaluate fluid challenges and patient responsiveness to circulatory volume challenges and have been studied extensively in surgical patients. The technique and equipment used in TED are simpler than transthoracic echocardiography but generally require that patients be sedated. The probe is inserted orally or nasally and advanced to the midthoracic region where the esophagus and the descending aorta are aligned. Adjustments are made in the calculation of blood flow since the distribution is generally 70% in the descending aorta and proprietary factoring of patient age, weight, height, and aortic cross-sectional area is converted to estimates of SV and CO (Schober, Loer, and Schwarte, 2009).

Phan *et al.* (2008) reviewed perioperative fluid optimization with TED in a meta-analysis of nine randomized controlled studies. In this analysis, patients had reduced lengths of stay, improved return of gastrointestinal function (in colorectal surgery patients), and reduced postoperative morbidity compared with controls who did not have fluid management by TED. Phan *et al.* (2008) promote the use of 250 ml boluses of colloids to treat low SVV. Parameters that are trended with TED include preload width (FTc), representing systolic flow time; peak velocity, reflective of contractility; and SVI. These continuously displayed values are analyzed following fluid boluses, with 10% improvement in SVV desired. When patients have less than 10% improvement, preload optimization is evidenced and further fluids are not indicated. Other trended values obtainable by esophageal Doppler methods include CO, preload, afterload, and left ventricular contractility (Vincent *et al.*, 2011).

The Agency for Healthcare Research and Quality (2007) issued a technology assessment on the use of TED and endorsed the effectiveness of this technology to guide fluid replacement during surgery with decreased surgical complications when compared with CVP monitoring, assigning strong evidence to these findings. While the insertion of the probe used to monitor TED and additional education to interpret data obtained by TED are necessary, this technique in critical care units holds promise for positively influencing critical care treatment and outcomes.

Volume responsiveness

While fluid challenges are often a first-line treatment for hemodynamic instability, the measurement of fluid responsiveness is often difficult given physiologic interactions within the thorax, compliance issues, and compensatory circulatory action. Approximately half of unstable critically ill patients will respond to a fluid challenge (Marik, Baram, and Vahid, 2008; Marik *et al.*, 2009; Michard and Teboul, 2002). The key to successful fluid responsiveness is optimizing fluid volume in patients whose ventricular function is responsive to fluids (on the ascending portion of the Frank–Starling curve), maximizing SV with additional fluids. Successful optimization of goal-directed fluid therapy is

especially effective using Doppler technology in high-risk surgical patients (Roche, Miller, and Gan, 2009).

Marik *et al.* (2009) found strong correlation of pulse pressure variation (PPV), SVV, and SPV changes on stroke index/CI values in a systematic review of dynamic changes in arterial waveform-derived variables. In 29 pooled studies, PPV performed the best in response to fluid challenge on the outcome variable, with 0.94 correlation and 0.94 area under the curve ($p < 0.001$). While these measures reflect volume responsiveness, clinicians must keep in mind the limitations of this technique, particularly the invalidation of calculations in patients with cardiac arrhythmias and variable spontaneous breathing patterns that influence venous return to the heart. In addition, the status of left ventricular function is not revealed by this technique so its application is limited to those with recruitable preload conditions (Marik *et al.*, 2009).

PPV is directly calculated by most arterial pressure-based systems by averaging the maximal pulse pressure minus the minimum pulse pressure divided by the average of these two (Wiesenack *et al.*, 2003). As a reflection of left ventricular stroke work, the PPV is less influenced by intrathoracic pressure changes.

Manoach, Weingart, and Charchaflieh (2012) reviewed the current literature on invasive monitoring and volume responsiveness during resuscitation, perioperative management, and in critical care. Manoach, Weingart, and Charchaflieh (2012) concluded that use of PAC may be helpful in patients with a number of conditions, including complex right and left cardiopulmonary disorders, pulmonary hypertension, and selected complex cardiac surgery, trauma, and high-risk surgical patients. Recommendations for application of CVP-based systems were supported in critically ill patients with left-sided heart failure, septic shock, ARDS and other subsets of critically ill patients (Manoach, Weingart, and Charchaflieh, 2012). Finally, arterial pulse pressure trending is recommended in patients in sinus rhythm with sufficient sedation to offset mechanically ventilated intrathoracic effects on venous return (Δ PP). Since spontaneous breathing lessens the predictive value of Δ PP to fluid responsiveness, and arrhythmias also invalidate values, the limitations in the use of these systems are evident. Manoach, Weingart, and Charchaflieh (2012) highlight many of the serious complexities inherent in managing hemodynamic monitoring in critically ill settings.

While many of the techniques for assessing fluid responsiveness are not accurate in spontaneously breathing patients, pulse oximetry plethysmography analysis may hold promise. Plethysmography analysis in anesthetized, controlled ventilation patients revealed that changes in pulse oximetry waveforms (Δ POP) were predictive of fluid responsiveness (Desebbe and Cannesson; Wyffels *et al.*, 2007). Changes in pulse oximetry waveforms (Δ POP) may be predictive of fluid responsiveness, enabling noninvasive trending of hemodynamic changes, but continued research is needed (Cannesson *et al.*, 2011).

Pulse contour analysis

Arterial waveform pulse contour analysis is a technique used for hemodynamic monitoring in critical care. Some systems on the market use a derivation based on pulsatile analysis from existing arterial pressure waveforms. Others use combined data obtained from CVC and arterial pressure monitoring, applying algorithms to analyze pulse contours and

intermittent thermodilution measures to derive CO. When combined with a CVC, these systems also allow for measurement of central venous oxygenation ($ScvO_2$) and left ventricular SV estimated by measurement of arterial pulse pressure, CCO, and SV. The magnitude of changes in the pulse pressure is reflective of changing SV affected by arterial compliance. A key element of this technology is the ability to evaluate responses to fluid challenge. Garcia and Pinsky (2011) noted that "volume responsiveness has been arbitrarily defined as ≥15% change in cardiac output in response to a 500 ml bolus fluid challenge" (p. 1) but cautioned that this is but one element of evaluating critically ill patients. Using measures of SV and oxygenation together provides guidance in critically ill patient management and strong trending data for more meaningful decision making (see Fig. 5.2). Reuter *et al.* (2002) found that SVV predicted preload changes and volume responsiveness in a study of 20 mechanically ventilated postoperative cardiac surgery patients. SVV is increasingly used to assess fluid responsiveness whether measured by arterial-based systems or by Doppler technologies (see Fig. 5.3).

Specific delivery systems for pulse contour analysis and measurement of SVV follow.

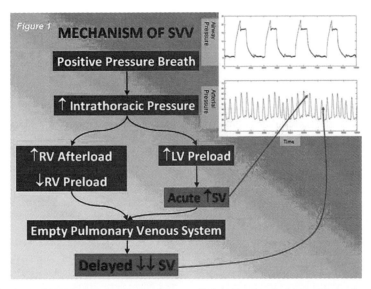

Figure 5.2 Mechanisms of SVV during positive pressure ventilation. Reprinted with permission from McGee (2009). A simple physiologic algorithm for managing hemodynamics using stroke volume and stroke volume variation: Physiologic optimization program. *Journal of Intensive Care Medicine*, **24**, 352–366. © SAGE.

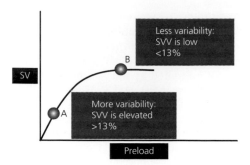

Figure 5.3 SVV and fluid responsiveness. Reprinted with permission from McGee (2009). A simple physiologic algorithm for managing hemodynamics using stroke volume and stroke volume variation: Physiologic optimization program. *Journal of Intensive Care Medicine*, **24**, 352–366. © SAGE.

FloTrac/Vigileo®

This method of hemodynamic analysis incorporates a FloTrac transducer in an arterial catheter system and a Vigileo monitor, calculating CCO by analysis of pulse pressure derived from arterial waveforms. Saraceni *et al.* (2011) found underestimation of CO compared with PAC thermodilution techniques but others have found acceptable agreement between FloTrac and PAC in cardiac surgery and critically ill ventilated patients (Mayer *et al.*, 2009; Senn *et al.*, 2009). The Vigileo monitor also tracks central venous oxygenation in the right atrium (RA) (ScvO$_2$) using a special CVC, based upon all venous admixture except that supplied by the coronary venous system. This allows for continuous ScvO$_2$, CO, and SVV displays.

Benes and colleagues (2010) found significantly lower rates of postoperative complications and lower lactate concentrations in high-risk patients undergoing major abdominal surgery managed with Vigileo/FloTrac monitoring compared with controls. Liu *et al.* (2010) compared the use of SVV and arterial-based calculations of CO with traditional PAC values in cardiac surgery patients, detecting strong correlation between arterial CO measures and CCO obtained from PACs. The experimental group had fluid management targeted to SVV<10%, using colloid boluses of 3 ml/kg. Patients in the Vigileo-managed group had significantly improved outcomes including fewer hypotensive epidodes, fewer complications, and reductions in serum lactate. Continuous trending to

guide interventions allows for rapid evaluation of patient changes and prevention of deterioration (Marik *et al.*, 2009). The FloTrac®/Vigileo system may not be useful in rapidly changing conditions, immediate post-cardiopulmonary bypass, aortic regurgitation, hepatic cirrhosis, or in patients undergoing intra-aortic balloon counterpulsation (Mayer *et al.*, 2009).

Takala *et al.* (2011) reported on early non-invasive CO monitoring in hemodynamically unstable medical-surgical patients in three ICUs in Switzerland. Patients were randomized to FloTrac arterial systems, or to a control group (total *n* = 386). Hemodynamic instability was identified by any of the following criteria: clinically relevant hypotension (<90 mmHg), evidence of cerebral hypoperfusion, or acute drops in urinary output following hypotension; clinical evidence of hypovolemia; oliguria; elevated blood lactate; or acute changes in mental status related to hemodynamic state. Although the intent of the study was that the experimental group would stabilize more rapidly, findings revealed no differences in patients reaching hemodynamic stability within 6 h and enrolled patients showed similar patterns of ICU and hospital length of stays. Research on outcomes is ongoing and definitive evidence on patient outcomes remains inconclusive, though promising, in targeted patient conditions.

Transpulmonary dilution techniques

The transpulmonary thermal-dye dilution techniques assess ventricular preload by estimation of intrathoracic blood volume (ITBV), global end-diastolic volume (GEDV), and extravascular lung water (EVLW). Measurements may be by temperature (e.g., PiCCO®, PULSION Medical Systems, Munich, Germany) or by lithium (e.g., LidCO® LidCO Group PLC, London, UK). These systems measure normovolemia and hypovolemia in a range of clinical applications (Benington, Ferris, and Nirmalan, 2009). They also estimate CCO and the major limitation involves changes induced by altered vascular compliance (Vincent *et al.*, 2011). EVLW has been shown to estimate pulmonary edema and values higher than 10 ml/kg are consistent with ARDS (Benington, Ferris, and Nirmalan, 2009). The pulse contour cardiac output (PiCCO) system continuously calculates and displays SVI and SVV, allowing for interventional assessment on these indicators. In a multisite noninterventional study, patient management and outcomes using PiCCO were compared to PAC use in over 300 critically ill patients from eight ICUs in four countries (Uchino *et al.*, 2006). While selection of monitoring systems was not controlled in this study, outcomes were compared and patients with PiCCO systems had fewer ventilator-free days and a higher positive fluid balance. Final multivariate analysis did not show significant differences between types of monitoring device and the authors primarily demonstrated that PACs were used more often in patients requiring inotropes and PiCCO was selected more often for patients exhibiting vasodilatory shock. While helpful in demonstrating the need for further controlled trials, conclusions remain elusive for patient outcomes in this study (Uchino *et al.*, 2006).

Berkenstadt *et al.* (2001) studied the effectiveness of the PiCCO system in 15 neurologic surgery patients undergoing brain tumor resection or aneurysm repair and reported successful SVV responsiveness detection to guide fluid management. The greatest drawback of the use of PiCCO is the requirement for repeated calibrations for accuracy. Research continues and published guidelines are not yet available to guide practitioners in the selection of patient conditions and treatment protocols for management of these systems.

Passive leg raising

Elevation of lower extremities results in a natural fluid bolus through venous return, potentially predicting responsiveness to a fluid bolus naturally. This technique involves elevating both lower extremities 45° for 4–5 min. Monnet *et al.* (2006) found that critically ill patients responded favorably to passive leg raising (PLR) techniques. In a study of 35 patients with circulatory failure, Jabot *et al.* (2009) identified stronger patient response to PLR when the patient moved from semirecumbant positions to supine with simultaneous leg raising rather than simple elevation of legs from the supine position. PLR was associated with significant changes in hemodynamic measurements assessed by the PiCCO system. This technique assesses fluid responsiveness in patients regardless of respiratory status or cardiac arrhythmias and is considered to estimate the result of a 300–500 ml fluid challenge. In a meta-analysis of nine studies, Cavallaro *et al.* (2010) verified the found correlation between improved CO following PLR and its ability to assess patient fluid responsiveness despite respiratory status or arrhythmias. Teboul and Monnet (2008) identified PLR as the only reliable method for assessing volume responsiveness in spontaneously breathing patients but recommended further study.

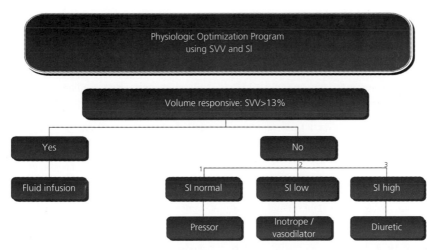

Figure 5.4 Physiologic optimization program using Stroke Volume Variation (SVV) and Stroke Index (SI). Reprinted with permission from McGee (2009). A simple physiologic algorithm for managing hemodynamics using stroke volume and stroke volume variation: Physiologic optimization program. *Journal of Intensive Care Medicine*, **24**, 352–366. © SAGE.

SVV protocols for management

McGee (2009) suggests that SVV greater than 13% indicates volume responsiveness and recommends that 1 liter of normal saline be administered over 10–15 min. Colloids or reductions in crystalloid may be clinically indicated based on the patient (McGee, 2009) and results of fluid challenges should be continuously monitored by stroke index or CO variables. The use of an algorithm for optimization of fluid based on stroke index is promoted (McGee, 2009). See Figure 5.4

In summary, protocols are emerging for monitoring patients with threats to tissue oxygen delivery. Many studies described in this chapter enrolled small numbers of patients and lack generalizability. The need for more controlled trials in this area is paramount to guide practice by identifying patient parameters in which optimization affects patient outcomes in a more predictable manner for critically ill adults admitted with complex pathologies. As recommended by Garcia and Pinsky (2011), collective measures of fluid status, responsiveness, and tissue oxygenation must be analyzed with clearly defined data assessing circulatory adequacy such as lactate or anion gap measurements to better define successful treatment end points. This goal continues.

References

Agency for Healthcare Research and Quality (2007) Esophageal Doppler ultrasound-based cardiac output monitoring for real-time therapeutic management of hospitalized patients. A review, Author, Rockville, pp. 1–131, https://www.ecri.org/Documents/EPC/Esophageal_Doppler_Ultrasound-Based_Cardiac_Output_Monitoring.pdf (accessed August 8, 2014).

Antonelli, M., Levy, M., Andrews, P.J.D. *et al.* (2007) Hemodynamic monitoring in shock and implications for management. *Intensive Care Medicine*, **33**, 575–590.

Baird, M. and Bethel, S. (2011) *Manual of Critical Care Nursing*, Elsevier, St. Louis.

Bendjelid, K. and Romand, J.A. (2003) Fluid responsiveness in mechanichally ventilated patients: a review of indices used in intensive care. *Intensive Care Medicine*, **29**, 352–360.

Benes, J., Chytra, I., Altmann, P. *et al.* (2010) Intraoperative fluid optimization using stroke volume variation in high risk surgical patients:

results of prospective randomized study. *Critical Care*, **14**, R118.

Benington, S., Ferris, P., and Nirmalan, M. (2009) Emerging trends in minimally invasive haemodynamic monitoring and optimization of fluid therapy. *European Journal of Anaesthesiology*, **26**, 893–905.

Berkenstadt, H., Margalit, N., Hadani, M. *et al.* (2001) Stroke volume variation as a predictor of fluid responsiveness in patients undergoing brain surgery. *Anesthesia Analgesia*, **92**, 984–989.

Bridges, E.J. (2008) Arterial pressure-based stroke volume and functional hemodynamic monitoring. *Journal of Cardiovascular Nursing*, **23**, 105–112.

Cannesson, M., Aboy, M., Hofer, C.K., and Rehman, M. (2011) Pulse pressure variation: where are we today? *Journal of Clinical Monitoring and Computing*, **25**, 45–56.

Cavallaro, F., Sandroni, C., Marano, C. *et al.* (2010) Diagnostic accuracy of passive leg raising for prediction of fluid responsiveness in adults: systematic review and meta-analysis of clinical studies. *Intensive Care Medicine*, **36**, 1475–1483.

Garcia, X. and Pinsky, M.R. (2011) Clinical applicability of functional hemodynamic monitoring. *Annals of Intensive Care*, **1**, 35.

Hadian, M. and Pinsky, M.R. (2007) Functional hemodynamic monitoring. *Current Opinions in Critical Care*, **13**, 318–323.

Harvey, S., Harrison, D.A., Singer, M. *et al.* (2005) Assessment of the clinical effectiveness of pulmonary artery catheters in management of patients in intensive care (PAC-Man): a randomized controlled trial. *Lancent*, **366**, 472–477.

Harvey, S., Rowan, K., Harrison, D., and Black, N. (2010) Using clinical databases to evaluate healthcare interventions. *International Journal of Technology Assessment in Health Care*, **26**, 86–94.

Isakow, W. and Schuster, D.P. (2007) Extravascular lung water measurements and hemodynamic monitoring in the critically ill: bedside alternatives to the pulmonary artery catheter. *American Journal of Physiology and Lung Cell Molecular Physiology*, **291**, L1118–L1131.

Jabot, J., Teboul, J.L., Richard, C., and Monnet, X. (2009) Passive leg raising for predicting fluid responsiveness: importance of the postural change. *Intensive Care Medicine*, **35**, 85–90.

Jellinek, H., Krafft, P., Fitgerald, R.D. *et al.* (2000) Right atrial pressure predicts hemodynamic response to apneic positive airway pressure. *Critical Care Medicine*, **28**, 672–678.

Kirov, M.Y., Kuzkov, V.V., and Moinar, Z. (2010) Perioperative haemodynamic therapy. *Current Opinion in Critical Care*, **16**, 384–392.

Kunde, L. (2012) *Arterial Lines: Management and Monitoring*, Joanna Briggs Institute, pp. 1–6.

Liu, H., Konia, M.R., Li, Z., and Fleming, N.V.V. (2010) The comparison of stroke volume variation and arterial pressure based cardiac output with standard hemodynamic measurements during cardiac surgery. *Internet Journal of Anesthesiology*, **22** (2), 1–11.

Manoach, S., Weingart, S.D., and Charchaflieh, J. (2012) The evolution and current use of hemodynamic monitoring for predicting volume responsiveness during resuscitation, perioperative, and critical care. *Journal of Clinical Anesthesia*, **24**, 242–250.

Marik, P.E., Baram, M., and Vahid, B. (2008) Does central venous pressure predict fluid responsiveness? A systematic review of the literature and the tale of seven mares. *Chest*, **134** (1), 172–178.

Marik, P.E., Cavallazzi, R., Vasu, T., and Hirani, A. (2009) Dynamic changes in arterial waveform derived variables and responsiveness in mechanically ventilated patients: a systematic review of the literature. *Critical Care Medicine*, **37**, 2642–2647.

Mathews, L. (2007) Paradigm shift in hemodynamic monitoring. *Internet Journal of Anesthesiology*, **11**, 1–33.

Mayer, J., Boldt, J., Poland, R. *et al.* (2009) Continuous arterial pressure waveform-based cardiac output using the FloTrac/Vigileo: a review and meta-analysis. *Journal of Cardiothoracic and Vascular Anesthesia*, **23** (30), 401–406.

McGee, W.T. (2009) A simple physiologic algorithm for managing hemodynamics using stroke volume and stroke volume variation: physiologic optimization program. *Journal of Intensive Care Medicine*, **24** (6), 352–360.

Michard, F. and Teboul, J.L. (2002) Predicting fluid responsiveness in ICU patients: a critical analysis of the evidence. *CHEST*, **121**, 2000–2008.

Monnet, X. and Teboul, J.L. (2008) Passive leg raising. *Intensive Care Medicine*, **34**, 659–663.

Monnet, X., Rienzo, M., Osman, D. *et al.* (2006) Passive leg raising predicts fluid responsiveness in the critically ill. *Critical Care Medicine*, **34**, 1402–1407.

Napoli, A.M. (2012) Physiologic and clinical principles behind noninvasive resuscitation techniques and cardiac output monitoring. *Cardiology Research and Practice*, **2012**, 1–12.

Osman, D., Ridel, C., Ray, P. *et al.* (2007) Cardiac filling pressures are not appropriate to predict hemodynamic response to volume challenge. *Critical Care Medicine*, **35** (1), 64–68.

Phan, T.D., Ismail, H., Heriot, A.G., and Ho, K.M. (2008) Improving perioperative outcomes: fluid optimization with the esophageal Doppler monitor, a metaanalysis and review. *Journal of the American College of Surgeons*, **207**, 935–941.

Pinsky, M.R. (2007) Hemodynamic evaluation and monitoring in the ICU. *CHEST*, **132**, 2020–2029.

Pinsky, M.R. and Payen, D. (2005) Functional hemodynamic monitoring. *Critical Care*, **9**, 566–572.

Rajaram, S.S., Desai, N.K., Kalra, A. *et al.* (2013) Pulmonary artery catheters for adult patients in intensive care. *Cochrane Database of Systematic Reviews*, **2**, CD003408.

Reuter, D.A., Felbinger, T.W., Schmidt, C. *et al.* (2002) Stroke volume variations for assessment of cardiac responsiveness to volume loading in mechanically ventilated patients after cardiac surgery. *Intensive Care Medicine*, **28**, 392–398.

Rivers, E.P., Katranji, M., Haehne, K.A. *et al.* (2012) Early interventions in severe sepsis and septic shock: a review of the evidence one decade later. *Minerva Anestesiologica*, **78**, 712–724.

Roche, A.M., Miller, T.E., and Gan, T.J. (2009) Goal-directed fluid management with trans-oesophageal Doppler. *Best Practice & Research Clinical Anaesthesiology*, **23**, 327–334.

Saraceni, E., Rocci, S., Persona, P. *et al.* (2011) Comparison of two methods for cardiac ouput measurement in critically ill patients. *British Journal of Anaesthesia*, **106** (5), 690–694.

Schober, P., Loer, S.A., and Schwarte, L.A. (2009) Perioperative hemodynamic monitoring with transesophageal Doppler technology. *International Anesthesia Research Society*, **109** (2), 340–353.

Senn, A., Button, D., Zollinger, A., and Hofer, C.K. (2009) Assessment of cardiac output changes using a modified FloTrac/Vigileo™ algorithm in cardiac surgery patients. *Critical Care*, **13**, R32.

Takala, J., Ruokonen, E., Tenhunen, J.J. *et al.* (2011) Early non-invasive cardiac output monitoring in hemodynamically unstable intensive care patients: a multi-center randomized controlled trial. *Critical Care*, **15**, R148, 1–9.

Tchorz, K.M., Chandra, M.S., Markert, R.J. *et al.* (2012) Comparison of hemodynamic measurements from invasive and noninvasive monitoring during resuscitation. *Journal of Trauma*, **72**, 852–860.

Teboul, J.L. and Monnet, X. (2008) Prediction of volume responsiveness in critically ill patients with spontaneous breathing activity. *Current Opinion in Critical Care*, **14**, 334–339.

The National Heart, Lung, and Blood Institute (NHLBI) Acute Respiratory Distress Syndrome (ARDS) Clinical Trials Network (2006) Pulmonary-artery versus central venous catheter to guide treatment of acute lung injury. *New England Journal of Medicine*, **354**, 2213–2224.

Uchino, S., Bellomo, R., Morimatsu, H. *et al.* (2006) Pulmonary artery catheter versus pulse contour analysis: a prospective epidemiological study. *Critical Care*, **10**, R174.

Vieillard-Baron, A., Prin, S., Chergui, K. *et al.* (2003) Hemodynamic instability in sepsis. Bedside assessment by Doppler echocardiography. *American Journal of Respiratory and Critical Care Medicine*, **168**, 1270–1276.

Vincent, J.L., Rhodes, A., Perel, A. *et al.* (2011) Clinical review: update on hemodynamic monitoring—a consensus of 16. *Critical Care*, **15**, 229.

Wiesenack, C., Passer, C., Rodig, G., and Keyl, C. (2003) Stroke volume variation as an indicator of fluid responsiveness using pulse contour analysis in mechanically ventilated patients. *Anesthesia Analgesia*, **96**, 1254–1257.

Wyffels, P.A., Dumez, P.J., Helderweirt, J. *et al.* (2007) Ventilation-induced plethysmographic variations predict fluid responsiveness in ventilated postoperative cardiac surgery patients. *Anesthesiology and Analgesia*, **105**, 448–452.

CHAPTER 6

Monitoring for neurologic dysfunction

Janice L. Hinkle[1] and Carey Heck[2]

[1] *Washington, DC, USA*
[2] *Jefferson School of Nursing, Philadelphia, PA., USA*

Physiological guidelines

Neurologic dysfunction can result from a variety of pathophysiologic changes. Causes include neurologic (head injury, stroke, brain tumors, encephalopathy, etc.), toxicological (drug overdose, alcohol intoxication, etc.), or metabolic (hepatic or renal failure, diabetic ketoacidosis, etc.) disruption. The wide variety of clinical problems that can lead to neurologic dysfunction in adult patients is part of what makes nursing surveillance in this population such a challenge.

Intact anatomic structures of the brain and spinal cord are needed for normal neurologic function. The two hemispheres of the cerebrum must communicate, via an intact corpus callosum, and the lobes of the brain (frontal, parietal, temporal, and occipital) must communicate and coordinate their specific functions. Other important brain structures include the cerebellum and the brain stem. The cerebellum has both excitatory and inhibitory actions and is largely responsible for coordination of movement. The brain stem contents are essential for brain and body functions with areas that control heart rate, respirations, and blood pressure (Smeltzer *et al.*, 2010).

The spinal cord is a long cylindrical structure that begins in the medulla and ends at the lumbar vertebrae L1–L2 (Bader and Littlejohns, 2004, 2010). It is the "main highway" for ascending and descending fiber tracts that connect the brain to the spinal nerves and is responsible for reflexes. Disruptions in the anatomic structures of the brain and spinal cord can result from trauma, edema, pressure from tumors, or other mechanisms, such as an increase or decrease in the circulation of blood or cerebrospinal fluid (CSF).

Increased intracranial pressure

The rigid cranial vault contains brain tissue (1400 g), blood (75 ml), and CSF (75 ml) (Smeltzer *et al.*, 2010). The volume and pressure of these three components are usually in a state of equilibrium and produce a normal ICP.

The Monro–Kellie hypothesis states that, because of the limited space for expansion within the skull (a closed box), an increase in any one of the components causes a change in the volume of the others (Bader, 2006a; Bader and Littlejohns, 2004, 2010). Because brain tissue has limited space to expand, compensation typically is accomplished by displacing or shifting CSF, increasing the absorption or diminishing the production of CSF, or decreasing cerebral blood volume. Without compensatory changes, ICP begins to rise. Under normal circumstances, minor changes in blood volume and CSF volume occur constantly as a result of alterations in intrathoracic pressure (coughing, sneezing, straining), posture, blood pressure, systemic oxygen and carbon dioxide levels (Hickey, 2009).

Increased intracranial pressure (ICP) occurs in many patients with acute neurologic conditions because pathologic conditions alter the relationship between intracranial volume and ICP. Although elevated ICP is most commonly associated with head injury, it may also be seen as a secondary effect in

Critical Care Nursing: Monitoring and Treatment for Advanced Nursing Practice, First Edition. Edited by Kathy J. Booker.
© 2015 John Wiley & Sons, Inc. Published 2015 by John Wiley & Sons, Inc.

other conditions, such as brain tumors, subarachnoid hemorrhage, as well as toxic and viral encephalopathies (Smeltzer et al., 2010). Increased ICP from any cause decreases cerebral perfusion, stimulates further swelling (edema), and may shift brain tissue, resulting in herniation, a dire and frequently fatal event (Smeltzer et al., 2010).

Decreased cerebral blood flow

Increased ICP may reduce cerebral blood flow (CBF) or decrease cerebral perfusion and this can result in ischemia and cell death (Patho puzzler, 2007). In the early stages of cerebral ischemia, the vasomotor centers are stimulated and the systemic pressure rises to maintain CBF. Usually, this is accompanied by a slow bounding pulse and respiratory irregularities. These changes in blood pressure, pulse, and respiration are important clinically because they suggest increased ICP (Smeltzer et al., 2010).

The concentration of carbon dioxide in the blood and in the brain tissue also plays an important role in the regulation of CBF. An increase in the arterial partial pressure of carbon dioxide ($PaCO_2$) causes cerebral vasodilation, leading to increased CBF and increased ICP. A decrease in $PaCO_2$ has a vasoconstrictive effect, limiting blood flow to the brain. Decreased venous outflow may also increase cerebral blood volume, thus raising ICP (Smeltzer et al., 2010).

Cerebral edema or swelling is defined as an abnormal accumulation of water or fluid in the intracellular space, extracellular space, or both, associated with an increase in the volume of brain tissue. Edema can occur in the gray, white, or interstitial matter. As brain tissue swells within the rigid skull, several mechanisms attempt to compensate for the increasing ICP. These compensatory mechanisms include autoregulation as well as decreased production and flow of CSF. Autoregulation (see Fig. 6.1) refers to the brain's ability to change the diameter of its blood vessels to maintain a constant CBF during alterations in systemic blood pressure. This complex mechanism can be impaired in patients who are experiencing a pathologic and sustained increase in ICP (Smeltzer et al., 2010).

Cerebral response to increased intracranial pressure

As ICP rises, compensatory mechanisms in the brain work to maintain blood flow and prevent secondary neurologic damage. The brain can maintain a steady perfusion pressure if the arterial systolic blood pressure is 50–150 mmHg and the ICP is less than 40 mmHg. Changes in ICP are closely linked with cerebral perfusion pressure (CPP). The CPP is calculated by subtracting the ICP from the mean arterial pressure (MAP). For example, if the MAP is 100 mmHg and the ICP is 15 mmHg, then the CPP is 85 mmHg. The normal CPP is 70–100 mmHg (Hickey, 2009). As ICP rises and the autoregulatory mechanism of the brain is overwhelmed, the CPP can increase to greater than 100 mmHg or decrease to less than 50 mmHg. Patients with a CPP of less than 50 mmHg experience irreversible neurologic damage. Therefore, the CPP must be maintained and monitored to ensure adequate blood flow to the brain. If ICP is equal to MAP, cerebral circulation ceases (Smeltzer et al., 2010).

A clinical phenomenon known as Cushing's response (or Cushing's reflex) is seen when CBF decreases significantly (Patho puzzler, 2007). When ischemic, the vasomotor center triggers an increase in arterial pressure in an effort to overcome the increased ICP. A sympathetically mediated response causes an increase in the systolic blood pressure with a widening of the pulse pressure and cardiac slowing. This response is seen clinically as an increase in systolic blood pressure, irregular respirations, and reflex slowing of the heart rate (bradycardia) (Andrews, 2011). It is a late sign requiring immediate intervention but perfusion may be recoverable if Cushing's response is treated rapidly (Smeltzer et al., 2010; Wyatt, Moreda, and Olson, 2009).

At a certain point, the brain's ability to autoregulate becomes ineffective and decompensation (ischemia and infarction) begins. When this occurs, the patient exhibits significant changes in mental status and vital signs. The bradycardia, hypertension, and bradypnea associated with this deterioration are known as Cushing's triad, a grave sign

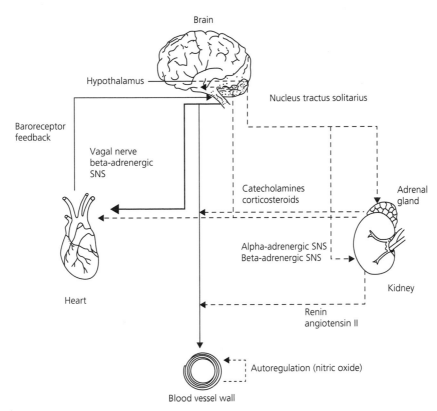

Figure 6.1 Cerebral autoregulation. The Major physiological system involved in the complex regulation of blood pressure. Dotted lines represent local autoregulation, solid lines represents neural influences, and dashed lines represents neuroendocrine influence. SNS, sympathetic nervous system. Adapted from figure 1.2 Cerebral autoregulation and blood flow at available www.electrical-res.com.

(Smeltzer *et al.*, 2010). At this point, herniation of the brain stem and occlusion of the CBF occur if therapeutic intervention is not initiated. Herniation refers to the shifting of brain tissue from an area of high pressure to an area of lower pressure. The herniated tissue exerts pressure on the brain area into which it has shifted, which interferes with the blood supply in that area. Cessation of CBF results in cerebral ischemia, infarction, and brain death.

While the following sections address various aspects of neurological monitoring individually, the advanced practice nurse needs to keep in mind that currently multimodal neuromonitoring is commonly used to guide therapy (Cecil *et al.*, 2011).

Rapid assessment of neurologic dysfunction in intensive care unit patients

Monitoring elements

It is vital for advanced practice nurses to identify the signs and symptoms of increased ICP early while treatments can still be effective. The first and perhaps most important early sign critical to nursing surveillance is decrease in the level of consciousness (LOC). The LOC is most often monitored with the Glasgow Coma Scale (GCS) (see Fig. 6.2).

Pupillary dysfunction (most often one larger and slower to react pupil), changes in vision and extraocular movements (EOMs), deteriorating motor function, headache, and/or

Scoring of eye opening

- 4 Opens eyes spontaneously when the nurse approaches
- 3 Opens eyes in response to speech (normal or shout)
- 2 Opens eyes only to painful stimuli (e.g., squeezing of nail beds)
- 1 Does not open eyes to painful stimuli

Scoring of best motor response

- 6 Can obey a simple command, such as "Lift your left hand off the bed"
- 5 Localizes to painful stimuli and attempts to remove source
- 4 Purposeless movement in response to pain
- 3 Flexes elbows and wrists while extending lower legs to pain
- 2 Extends upper and lower extremities to pain
- 1 No motor response to pain on any limb

Scoring of best verbal response

- 5 Oriented to time, place, and person
- 4 Converses, although confused
- 3 Speaks only in words or phrases that make little or no sense
- 2 Responds with incomprehensible sounds (e.g., groans)
- 1 No verbal response

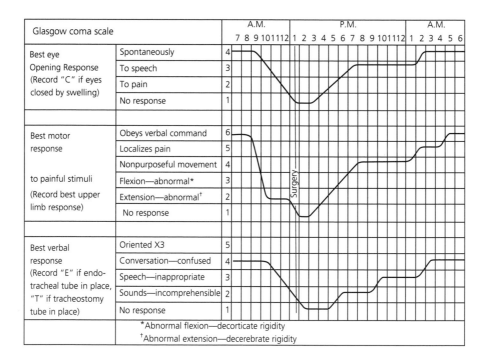

Figure 6.2 Glasgow Coma Scale and application. From Hickey (2009). © LWW.

vomiting (Wyatt, Moreda, and Olson, 2009) are additional signs of decreasing LOC. Changes in the vital signs, especially those associated with blood pressure, are considered a late sign reflecting pressure on the brain stem (Wyatt, Moreda, and Olson, 2009).

Evidence-based treatment guidelines

Advanced practice nurses often begin care in the Emergency Department (ED) and there are published guidelines for nursing surveillance of the neurological system of the patient in the ED

Item tested	Title/domain	Response/score
1A	LOC	0-alert 1-drowsy 2-obtunded 3-coma/unresponsive
1B	Orientation	0-answers both correctly 1-answers one correctly 2-answers none correctly
1C	Response/ two questions	0-performs both correctly 1-performs one correctly 2-performs none correctly
2	Gaze	0-normal horizontal movements 1-partial palsy 2-complete gaze palsy
3	Visual fields	0-no visual field defect 1-partial hemianopia 2-complete hemianopia 3-bilateral hemianopia
4	Facial movement	0-normal 1-minor facial weakness 2-partial facial weakness 3-complete unilateral palsy
5	Motor Function (arm) (a) left____ (b) right____	0-no drift 1-drift before 5 s 2-falls before 10 s 3-no effort against gravity 4-no movement
6	Motor Function (leg) (a) left____ (b) right____	0-no drift 1-drift before 5 s 2-falls before 10 s 3-no effort against gravity 4-no movement
7	Limb ataxia	0-no ataxis 1-ataxis in one limb 2-ataxis in two limbs
8	Sensory	0-no sensory deficit 1-mild sensory loss 2-severe sensory loss
9	Best language	0-normal 1-mild aphasia 2-severe aphasia 3-mute or global aphasia
10	Articulation dysarthria	0-normal 1-mild dysarthria 2-severe dysarthria
11	Extinction or inattention	0-absent 1-mild (loss of one sensory modality) 2-severe (loss of two sensory modalites)

Total NIHSS Score _____(0–42)

LOC, level of consciousness.
National Institute of Health Stroke Scale (NIHSS). From the National Institute of Neurological
Disorders and Stroke at the National Institutes of Health, Bethesda, MD.

Figure 6.3 National Institute of Health Stroke Scale (NIHSS).

who has evidence of cerebral contusion, sub-dural, epidural, subarachnoid hemorrhage, or other intracranial injury identified on computed tomography (CT) scan. These guidelines state that neurological checks must be performed and documented on a neurological flow sheet (Neurological Monitoring Guideline, 2010). Monitoring of the GCS, pupils, and grips/grasps should occur every 15 min for the first hour and then every 30 min for the next 6 h and hourly there after (Neurological Monitoring Guideline, 2010).

Best practice guidelines for nursing surveillance of the neurological system of patients with head injuries and other intracranial injury once they reach the ICU include serial GCS (recognizing the limitations of this technique) plus inclusion of other neurological data (Rauen *et al.*, 2008). Other recommended data include assessment of brain stem reflexes, eye

---

Clinical Pearls—Patient Management and Treatment

Some advanced practice nurses responsible for the orientation and ongoing education of staff in neurological intensive care units (ICUs) use laminated "BRAIN cards" (Presciutti and Finck, 2011). BRAIN stands for Brain Resuscitation: Advanced Indicators in Neuromonitoring. The cards are a reference for registered nurses at the bedside to quickly access information that may help novice nurses become familiar with therapies and parameters. Experienced nurses may use it as a teaching tool. Figure 6.4 contains the basic resuscitation as well as the basic and advanced neuromonitoring parameters that appear on the card.

A relatively new device, the pupillometer, is being used for nursing surveillance of pupil reactions (Bader, 2006a; Cecil *et al.*, 2011). A pupillometer is a handheld battery-operated device about the size of a mobile phone. A microprocessor-based optical scanner captures and analyzes pupil dynamics. The device displays the maximum and minimum aperture of the pupil before and after a light stimulus, the percentage change in the pupil, and several velocities (Bader, 2006a). Preliminary research indicates that the pupillometer is an easy and rapid adjunct to assess neurological changes of the pupils in patients with traumatic brain injury (TBI) (Cecil *et al.*, 2011) but insufficient evidence exists to warrant the widespread application of this device.

Some recommend the rapid assessment of neurological dysfunction compromised by depressed LOC or concurrent drug therapy be supplemented. Neuroimaging and neurophysiological evaluation (electroencephalographic) are the recommended forms of supplemental monitoring (Rauen *et al.*, 2008).

Brain Resuscitation

- Airway/breathing/brain/circulation
- Vital signs:

    Airway/oxygenation/ventilation

    Blood pressure

    Temperature
- Level of consciousness (LOC)
- Glasgow coma scale (GCS)
- Cranial nerves
- Motor examination

Basic and advanced neuromonitoring techniques

- ICP < 20 mmHg.
- CPP

    50 to 70 mmHg.

    70 mmHg.

    Confirm with MD if autoregulation intact for which CPP value to use
- $PbtO_2 > 15$ mmHg.
- $SjvO_2 > 55\%$

The adaptation from Presciutti, M., & Finck, A. (2011).

Figure 6.4 Two sections of BRAIN card.

examination (pupil reactions and EOMs), vital signs (respiration depth, rate, and pattern). Best practices also include consideration of clinical state, concurrent injury, and drug use (Rauen *et al.*, 2008).

Best practices for the rapid assessment of neurologic dysfunction in patients who have had an acute ischemic stroke recommend the use of the National Institute of Health Stroke Scale (NIHSS) (see Fig. 6.3) (Gocan and Fisher, 2008; Summers *et al.*, 2009). A complete NIHSS is recommended upon admission to the ICU and an abridged version can be performed when more frequent assessment is needed (Summers *et al.*, 2009).

Intracranial pressure monitoring

Monitoring elements

Nursing surveillance of ICP can be accomplished using a variety of devices including a ventriculostomy, a parenchymal catheter, a subarachnoid screw or bolt, a subdural device, an epidural device, or a hybrid or combination of these that are placed inside the cranial vault (Bader, 2006a). Table 6.1 provides an overview of the advantages and disadvantages of ICP devices (Bader and Littlejohns, 2004, p. 201). These devices make use of a variety of technologies to measure the pressure including pneumatic transducers, microchip transducers, fiber-optic technology, or an air pouch (Bader and Littlejohns, 2004). Some consider "normal" ICP to be 0–10 mmHg (Moreda, Wyatt, and Olson, 2009) with 15 mmHg as the upper limit of normal (Hickey, 2009); other authors state 10–20 mmHg is "normal" (Patho puzzler, 2007).

Evidence-based treatment guidelines

The Neuro-Intensive Care and Emergency Medicine (NICEM) section of the European Society of Intensive Care Medicine states that there are insufficient data to recommend ICP monitoring and management as a standard of care in all brain-injured patients (Andrews

Table 6.1 Intracranial pressure monitoring options.

Monitoring Device	Transducer Type	Advantages	Disadvantages
Ventriculostomy -	ESG ISG F	Gold standard Allows CSF drainage	Most difficult to insert—small ventricle or ventricular shift Good waveform May occlude F—may malfunction ISG and F—unable to rezero
Parenchymal	ISG F	Quick insertion Low complication rate	Good waveform F—catheter breakage ISG—catheter displacement ISG and F—unable to rezero
Subarachnoid screw	ESG F	Quick insertion	Fair waveform Occlusion of device—debris in device (brain, dura, clot) CSF leak
Epidural	ESG F	Extradural Easy insertion	Indirect measure Poor waveform Poor accuracy
Subdural	ESG ISG F	Tunnel system May be inserted postoperatively through craniotomy	Poor waveform Poor accuracy May be compressed as brain swells

From March K: Intracranial pressure monitoring and assessing intracranial compliance in brain injury, *Crit Care Nurs Clin North Am* 12(4):429–36, 2000.
CSF, Internal strain gange; *ESG,* external strain gauge; *F,* fiberoptic; *ISG,* internal strain gauge. Bader, M. K., & Littlejohns, L. R. (Eds.)· (2004). *AANN core curriculum for neuroscience nursing* (4th ed.). St. Louis: Elsevier. used with permission
From Bader and Littlejohns (2004). © Elsevier.

et al., 2008). However, the evidence is "good enough" to recommend ICP monitoring in all potentially salvageable patients with a severe TBI (defined as GCS ≤ 8) with abnormal findings on CT scan (Andrews *et al.*, 2008). Other summaries support ICP monitoring in severe TBI (Littlejohns and Bader, 2009). There are much lower levels of evidence for

---

Clinical Pearls—Patient Management and Treatment

A common concern of ICU nurses caring for patients with ICP monitoring is how nursing interventions affect ICP. The ICP reference range should be determined for each patient taking into consideration the physician's orders, the underlying pathology, and the plan of care (Bell, 2009). The nurse should monitor pulmonary hygiene and the effects of interventions, such as suctioning and patient positioning on ICP (Bell, 2009). Current research shows that the routine chest percussion therapy (using specialty beds) is safe to perform in patients with monitoring in place (Olson *et al.*, 2009a, 2010). One study reported that a small number of patients had ICP values greater than 20 mmHg but there was no trend toward overall worsening of ICP immediately after oral care (Prendergast *et al.*, 2009). Regular oral care is known to decrease the incidence of ventilator-assisted pneumonia but larger well-designed studies are needed to fully understand ICP and oral care. It is recommended that nursing care be planned at intervals to allow patients with elevated ICP to stabilize (Bell, 2009).

Elevating the head-of-bed (HOB) should be based on the underlying disease process of the patient to help control ICP (Bell, 2009). Much research has gone into HOB elevation and ICP but still there are not high levels of evidence to support practices (Littlejohns and Bader, 2009). Patients who have had a stroke are thought to benefit from horizontal backrest positions to optimize CPP (Littlejohns and Bader, 2009). Maintaining the HOB at 30° reduces ICP and improves CPP without concomitant decrease in cerebral oxygenation in patients who have had a TBI (Littlejohns and Bader, 2009). In patients with other neurological injuries, ICP is improved with HOB at 30° but the CPP is not improved (Littlejohns and Bader, 2009).

As mentioned in the section on rapid neurological assessment, the monitoring of pupils is being conducted in some institutions with a new device, the pupillometer. Preliminary research indicates that the monitoring of constriction velocities and pupil reactivity aids in the detection of increased ICP (Cecil *et al.*, 2011).

There is also preliminary research on the analysis of ICP waveforms to measure cerebral compliance (Fan, 2006; Fan *et al.*, 2008; Hickey, Olson, and Turner, 2009). With additional research these techniques may prove useful as a clinical tool to measure compliance and detect early deterioration in those with neurological injury.

ICP monitoring in patients with intracranial hemorrhage, subarachnoid hemorrhage, hydrocephalus, sylvian arachnoid cysts, cerebral fat embolism, fulminant hepatic failure, acute ischemic stroke, or meningitis (Littlejohns and Bader, 2009).

Several authors mention the ventriculostomy as the "gold standard" or the most accurate for ICP monitoring (Andrews *et al.*, 2008; Bader and Littlejohns, 2004; Brain Trauma Foundation, 2007; Littlejohns and Bader, 2009). The NICEM consensus stated that "in general, ICP and CPP target values should be ≤20 mmHg and ≥50–70 mmHg respectively" (Andrews *et al.*, 2008, p. 1365) and others concurred (Brain Trauma Foundation, 2007; Littlejohns and Bader, 2009). Others suggest ICP should be ≤20–25 mmHg (Bader, 2006a; Blissitt, 2006; Cecil *et al.*, 2011) and CPP 60–70 mmHg (Blissitt, 2006). Clear guidelines remain elusive and further research is needed.

Measuring brain temperature

Fever (temperature ≥38.3 °C) is known to exacerbate secondary neuronal damage in all forms of brain injury and has been shown to adversely affect neurologic outcomes (Badjatia, 2009). A more aggressive approach to actively controlling patient temperature is supported by studies that appear to show improved outcomes when normothermia is maintained (Polderman and Herold, 2009). Brain temperatures exceed core body temperatures (Bader and Littlejohns, 2010, p. 192) and so there may be a benefit to monitoring brain temperatures in addition to core temperatures (see Table 6.2). Monitoring brain temperature using an invasive device, such as a thermistor, may detect

Table 6.2 Differences in brain and body temperatures.

Brain temperature 0.5–1 °C higher than core and jugular
Brain temperature 0.3–1.9 °C higher than bladder
Brain temperature 0.1–2 °C higher than rectal
Deep white matter 0.5–1 °C higher than cortical
There are greater differences with temperatures higher than 38 °C

Adapted from Bader and Littlejohns (2010). © American Association of Neuroscience Nursing.

episodes of neural hyperthermia, which, if untreated, could lead to further neurological injury (Mcilvoy, 2007). One literature review suggested that brain temperature is higher than core temperature and without monitoring brain temperature, detection of fever and its effects may be limited (Mcilvoy, 2007). Monitoring brain temperature may provide the clinician with additional information that has the potential to improve patient outcomes.

Evidence-based treatment guidelines

No evidence-based treatment guidelines to support the use of the routine measurement of brain temperature were identified.

> **Clinical Pearls—Patient Management and Treatment**
>
> Brain temperature monitoring is relatively easy as it is included in several multimodality systems. Some suggest preventing brain hyperthermia (>38.5 °C) with cooling interventions following TBI (Cecil et al., 2011).

Brain tissue O_2 monitoring

Monitoring elements

Two methods exist to measure brain tissue oxygenation: jugular venous saturation (SjO$_2$) and partial pressure brain tissue oxygen (PbtO$_2$). The former measures the oxygen saturation of hemoglobin as it exits the cerebral circulation via a catheter in the internal jugular vein and provides a means of identifying global cerebral oxygenation (Bader, 2006b). Normal findings for SjO$_2$ are 55–75% saturation (Bader and Littlejohns, 2004; Wiegand and American Association of Critical Care Nurses [AACN], 2011). The latter method monitors the balance between cerebral oxygen delivery and oxygen consumption and is obtained by the placement of a catheter within the brain parenchyma. This method has the ability to detect regional cerebral oxygenation (Andrews et al., 2008; Bader and Littlejohns, 2004). Normal values for PbtO$_2$ are between 25 and 35 mmHg (Bader and Littlejohns, 2004).

Evidence-based treatment guidelines

There are limited clinical studies supporting the use of cerebral tissue oxygenation monitoring (Littlejohns and Bader, 2009). However, several authors recommend initiating treatment for SjO$_2$ < 50% and PbtO$_2$ < 20 mmHg (Bader, 2006b; Bader and Littlejohns, 2004; Brain Trauma Foundation, 2007).

> **Clinical Pearls—Patient Management and Treatment**
>
> Changes seen in oxygen delivery and consumption in the brain may occur before clinical signs are seen in the patient. Careful and diligent monitoring of changes and trends will provide the nurse with information that can be used to guide treatment and prevent hypoxia and subsequent cerebral ischemia. SjO$_2$ < 40% represents global cerebral ischemia and has been associated with poor outcomes (Wiegand and AACN, 2011). Cerebral tissue hypoxia is seen in PbO$_2$ < 15 mmHg with cerebral tissue death occurring at 5 mmHg (Bader and Littlejohns, 2004; Wiegand and AACN, 2011).

Microdialysis

Monitoring elements

Microdialysis allows for the continuous measurement of tissue chemistry across a semipermeable membrane in the extracellular space of the brain (Andrews et al., 2008; Bader and Littlejohns, 2004, 2010). Biochemical markers including the lactate/pyruvate ratio, glucose, and glutamate levels are monitored. Changes in these biomarkers are early indicators of cerebral hypoxia and ischemia (Andrews et al., 2008; Bader and Littlejohns, 2004, 2010).

Evidence-based treatment guidelines

No evidence-based treatment guidelines were identified to support the routine use of cerebral microdialysis. However, several authors have recommended the use of microdialysis in patients with TBI who require intracranial monitoring (Bellander et al., 2004; Cecil et al., 2011).

Clinical Pearls—Patient Management and Treatment

There is currently a lack of consensus regarding treatment parameters and indications for use of cerebral microdialysis (Bader and Littlejohns, 2004, 2010). This monitoring modality has been studied in neurological patients with TBI (Cecil et al., 2011), subarachnoid hemorrhage (SAH), epilepsy, and stroke (Bader, 2006a). When considering adding microdialysis to the nursing surveillance, the individual patient's clinical course, the overall treatment goals, outcomes, and risk/benefit status must be considered.

Electrophysiological monitoring

Monitoring elements

Electroencephalography (EEG) is a technology used to measure cerebral electrical activity as an electrochemical phenomenon and reflects the metabolic and physiological state of cerebral tissue (Bader and Littlejohns, 2010). The placement of multiple surface electrodes detects electrical impulses that generate a waveform reflecting chemical events at the tissue and cellular levels (Bader and Littlejohns, 2010).

Evidence-based treatment guidelines

Surprisingly there are very few evidence-based guidelines for EEG monitoring. The evidence-based guidelines for the management

Clinical Pearls—Patient Management and Treatment

There are a number of clinical indications for nursing surveillance of the neurologic system using EEG monitoring. It is used mainly for the evaluation of unconscious patients to detect subclinical seizure activity and to monitor the onset and/or progression of cerebral ischemia (Bader and Littlejohns, 2010). It is used to evaluate patients post cardiac arrest as well as patients in coma states including barbiturate coma (Bader and Littlejohns, 2010). It is also used as a cerebral evaluation of pharmacologically paralyzed states. One study suggested that a mathematical model of EEG recording might be useful in differentiating between patients in a vegetative state and those with a higher LOC following severe brain injury (Boly et al., 2011).

of spontaneous intracerebral hemorrhage (ICH) state that "continuous EEG monitoring is probably indicated in ICH patients with depressed mental status that is out of proportion to the degree of brain injury" (Morgenstern et al., 2010, p. 2116). Further, the guidelines state that those patients with seizures identified on EEG need to be treated with antiepileptic drugs (Morgenstern et al., 2010).

The BiSpectral index monitoring

Monitoring elements

BiSpectral ndex (BIS) monitoring was originally developed for use during surgery as an adjunct to sedation monitoring for general anesthesia but has been shown to be a useful tool in managing the sedation levels of the general critical care patient. The BIS monitor is a processed EEG-based parameter used to assess individual LOC and sedation (Arbour et al., 2009; Bader and Littlejohns, 2010). Through the application of a sensor placed on the individual's forehead, information obtained is calculated into a numeric value correlating with the patient's LOC. Many factors may affect BIS readings so an understanding of the significance of the parameters obtained is crucial for data interpretation. Factors such as analgesic and neuromuscular blockade administration, pain, muscle artifact, sleep patterns, or altered neurologic states due to a variety of pathologies have the potential to increase or decrease this value (Fraser and Riker, 2005; Sessler, Grap, and Ramsay, 2008).

Evidence-based treatment guidelines

Several studies evaluating sedation levels of patients in the ICU have shown BIS monitoring to be an effective adjunct tool in decreasing the use of sedative medications without increasing patient complications. However, research to date does not support the use of BIS monitoring alone for the management of sedation in the critically ill patient (Arbour et al.,

Table 6.3 BIS values and corresponding levels of sedation

BIS value	Corresponding level of sedation
100	Awake state, patient able to respond appropriately to verbal stimulation
80	Patient able to respond to loud verbal or limited tactile stimulation such as mild prodding or shaking
60	Low probability of explicit recall, patient unresponsive to verbal stimulation
40	Patient unresponsive to verbal stimulation, less responsive to physical stimulation
20	Minimal responsiveness
0	No responsiveness mediated by brain function, spinal reflexes may be present

Adapted from Bader and Littlejohns (2004). © Elsevier.

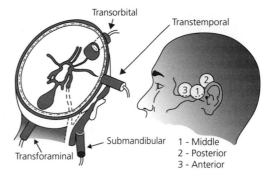

Figure 6.5 The image on the left shows 4 windows of transcranial Doppler insonation. Clockwise these are orbital, temporal, submandifular, and foraminal. The image on the right shows the 3 aspects of the temporal window: 1) middle; 2)posterior; and 3)anterior. Adapted with permission from Wiegand, D.J.L., and the American Association of Critical-Care Nurses (AACN) (2011).

intracranial stenoses or occlusions, detection of cerebral emboli, monitoring of hemodynamic changes with impaired intracranial perfusion, and assessment of therapeutic interventions on intracranial hemodynamics (Wiegand and AACN, 2011, p. 849).

Evidence-based treatment guidelines

No evidence-based treatment guidelines were identified for TCD use. Evidence for the procedure comes from case studies, expert opinion, or professional organization standards without

2009; Weaver *et al.*, 2007). No evidence-based treatment guidelines were identified for BIS monitoring.

Transcranial Doppler ultrasonograpy

Monitoring elements

Transcranial Doppler (TCD) ultrasonograpy is a valuable technique for the advanced practice nurse to have in the nursing surveillance arsenal as it provides an indirect measure of CBF by measuring the CBF velocity and can be carried out at the bedside of the patient (Littlejohns and Bader, 2009). TCD measures blood flow velocities in the major branches of the circle of Willis through bone windows in an intact skull (see Fig. 6.5) (Wiegand and AACN, 2011). This measure supports the assessment and monitoring of vasospasm severity, localization of clinical studies to support the recommendations (Wiegand and AACN, 2011). The evidence for the use of TCDs in patients with fulminant hepatic failure is an active area of research (Bindi *et al.*, 2008; Kawakami, Koda, and Murawaki, 2010).

Shunts

Monitoring elements

Shunts are small tubes made of Silast that divert CSF from the ventricles or subarachnoid space within the brain into other body cavities to treat hydocephalus. The insertion of shunts is one of the most common procedures performed in many neurosurgical centers (Bader and Littlejohns, 2010). Types include ventriculoperitoneal, ventriculoatrial, ventriculopleural, and lumbar peritoneal shunts (Bader and Littlejohns, 2010).

Evidence-based treatment guidelines

No evidence-based treatment guidelines could be located for routine postoperative monitoring of a newly placed shunt or to determine whether a shunt is malfunctioning or not.

> **Clinical Pearls—Patient Management and Treatment**
>
> Frequent vital signs and neurological checks are needed in patients who have had a newly inserted shunt to assess for complications of intracerebral or subdural hematoma, meningitis, or peritonitis (Bader and Littlejohns, 2010). The cranial and peritoneal (or alternate catheter site) incision needs to be assessed for signs and symptoms of wound infection (Bader and Littlejohns, 2010).
>
> Routine strategies for detecting shunt malfunction include clinical neurological assessment, neuropsychological testing, and neuroimaging (Petrella *et al.*, 2009). One study reported that *in vivo* shunt testing using a constant rate infusion of normal saline was easy, safe, and clinically useful, especially when shunt malfunction was suspected but not certain (Petrella *et al.*, 2009).

Neuromuscular transmission

Monitoring elements

Neuromuscular transmission, or stimulation, is used to assess evoked responses (Bader and Littlejohns, 2010). The main types include the supramaxial stimulation to assess a single twitch, the "train-of-four," which comprises four stimuli over 2s, the double-burst stimulation, and the titanic stimulation (Bader and Littlejohns, 2004, 2010). The primary indication is to monitor the peripheral nervous system.

Evidence-based treatment guidelines

No evidence-based treatment guidelines could be located for neuromuscular stimulation.

> **Clinical Pearls—Patient Management and Treatment**
>
> The interpretation of evoked responses (to stimulation) requires specialized training and must be interpreted within the context of other clinical assessment findings.

Management of cervical stabilization devices

Monitoring elements

Cervical instability can result from many causes including trauma, degenerative changes, infectious causes, or neoplastic disease. Depending upon the cause of the cervical instability, treatment varies. Options include surgical or nonsurgical interventions. Decisions for treatment are made based on several considerations including patient presentation, the underlying cervical pathology, mechanical and technical considerations of treatment, patient preference, and surgeon expertise and experience (American Association of Neuroscience Nurses [AANN], 2007; Bader and Littlejohns, 2010). Nonsurgical management for cervical instability as a result of traumatic or nontrauma pathologies may include application of a hard cervical collar or halo brace. These may be used as an alternative to surgery in the case of some vertebral fractures or as an adjunct to surgery when placed post-operatively to facilitate bony healing (Bader and Littlejohns, 2010; Sarro *et al.*, 2010). Surgical management for cervical instability will vary greatly from patient to patient (see Fig. 6.6). Extensive pathology may require a combined anterior/posterior approach while other presentations may require only one of these approaches

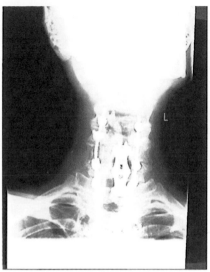 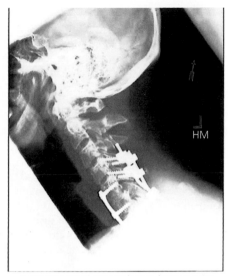

• Anterior/posterior cervical spine decompression and fusion, A/P X ray

• Anterior/posterior cervical spine decompression and fusion, lateral X ray

Figure 6.6 Cervical spine stabilization from AANA (2007). Cervical Spine Surgery. A Guide to Preoperative Patient Care. Used with permission from AANA.

(AANN, 2007). The use of instrumentation (e.g., plates, wires, cages, or screws) to provide internal fixation and stabilization promotes bony healing and may be part of a surgical treatment plan (AANN, 2007). Atlantoaxial instability (C1–C2 instability), often the result of degenerative, infectious, or neoplastic causes, is typically treated with surgery and instrumentation (Nockels *et al.*, 2007).

Evidence-based treatment guidelines

Recommendations for the management of cervical instability due to traumatic injuries are made in *Early Acute Management in Adults with Spinal Cord Injury: A Clinical Practice Guideline for Health-Care Providers* authored by the Consortium for Spinal Cord Medicine (2008) and in the *Advanced Trauma Life Support* guidelines (American College of Surgeons Committee on Trauma, 2012). These guidelines recommend initial immobilization of the neck in a hard collar for all patients with a suspected cervical spine injury until definitive diagnosis is established. Several authors have recommended early surgical intervention in traumatic spinal cord injuries (SCIs) to improve neurologic outcomes (Consortium for Spinal Cord Medicine, 2008).

Others conclude that the current evidence does not allow decisions to be drawn regarding the potential benefits or harms of spinal fixation surgery in patients with traumatic spinal cord injury (Bagnall *et al.*, 2009). Review of the literature concerning surgery for cervical instability due to causes other than trauma reveals numerous small studies and case reports of interventions and so evidence-based recommendations for practice cannot be made at this time.

Literature is limited concerning evidenced-based management of halo devices and reveals the need for standardization of care regarding

> **Clinical Pearls—Patient Management and Treatment**
>
> Regardless of the cause of cervical instability, the importance of serial examinations to detect motor and/or sensory changes cannot be stressed enough. A complete motor and sensory exam must be performed after any application, removal, or manipulation of stabilization device (Bader and Littlejohns, 2010). Changes in a patient's clinical exam must be reported promptly to the physician or advanced practice clinician.
>
> There exists an increased potential for skin breakdown due to orthotic devices. Meticulous care and inspection of areas at high risk for skin breakdown (i.e., occiput) are of paramount importance in any patient evaluation (AANN, 2007; Bader and Littlejohns, 2010).

these devices (Sarro *et al.*, 2010). Inspection of pin sites for signs of infection, loosening of pins, or halo ring movement are all considered to be standard aspects of nursing management of halo devices (AANN, 2007; Sarro *et al.*, 2010).

Induced coma and sedation protocols

Monitoring elements

Therapeutic interventions provided in the ICU may result in anxiety, pain, and agitation in the critically ill patient, which can increase ICP and adversely affect outcomes. The use of analgesics and sedatives to ameliorate these unintended side effects of care are a common management strategy for ICP control and are vital for the comfort and safety of patients (Bader and Littlejohns, 2010; Brain Trauma Foundation, 2007; Rangel-Castillo, Gopinath, and Robertson, 2008; Wunsch and Kress, 2009). Inadequate or excessive sedation, however, has been shown to lead to significant patient complications and therefore must be avoided (Sessler, Grap, and Ramsay, 2008; Sessler and Pedram, 2009). The neurologically impaired patient requires frequent neurologic assessment and the practitioner must take this into consideration when choosing agents for sedation. The use of sedation in all patients, but particularly in the neurologic patient, should be based on patient needs and the indications for their use reassessed regularly (Wyatt, Moreda, and Olson, 2009).

High-dose barbiturate coma has been used as a management strategy for reducing ICP refractory to maximal medical and/or surgical intervention (Bader and Littlejohns, 2010; Brain Trauma Foundation, 2007). The mechanism of action is a reduction of cerebral metabolic demand through cerebral vasoconstriction and blood flow, which results in decreased ICP (Hickey, 2009; Wyatt, Moreda, and Olson, 2009). Significant side effects of barbiturate coma may occur including cardiac depression, hypotension, hypothermia, and immunosuppression, and careful monitoring for these complications must be ongoing (Bader and Littlejohns, 2010; Tobias, 2008). Due to the loss of neurologic exam with induction of barbiturate coma, several authors recommend neurophysiologic monitoring to evaluate burst suppression activity since the physical exam is of limited value in detecting changes (Brain Trauma Foundation, 2007; Tobias, 2008; Rangel-Castillo, Gopinath, and Robertson, 2008).

Evidence-based treatment guidelines

There are no evidenced-based protocols for the management of sedation for neurologic conditions. Selection of agents is guided by the individual practitioner's judgment based on the patient's condition and treatment goals (Brain Trauma Foundation, 2007; Rangel-Castillo, Gopinath, and Robertson, 2008). Some authors have recommended the use of short-acting agents, which allow brief interruptions of sedation to evaluate neurologic status (Rangel-Castillo, Gopinath, and Robertson, 2008). When utilized, attention must be paid to potential undesirable side effects, such as hypotension, that may contribute to secondary injury (Brain Trauma Foundation, 2007; Tobias, 2008). Although barbiturate coma reduces ICP, it has not been shown to improve outcomes and therefore recommendations for use as a first-line treatment choice are not indicated (Bader and Littlejohns, 2010; Roberts and Syndenham, 2009).

> **Clinical Pearls—Patient Management and Treatment**
>
> The use of sedation clearly has advantages in this population, particularly when increased ICP is a concern. Care must be taken to manage the deleterious effects of agitation and pain on ICP, yet at the same time avoiding oversedation. Oversedation can mask a deteriorating neurologic exam, which, if not recognized and acted upon appropriately, could result in unfavorable patient outcomes.

Research-based neurologic protocols

Many of the clinical guidelines mentioned in this chapter are research-based and contain recommendations for monitoring neurological conditions such as TBI (Brain Trauma Foundation,

2007) and SCI (AANN, 2007; Consortium for Spinal Cord Medicine, 2008). However, no specific research-based protocols for neurological monitoring were located. Neurologic injury and trauma induce multiple changes that are difficult to control, thus randomized control trials remain difficult to design and complete. However, continued research is under way on many of the techniques discussed within this chapter.

References

American Association of Neuroscience Nurses (AANN) (2007) *Cervical Spine Surgery. A Guide to Preoperative and Postoperative Patient Care.* AANN, Glenview.

Andrews, P.J.D., Citerio, G., Longhi, L., Polderman, K., Sahuquillo, J., and Vajkoczy, P. (2008) NICEM consensus on neurological monitoring in acute neurological disease. *Intensive Care Medicine,* **34** (8), 1362–1370.

Andrews, P.L. (2011) Quick guide to clinical assessment findings. *American Nurse Today,* **6** (5), 8–10.

Arbour, R., Waterhouse, J., Seckel, M.A., and Bucher, L. (2009) Correlation between the sedation-agitation scale and the bispectral index in ventilated patients in the intensive care unit. *Heart & Lung,* **38** (4), 336–345.

Bader, M.K. (2006a) Gizmos and gadgets for the neuroscience intensive care unit. *Journal of Neuroscience Nursing,* **38** (4), 248–260.

Bader, M.K. (2006b) Recognizing and treating ischemic insults to the brain: the role of brain tissue oxygen monitoring. *Critical Care Nursing Clinics of North America,* **18** (2), 243–256.

Bader, M.K. and Littlejohns, L.R. (eds) (2004) *AANN Core Curriculum for Neuroscience Nursing,* 4th edn. Elsevier, St Louis.

Bader, M.K. and Littlejohns, L.R. (eds) (2010) *AANN Core Curriculum for Neuroscience Nursing,* 5th edn. AANN, Glenview.

Badjatia, N. (2009) Hyperthermia and fever control in brain injury. *Critical Care Medicine,* **37** (7), S270–S257.

Bagnall, A., Jones, L., Duffy, S., and Riemsma, R.P. (2009) Spinal fixation surgery for acute Traumatic spinal cord injury. *Cochrane Injuries Group Cochrane Database of Systematic Reviews,* **2**, CD004725.

Bell, L. (2009) Nursing care and intracranial pressure monitoring. *American Journal of Critical Care,* **18** (4), 338.

Bellander, B.M., Cantais, E., Enblad, P. *et al.* (2004) Consensus meeting on microdialysis in neurointensive care. *Intensive Care Medicine,* **30**, 2166–2169.

Bindi, M.L., Biancofiore, G., Esposito, M. *et al.* (2008) Transcranial doppler sonography is useful for the decision-making at the point of care in patients with acute hepatic failure: a single centre's experience. *Journal of Clinical Monitoring and Computing,* **22** (6), 449–452.

Blissitt, P.A. (2006) Hemodynamic monitoring in the care of the critically ill neuroscience patient. *AACN Advanced Critical Care,* **17** (3), 327–340.

Blissitt, P.A., Mitchell, P.A., Newell, D.W., Woods, S.L., and Belza, B. (2006) Cerebrovascular dynamics with head-of-bed elevation in patients with mild or moderate vasospasm after aneurysmal subarachnoid hemorrhage. *American Journal of Critical Care,* **15** (2), 206–216.

Boly, M., Garrido, M.I., Gosseries, O. *et al.* (2011). Preserved feedforward but impaired top-down processes in the vegetative state. *Science,* **332**, 858–861.

Brain Trauma Foundation (2007) Guidelines for the management of severe traumatic brain injury. *Journal of Neurotrauma,* **24** (8), S1. doi:10.1089/neu.2007.9999.

Cecil, S., Chen, P.M., Callaway, S.E. *et al.* (2011). Traumatic brain injury: advanced multimodal neuromonitoring from theory to clinical practice. *Critical Care Nurse,* **31** (2), 25–37. doi:10.4037/ccn2010226.

Consortium for Spinal Cord Medicine (2008) Early acute management in adults with spinal cord injury: a clinical practice guideline for health-care professionals. *Journal of Spinal Cord Medicine,* **31** (4), 403–479.

Darwish, R.S., Ahn, E., and Amiridze, N.S. (2008) Role of transcranial doppler in optimizing treatment of cerebral vasospasm in subarachnoid hemorrhage. *Journal of Intensive Care Medicine,* **23** (4), 263–267.

Fan, J. (2006) Intracranial pressure waveform analysis in individual with traumatic brain injury. *Communicating Nursing Research,* **39**, 416.

Fan, J., Kirkness, C., Vicini, P., Burr, R., and Mitchell, P. (2008) Intracranial pressure waveform morphology and intracranial adaptive capacity. *American Journal of Critical Care,* **17** (6), 545–554.

Fraser, G.L. and Riker, R.R. (2005) Bispectral index monitoring in the intensive care unit provides more signal than noise. *Pharmacotherapy,* **25** (5 Pt 2), 19S–27S.

Gocan, S. and Fisher, A. (2008) Neurological assessment by nurses using the national institutes of health stroke scale: implementation of best practice guidelines. *Canadian Journal of Neuroscience Nursing,* **30** (3), 31–42.

Hickey, J.V. (2009) *The Clinical Practice of Neurological and Neurosurgical Nursing,* 6th edn. Lippincott Williams & Wilkins, Philadelphia.

Hickey, J.V., Olson, D.M., and Turner, D.A. (2009) Intracranial waveform analysis during rest and suctioning. *Biological Research in Nursing*, **11** (2), 174–186. doi:10:1177/1099800409332902

Kawakami, M., Koda, M., and Murawaki, Y. (2010) Cerebral pulsatility index by transcranial doppler sonography predicts the prognosis of patients with fulminant hepatic failure. *Clinical Imaging*, **34** (5), 327–331. doi:10.1016/j.clinimag.2009.09.006.

Littlejohns, L.R. and Bader, M.K. (eds) (2009) *AACN-AANN Protocols for Practice: Monitoring Technologies in Critically Ill Neuroscience Patients*, 1st edn. Jones and Bartlett Publishers, Sudbury.

Mcilvoy, L. (2007). The impact of brain temperature and core temperature on intracranial pressure and cerebral perfusion pressure. *Journal of Neuroscience Nursing*, **39** (6), 324–331.

Moreda, M., Wyatt, A.H., and Olson, D.W. (2009) Keeping the balance: understanding intracranial pressure monitoring. *Nursing Critical Care*, **4** (6), 42–47. doi:10.1097/01.CCN.0000363762.63507.00.

Morgenstern, L.B., Hemphill III, J.C., Anderson, C. *et al.* (2010) Guidelines for the management of spontaneous intracerebral hemorrhage: a guideline for healthcare professionals from the American heart Association/American stroke association. *Stroke: Journal of Cerebral Circulation*, **41** (9), 2108–2129. doi:10.1161/STR.0b013e3181ec611b.

Neurological Monitoring Guideline (2010) *ED Nursing*, http://search.ebscohost.com/login.aspx?direct=true&db=cin20&AN=2010692647&site=ehost-live&scope=site (accessed July 23, 2014).

Nockels, R.P., Shaffrey, C.I., Kanter, A.S. *et al.* (2007) Occipitocervical fusion with rigid internal fixation: long-term follow-up data in 69 patients. *Journal of Neurosurgery Spine*, **7** (2), 117–123.

Olson, D.M., Thoyre, S.M., Bennett, S.N. *et al.* (2009a) Effect of mechanical chest percussion on intracranial pressure: a pilot study. *American Journal of Critical Care*, **18** (4), 330–335.

Olson, D.M., Thoyre, S.M., Peterson, E.D., and Graffagnino, C. (2009b) A randomized evaluation of bispectral index-augmented sedation assessment in neurological patients. *Neurocritical Care*, **11** (1), 20. doi:10.1007/s12028-008-9184-6.

Olson, D.M., Bader, M.K., Dennis, C. *et al.* (2010) Multicenter pilot study: safety of automated chest percussion in patients at risk for intracranial hypertension [corrected] [published erratum appears in J NEUROSCI NURS 2010 aug;42(4):180]. *Journal of Neuroscience Nursing*, **42** (3), 119–127. doi:10.1097/JNN.0b013e3181d4a3aa.

Patho puzzler: Don't let your head explode over increased ICP (2007) *Nursing Made Incredibly Easy*, **5** (2), 21, http://search.ebscohost.com/login.aspx?direct=true&db=cin20&AN=2009528257&site=ehost-live&scope=site (accessed July 23, 2014).

Petrella, G., Czosnyka, M., Smielewski, P. *et al.* (2009) In vivo assessment of hydrocephalus shunt. *Acta Neurologica Scandinavica*, **120** (5), 317–323.

Polderman, K.H. and Herold, I. (2009) Therapeutic hypothermia and controlled normothermia in the intensive care unit: practical considerations, side effects, and cooling methods. *Critical Care Medicine*, **37**, 1101–1120.

Prendergast, V., Hallberg, I.R., Jahnke, H. *et al.* (2009) Oral health, ventilator-associated pneumonia, and intracranial pressure in intubated patients in a neuroscience intensive care unit. *American Journal of Critical Care*, **18** (4), 368–376.

Presciutti, M. and Finck, A. (2011) BRAIN: brain resuscitation advanced indicators in neuromonitoring. Poster presentation at the 43rd Annual Educational Meeting, New Relevance in Neuroscience Nursing, at the Kansas City Convention Center, Kansas City, MO.

Rangel-Castillo, L., Gopinath, S., and Robertson, C.S. (2008) Management of intracranial hypertension. *Critical Care Clinics*, **22** (4), 713–732.

Rauen, C.A., Chulay, M., Bridges, E. *et al.* (2008) Seven evidence-based practice habits: putting some sacred cows out to pasture. *Critical Care Nurse*, **28** (2), 98.

Roberts, I. and Syndenham, E. (2009) Barbiturates for acute traumatic brain injury. *Cochrane Database of Systematic Reviews*, **3**, CD000033.

Sarro, A., Anthony, T., Magtoto, R., and Mauceri, J. (2010). Developing a standard of care for halo vest and pin site care including patient and family education: a collaborative approach among three greater Toronto area teaching hospitals. *Journal of Neuroscience Nursing*, **42** (3), 169–173.

Sessler, C.N. and Pedram, S. (2009) Protocolized and target-based sedation and analgesia in the ICU. *Critical Care Clinics*, **25** (3), 489–513.

Sessler, C.N., Grap, M.J., and Ramsay, M.A. (2008) Evaluating and monitoring analgesia and sedation in the intensive care unit. *Critical Care*, **12** (Suppl 3), S2.

Smeltzer, S.C., Bare, B.G., Hinkle, J.L., and Cheever, K.H. (eds) (2010) *Brunner & Suddarth's Textbook of Medical-Surgical Nursing*, 12th ed. Lippincott Williams & Wilkins, Philadelphia.

Summers, D., Leonard, A., Wentworth, D. *et al.* (2009) Comprehensive overview of nursing and interdisciplinary care of the acute ischemic stroke patient: a scientific statement from the American Heart Association. *Stroke*, **40** (8), 2911–2944. doi:10.1161/STROKEAHA.109.192362.

Tobias, J.D. (2008) Bispectral index monitoring documents burst suppression during pentobarbital coma. *Journal of Intensive Care Medicine*, **23** (4), 258–262.

Weaver, C.S., Hauter, W.H., Duncan, C.E. *et al.* (2007) An assessment of the association of bispectral index with 2 clinical sedation scales for monitoring depth of procedural sedation. *American Journal of Emergency Medicine*, **25** (8), 918–924.

Wiegand, D.J.L., and American Association of Critical-Care Nurses (AACN) (2011) *AACN Procedure Manual for Critical Care*, 6th edn. Elsevier/Saunders, St. Louis.

Wunsch, H. and Kress, J.P. (2009) A new era for sedation in ICU patients. *Journal of the American Medical Association*, **301** (5), 542–544.

Wyatt, A.H., Moreda, M.V., and Olson, D.M. (2009) Keeping the balance: understanding intracranial pressure. *Nursing Critical Care*, **4** (5), 18–23. doi:10.1097/01.CCN.0000360668.99971.a5.

CHAPTER 7

Monitoring for renal dysfunction

Dawn Cooper

Medical Intensive Care Unit, Yale New Haven Hospital, New Haven, CT., USA

Renal dysfunction in critically ill patients may lead to catastrophic consequences. The incidence of acute kidney injury (AKI) occurs in over 20% of critically ill patients (Thakar *et al.*, 2009). The mortality rate of patients with AKI in the critical care unit is 59%, with another 8% who die before leaving the hospital (Uchino *et al.*, 2005). Unlike community-acquired AKI, AKI in critically ill patients is most often associated with more than a single insult (Dennen, Douglas, and Anderson, 2010). The most common causes of AKI in the critical care unit are sepsis, followed by major surgery, low cardiac output, hypovolemia, and medications. Other causes of AKI are hepatorenal syndrome, trauma, cardiopulmonary bypass, abdominal compartment syndrome, rhabdomyolysis, and obstruction (Uchino *et al.*, 2005). AKI negatively impacts clinical outcomes, prolongs hospitalization, and can eventually lead to the need for dialysis. The advanced practice nurse plays a pivotal role in prevention, early recognition, and prompt intervention of renal dysfunction to optimize patient outcomes.

Acute kidney injury

The term acute kidney injury (AKI) is used to describe several clinical conditions causing acute kidney dysfunction. Prior to 2004, the term "acute renal failure" was used to describe acute kidney impairment. Acute renal failure was a broad term that never had a standardized definition, diagnosis criteria, or disease stratification. The Acute Dialysis Quality Initiative (ADQI) group began the formal work of developing a consensus definition of acute renal failure that eventually led to a definition of AKI. The risk, injury failure, loss, and end-stage renal disease (RIFLE) criteria stratified the phases of AKI (Bellomo *et al.*, 2004). The RIFLE criteria are based on two categories: creatinine and urinary output (see Fig. 7.1).

A patient can fulfill the criteria though a change of one or both criteria in each category. The patient is classified by the criterion that falls in the most severe category. The Acute Kidney Injury Network (AKIN) later developed the definition of AKI as "a common clinical problem defined by an abrupt (within 48 h) increase in serum creatinine, resulting from an injury or insult that causes a functional or structural change in the kidney" (Molitoris *et al.*, 2007 p. 439). They later developed a staging system of AKI. Table 7.1 identifies the stages of AKI (Bellomo *et al.*, 2004). The spectrum of AKI ranges from the most subtle changes in renal function to the most severe.

The Kidney Disease: Improving Global Outcomes (KDIGO) workgroup recognized that variablity in the recognition and treatment of AKI continued despite the validation of the RIFLE and AKIN (Acute Kidney Injury Work Group, 2012). This group also developed a staged approach to classifying AKI since it has been widely identified that the risk for death and the need for renal replacement therapy increase as kidney disease progresses. The classification and prevention areas of these guidelines are more widely accepted, but treatment for AKI and recommendations for renal replacement are controversial because of minimal supporting evidence (James *et al.*, 2013; Palevsky *et al.*, 2013).

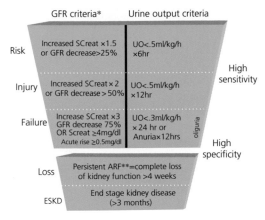

Figure 7.1 RIFLE classification/staging system for AKI. Used with permission by Mehta *et al.* (2007). © BioMed Central.
*GFR: Glomerular Filtration Rate.
** ARF: Acute Renal Failure.
SCreat: Serum Creatinine, UO: Urinary output.

Table 7.1 AKIN Classification/Staging System for Acute Kidney Injury.

Stage	Serum creatinine criteria	Urine output criteria
1	Increase in serum creatinine ≥0.3 mg/dl (>26.4 µmol/l) or increase to ≥150% to 200% to 300% (>1.5–2 times) from baseline	Less than 0.5 ml/kg/h for more than 6 h
2*	Increase in serum creatinine to >200–300% (>2–3 times) from baseline	Less than 0.5 ml/kg/h for more than 12 h
3†	Increase in serum creatinine to >300% (>3 times) from baseline (or serum creatinine ≥4.0 mg/dl (>354 µmol/l)	Less than 0.3 ml/kg/h to 24 h to anuria for 12 h

Used with permission by Mehta *et al.* (2007). © BioMed Central.
*200–300% increase=two- to threefold increase.
†Given wide variation in indications and timing of initiation of renal replacement therapy (RRT), individuals who receive RRT are considered to have met the criteria for stage 3 irrespective of the stage they are in at the time of RRT.

AKI is classified in one of three stages based on severity. Staging is based on criteria that will give the patient the highest stage. These three stages are defined based on serum creatinine levels and urinary output. For stage 1, serum creatinine rises to 1.5–1.9 times baseline or urinary output of <0.5 ml/kg/h for 6–12 h; stage 2 is characterized by rising creatinine 2.0–2.9 times baseline or urinary output of <0.5 ml/kg/h for ≥12 h; and stage 3 is identified as 3.0 times baseline creatinine or urinary output of <3.0 ml/kg/h for ≥24 h or anuria for ≥12 h (KDIGO, 2012).

The need for renal replacement and risk of death increase with increased stage. Despite the method used to classify and stage AKI, early recognition of renal impairment is essential to prevent long-term renal impairment and prevent complications. To date, there is no classification or staging system of AKI that has been proven to identify all patients with AKI. Clinical judgment also plays a dominent role in identifying patients at risk or with AKI.

Physiological guidelines

AKI is attributed to prerenal, intrarenal, or postrenal pathology. Regardless of the etiology, there are complex interactions between vascular, tubular, and inflammatory factors. The outcome is vasoconstriction, endothelial injury, and activation of an inflammatory response (Bagshaw *et al.*, 2010). Identifying the cause is critical to prevent or minimize renal injury.

Prerenal injury
Prerenal injury is a consequence of renal hypoperfusion from factors outside of the kidney (Table 7.2). Under normal conditions, about 20–25% of cardiac output, or 1100 ml/min is received by the kidneys (Hall, 2011). Autoregulatory mechanisms keep blood flow and pressure constant to maintain adequate renal tissue oxygenation. The autoregulatory properties of the kidney can tolerate a large reduction in perfusion before ischemic changes occur (Hall, 2011). The autoregulatory response can be negatively affected by many conditions that include atherosclerosis, hypertension, advanced age, and the presence of chronic kidney disease (Longo *et al.*, 2012). Medications, such as angiotension-converting enzyme (ACE) inhibitors and angiotension receptor blockers (ARB) cause decreased efferent vessel constriction and put the kidney at risk of injury in low renal perfusion states (Longo *et al.*, 2012).

Table 7.2 Etiologies of prerenal injury.

Intravascular volume depletion
   Dehydration
   Hypovolemic shock
   Hemorrhage
   Burns
   Diuretic overuse
   Gastrointestinal losses
   Diaphoresis
   Fluid shift to third space
   Ascites
Decreased cardiac output
   Heart failure/cardiogenic shock
   Myocardial infarction
   Cardiomyopathy
   Dysrhythmias
   Thrombus (pulmonary embolism, arterial or venous thrombus)
   Vasoactive medications
Decreased systemic vascular resistance
   Sepsis/septic shock
   Anaphylaxis
   Neurogenic shock
   Antihypertensive medication overuse
   Liver failure
   Multiple organ dysfunction syndrome
   Anesthesia
Other
   Vasculitis
   Eclampsia
   Disseminated intravascular coagulation
   Tumor
   Renal artery stenosis
   Nonsteroidal anti-inflammatory drugs

Table 7.3 Common causes of intrarenal failure.

Ischemic
   Shock
   Renal artery thrombosis
   Prolonged hypoperfusion
   Excessive fluid losses
   Sickle cell disease
Nephrotoxic
   Medications (such as aminoglycosides, amphotericin B, tetracyclines, vancomycin, rifampin, penicillins, cephalosporins, quinolones, sulfonamides, chemotherapeutic agents, anesthetic agents)
   Radiographic contrast dye
   Pesticides
   Fungicides
   Ethylene glycol
   Heavy metals (such as mercury and lead)
   Carbon tetrachloride
   Myloglobin
   Hemoglobin
   Uric acid
   Myeloma light chain proteins
Inflammatory
   Vasculitis
   Glomerulonephritis
   Acute pyelonephritis
   Blood transfusion reaction
   Allergic nephritis

Nonsteroidal anti-inflammatory drugs (NSAIDs) may also decrease perfusion, leading to prerenal failure (Lamiere, Biesen, and Vanholder, 2005). Metabolic processes of the kidney are oxygen-dependent; therefore, any interruption of the flow of oxygenated blood to nephrons makes the kidney susceptible to ischemic injury.

Decreased renal perfusion leads to a reduction in glomerular filtration rate (GFR) and increased sodium and water reabsorption. As the GFR decreases, less oxygen is required since the overall filtration of sodium chloride is reduced. The filtration of sodium chloride contributes to most of the consumption of oxygen and energy produced by the kidney. Prerenal failure is reversible as long as the renal blood flow does not decrease to less than 20–25% of normal and damage to the renal cells has not occurred. As the GFR approaches zero, renal oxygen consumption is minimized to the point needed to keep renal cells alive. Prerenal failure is reversible with early intervention to restore renal perfusion but otherwise it will progress to intrinsic injury within a few hours (Hall, 2011).

Intrarenal injury

Intrarenal, or intrinsic injury, is due to structural damage to the glomerulus, vessels, or kidney tubules. Intrinsic injury is caused by ischemic, nephrotoxic, or inflammatory factors (Carlson, 2009). Table 7.3 summarizes the etiologies of intrarenal failure.

Acute tubular necrosis

Acute tubular necrosis (ATN) is the most common cause of intrinsic injury (Lamiere, Biesen, and Vanholder, 2005). In the critical care unit, 35–50% of all ATN is caused by sepsis, and 20–25% of ATN is associated with surgery. Postoperative ATN is often a consequence of preexisting renal impairment, hypertension, cardiac disease, peripheral vascular disease, diabetes mellitus, jaundice, or advanced age. Radiocontrast nephropathy accounts for the third most common cause of ATN in hospitalized patients (Lamiere, Biesen, and Vanholder, 2005).

Conditions that impair blood flow to the kidney impede the delivery of oxygen and nutrients to renal cells. If adequate blood flow is not restored, epithelial cells in the tubules begin to die. The sloughing off of the dead epithelial cells fills the tubules with debris and impedes urine flow. Oliguria, which may evolve to anuria, along with electrolyte imbalance and acidosis, will develop (Hall, 2011).

A variety of medications or toxins may induce ATN. The large volume of blood that is filtered through the kidneys results in increased susceptibility to damage as blood is filtered and filtrate is reabsorbed. Moreover, the generation of toxic metabolites from certain medications makes the kidneys vulnerable to injury (Carlson, 2009). Renal cells are destroyed through various mechanisms including vasoconstriction, direct damage to tubular cells, or intratubular obstruction (Yaklin, 2011). Regardless of the cause, epithelial cells slough from the basement membrane, causing plugging of the tubules. New tubular epithelial cells can grow along the basement membrane allowing the tubule to heal within 10–20 days as long as the agent that precipated the damage is removed and there is no further injury to the kidney (Hall, 2011).

Radiographic contrast agents are particularly nephrotoxic to the kidneys if preexisting kidney disease is present (Longo *et al.*, 2012). Preexisting chronic kidney impairment makes the kidney more vulnerable to injury to contrast-induced nephropathy (CIN). Conditions such as diabetic nephropathy, chronic low cardiac output states, and multiple myeloma (Longo *et al.*, 2012) place patients at risk. Other risk factors for CIN include age greater than 70 years, dehydration, heart failure, and concurrent use of nephrotoxic agents (Naughton, 2008). If an AKI is caused by radiographic contrast agents, it usually evolves within 3 days after administration. Creatinine typically begins to increase within 24 h and peaks in 5 days (Bentley, Corwin, and Dasta, 2010).

Acute intersitial nephritis

Acute interstitial nephritis (AIN) is caused from NSAIDs, antibiotics, and other agents (Yaklin, 2011). AIN is believed to be the result of an allergic response to the suspected drug, and is not dose-dependent. In the kidney, medications causing AIN may bind to antigens or act as antigens that are deposited into the interstitium, causing a hypersenitivity reaction. Typical symptoms of an allergic response, such as fever, rash, and release of eosinophils, are not usually reported (Naughton, 2008). Table 7.4 lists common drugs that may cause AIN.

Progression of AIN has three stages including initiation, maintenance, and recovery (Yaklin,

Table 7.4 Drugs causing acute interstitial nephritis.

Allopurinol
Antibiotics
Beta lactams
Quinolones
Rifampicin
Sulfonamides
Vancomycin
Antivirals
Acyclovir
Indinavir
Diuretics
Loop
Thiazide
NSAIDs
Phenytoin
Proton pump inhibitors
Omeprazole
Pantoprazole
Lanoprazole
H_2 Blockers
Ranitidine

Adapted from Naughton (2008).

2011). It is important to keep in mind that all patients do not progress to the recovery stage, and the end result for that group of patients is chronic renal insufficiency or end-stage renal disease. During the initiation phase, blood urea nitrogen (BUN) and creatinine increase. Urinary output declines but not all patients progress to anuria. The maintenance phase usually lasts about 7–21 days, and often renal replacement therapy is required during this phase to maintain fluid, electrolyte, and acid–base balance. The recovery phase begins when there is a significant increase in urinary output and a decline in BUN and creatinine. As the epithelial cells in the tubules regenerate, the kidneys regain their ability to concentrate urine and maintain adequate electrolyte and acid–base balance (Yaklin, 2011).

Post renal injury

Post renal injury is caused by a partial or complete obstruction of urine flow at any point in the urinary drainage pathway from the kidney to the urethra. The cause of the obstruction may be from blood clots, calculi, strictures, benign prostatic hypertrophy, malignancies, or pregnancy (Yaklin, 2011). Other factors such as fibrosis, neurogenic disorders, or even urinary catheter obstruction can contribute to post renal injury. The amount of damage to the kidneys is determined by the location, duration, and amount of obstruction (Carlson, 2009).

When urinary flow becomes obstructed, the ureters and renal pelvis dilate. Eventually, intratubular pressure will exceed glomerular pressure. Complete obstruction causes a complete cessation of filtration, while a partial obstruction will decrease GFR but may not necessarily cause a total cessation of filtration. The tubules will respond by increasing water and sodium reabsorption. If the obstruction continues, the tubules become damaged and are unable to reabsorb water and sodium. If the obstruction is not corrected or removed, permanent renal damage can result (Carlson, 2009; Yaklin, 2011). If the obstruction is removed or corrected, a post-obstructive diuresis will occur during the next 24 h if the damage has not progressed to end-stage renal disease (Yaklin, 2011).

Monitoring elements

Specific diagnostic tests or physical assessment findings do not conclusively indicate AKI. A thorough patient history, physical examination, interpretation of laboratory, ultrasonographic, and radiological data all provide important information that contributes to the diagnosis (Bentley, 2011).

History and physical assessment

A thorough patient history and physical assessment findings are important for the diagnosis of AKI. Patient history should include both family and past medical history. Family history should examine any genetic factors that could contribute to AKI such as tubular metabolic anomalies, polycystic kidneys, unusual types of nephritis, or vascular or coagulation defects. Patient history includes any possible conditions of past or recent kidney injury such as infections, injuries, exposure to toxic agents or drugs, diabetes mellitus, hypertension, or autoimmune disorders that may make the patient more susceptible to AKI (Vincenti and Amend, 2008).

Physical assessment findings of AKI are often related to the etiology (Table 7.5). Prerenal failure is caused by hypovolemia, decreased systemic vascular resistance, or insufficient cardiac output. Assessment findings from hypovolemia may include tachycardia, hypotension, flat neck veins, dry mucous membranes, and decreased mental status. On the other hand, physical assessment findings from decreased systemic vascular resistance reveal signs similar to hypovolemia although systemic edema may be present (Carlson, 2009). The patient may be total

Table 7.5 Physical assessment findings in prerenal failure.

Hypovolemia/decreased intravascular resistance	Decreased cardiac output
Oliguria	Oliguria
Tachycardia	Tachycardia
Hypotension	Hypotension
Flat neck veins	Distended neck veins
Dry mucous membranes	
Decreased mental status	

Adapted from Carlson (2009).

body fluid overloaded but intravascularly depleted due to third spacing of fluid. If prerenal failure is from decreased cardiac output caused by cardiac failure, assessment findings such as oliguria, edema, distended neck veins, and hypotension are common.

Physical assessment findings for intrarenal failure are dependent upon the etiology. If the cause is ischemic from hypoperfusion, the signs are similar to the findings of hypovolemia or decreased intravascular resistance due to prerenal failure (Carlson, 2009). If failure is from other causes, signs such as oliguria or anuria, edema, distended neck veins, and other signs of fluid overload and deterioration of mental status may be noted.

Post renal failure physical assessment findings reveal anuria along with signs of fluid overload. The extent of fluid overload depends on the length of time and amount of fluid intake while the obstruction is present.

Laboratory analysis and data trending

Alterations in urine volume, urine specific gravity, urine osmolality, serum BUN, serum creatinine, serum BUN/creatinine ratio, urine sodium, and the fractional excretion of sodium (FENa) are laboratory studies that provide data for the practitioner to diagnose AKI and its etiology (Table 7.6).

Electrolyte imbalances are also a common finding in AKI. Of particular concern to the practitioner is the development of hyperkalemia, which, if not promptly acted upon, may result in life-threatening dysrhythmias. Signs of hyperkalemia include decreased reflexes, tachycardia, confusion, hypotension, anorexia, muscle weakness, and paresthesia. Electrocardiogram (ECG) changes associated with hyperkalemia are peaked T waves and widened QRS complexes. If not appropriately treated, ventricular fibrillation may result (Lippincott Manual of Nursing Practice, 2007). Other electrolytes that may be affected by AKI are sodium, magnesium, calcium, and phosphate. Table 7.7 lists electrolyte imbalances related to AKI.

The kidneys play an important role in acid–base regulation. Organic anions, such as phosphate, begin to accumulate when renal function is impaired. Bicarbonate production decreases in the proximal tubules along with decreased reabsorption. Patients with renal impairment tend to be hypoalbuminemic, causing a reduced protein-buffering capacity, contributing to metabolic acidosis. It is also important to keep in mind that conditions such as lactic acidosis, respiratory acidosis, shock, or others may also increase the severity of acidosis (Carlson, 2009).

Urinalysis is an important tool to diagnose AKI. The presence of urinary sediment is indicative of AKI, and provides insight for the practitioner into its etiology. Table 7.8 outlines urine findings in AKI.

Biomarkers reveal changes at the molecular–cellular level that may detect AKI in its earliest stages (Bentley, 2011). Cystatin C, an endogenous protease inhibitor measured in the serum, is a marker of AKI. Cystatin C has shown

Table 7.6 Differential laboratory diagnosis of renal dysfunction.

	Normal	Prerenal	Intrarenal	Postrenal
Urine volume	1–1.5 l/day	<400 ml/day	<400 ml/day	Variable
Urine specific gravity	1.010–1.020	1.020 or greater	Fixed (1.010 or less)	Fixed (1.010 or less)
Urine osmolality	500–850 mOsm/l	>500 Osm/l	<350 mOsm/l	≤350 mOsm/l
Serum BUN	10–20 mg/dl	>25 mg/dl	>25 mg/dl	<25 mg/dl
Serum creatinine	0.8–1.2 mg/dl	Normal to slightly elevated	>1.2 mg/dl	>1.2 mg/dl
Serum BUN: creatinine ratio	10:1	20:1 or greater	(10–15):1; both elevated but ratio remains constant	(10–15):1; both elevated but ratio remains constant
Urine sodium		<20 mEq/l	>40 mEq/l	>40 mEq/l
FENa		<1%	>1%*	>1%

Adapted from Carlson (2009, p. 890).
*When the patient is not under the influence of diuretics.
BUN, blood urea nitrogen; FENa, fractional excretion of sodium.

Table 7.7 Electrolyte imbalances related to AKI.

	Normal value	Abnormal value due to AKI	Comments
Calcium	Serum 8.2–10 mg/dl Ionized 4.65–5.68 mg/dl	Serum < 8.2 mg/dl Ionized < 4.65 mg/dl	
Magnesium	Serum 1.3–2.1 mg/dl	Serum > 2.1 mg/dl	
Phosphate	Serum 2.7–4.5 mg/dl	Serum > 4.5 mg/dl	
Potassium	Serum 3.5–5.0 mg/dl	Serum > 5.5 mg/dl	
Sodium	Serum 135–145 mg/dl	Variable	Urine sodium levels are more sensitive to changes in sodium balance and should be monitored along with serum sodium levels. The administration of diuretics makes the urine sodium less reliable

Compiled from Lippincott Manual of Nursing Practice Series: Diagnostic Tests (2007).

Table 7.8 Urinary findings in acute kidney injury.

Etiology	Sediment	FENa Fe-urea	Proteinuria
Prerenal azotemia	Few hyaline casts	<1–3	None or trace
Ischemia	Epithelial cells, muddy-brown casts, pigmented granular casts	>2–50	Trace to mild
Acute interstitial nephritis	White blood cells (WBCs), WBC casts, pigmented granular casts	>1	Mild to moderate
Acute glomerulonephritis	Dysmorphic red blood cells (RBCs), RBC cast	<1 early	Moderate to severe
Postrenal	Few hyaline casts, possibly RBC	<1 early >1 late	None or trace
Tumor lysis	Uric acid crystals		None or trace
Arterial/venous thrombosis	RBCs		Mild to moderate
Ethylene glycol	Calcium oxalate crystals		Trace to mild

Reproduced with permission from Yaqub and Molitoris (2009). © McGraw-Hill.

promise for identifying AKI 1–2 days earlier than the RIFLE criteria (Herget-Rosenthal *et al.*, 2004). It is produced at a constant rate by nucleated cells, but not produced by kidney tubules. While creatinine values are affected by age, muscle mass, diet, and sex, cystatin C is not (Dirkes, 2011). When the tubules are functioning normally, cystatin C is reabsorbed and eventually metabolized (Yaqub and Molitoris, 2009). As GFR decreases, cystatin C levels rise. This marker is considered a more sensitive indicator of AKI, especially in the elderly (Coca, 2010; Yaklin, 2011) but it is not yet routinely used in most medical centers.

Other novel biomarkers are now being evaluated for prediction and early detection of AKI. Biomarkers that have recently been under scrutiny are neutrophil gelatinase–associated lipocalin (NGAL), kidney injury molecule-1 (KIM-1), and interleukin (IL)-18.

These biomarkers are more specific for AKI than traditional markers and their routine use in the future is promising.

NGAL protein is detected early in AKI in animal models (Devarajan, 2011). It is present in the kidneys, lungs, stomach, and colon at low levels. Injured epithelium releases NGAL in conditions such as acute bacterial infections, asthma, and pulmonary disease. NGAL is present in both blood and urine more often than traditional markers in animal models (Dirkes, 2011). Urine NGAL is a reliable measure to distinguish between prerenal azotemia and intrarenal failure and chronic kidney disease (Nickolas *et al.*, 2008). Studies have shown that plasma or urinary elevations of NGAL 1–3 days after cardiac surgery were associated with postoperative AKI (Hassse-Fielitz *et al.*, 2009). Urine NGAL collected on the day of kidney transplant successfully identified patients who developed delayed graft function and required dialysis within the first week after transplant (Hall *et al.*, 2010).

KIM-1 is a transmembrane protein that becomes unregulated in proximal tubule cells after ischemic or nephrotoxic injury (Devarajan, 2011). KIM-1 appears to be more specific to ischemic or nephrotoxic injury, and is not significantly increased in chronic kidney disease or urinary tract infection (Dirkes, 2011). Urinary KIM-1 levels have been shown to predict adverse clinical outcomes and mortality of patients with AKI (Liangos *et al.*, 2007).

IL-18 is a proinflammatory mediator released in the proximal tubule after AKI. Urinary levels of IL-18 increase in ischemic injury (Parikh and Devarjan, 2008). IL-18 is a marker of AKI in patients with adult respiratory distress syndrome (ARDS) and elevated urinary levels predicted the development of AKI within 24 h. In addition, the level of IL-18 at initiation of mechanical ventilation was predictive of mortality independent of severity of illness, urine creatinine, and urinary output in one study (Parikh *et al.*, 2005). While these biomarkers appear promising, further study is needed to determine their sensitivity and specificity to AKI, and to determine if combinations of these biomarkers at specific levels are clinically significant (Lamiere, Biesen, and Vanholder, 2005).

Diagnostic imaging

Imaging is an essential part of the diagnostic work-up for AKI. A renal ultrasound reveals the size, position, internal structures, and perirenal tissues. It also detects urinary or perirenal obstruction. Fluid collections within or around the kidney can be identified that are indicative of urinary obstruction. It is important to note that false negative findings are possible in the earliest stages of urinary obstruction. Renal doppler ultrasound can evaluate blood flow to the kidneys. Abnormal blood flow to the kidneys can indicate obstruction, hypertension, or other acute or chronic kidney injury (Yaklin, 2011).

Computerized tomography (CT) scans can be used to visualize the kidneys and collecting system, but radiocontrast agents should be avoided. Without the use of a contrast agent, visualization of the collecting system may be suboptimal; CT scans without contrast are helpful to identify obstructing ureteral calculi (Sharfuddin *et al.*, 2012). Other diagnositic imaging that requires radiocontrast agents is usually avoided to prevent further progression of AKI. Table 7.9 summarizes diagnostic imaging findings and their implications.

Renal biopsy

Renal biopsy is not a first-line diagnostic tool to idenfy AKI. Prerenal and postrenal causes of AKI must be first ruled out. Renal biopsy is used only if the cause of intrarenal failure cannot be determined. Its use should be limited to intrinsic renal failure that is not due to ischemic or nephrotoxic injury (Sharfuddin *et al.*, 2012). Possible findings from renal biopsy are glomerulonephritis, vasculitis, or malignancy (Yaklin, 2011).

Table 7.9 Diagnostic imaging in acute kidney injury.

Imaging	Normal findings	Abnormal findings	Implications
Renal ultrasound	Kidneys located between the iliac crests and diaphragm, normal size, shape, and structure	Cysts, tumors, hydronephrosis, obstruction of ureters, calculi	May show renal obstruction
Renal Doppler ultrasound	Normal blood flow to both kidneys	Decreased blood flow to one or both kidneys	Possible obstruction, hypertension, or acute or chronic kidney injury
Computerized tomography (CT) scan	Kidneys located between the iliac crests and diaphragm, normal size, shape, and urinary collection system	Cysts, tumors, hydronephrosis, obstruction of ureters, calculi	May show renal obstruction; however, it is useful only if contrast media is contraindicated

Evidenced-based treatment guidelines

At this time, there is no specific treatment for AKI (Bagshaw *et al.*, 2010; Calzavacca, Licari, and and Bellomo, 2010; Dirkes, 2011; Sharfuddin *et al.*, 2012; Yaklin, 2011). The goals of therapy are to prevent AKI, minimize fluid and electrolyte imbalance if it should occur, and prevent uremic complications (Sharfuddin *et al.*, 2012). Preventative measures should be rapidly implemented for any critically ill patient at risk for AKI to prevent renal injury and complications associated with renal failure. Strategies to prevent or mitigate AKI must be individualized for each patient's unique clinical situation (Bagshaw *et al.*, 2010).

Prevention

Early recognition of patients at risk is a first-line intervention to prevent AKI. The RIFLE criteria (Fig. 7.1) present an important tool to identify patients at risk or those at the early stages of AKI (Bellomo *et al.*, 2004). Other risk scales for AKI are available for patients undergoing procedures such as cardiac catherization or cardiac surgery (Mehran *et al.*, 2004; Thakar *et al.*, 2005). Maintenance of adequate renal perfusion, avoidance of nephrotoxic drugs, and radiographic contrast whenever possible are important interventions for high-risk patients. Careful monitoring of drug levels has been demonstrated to reduce the risk of AKI with aminoglycosides (Appel, 1990; Blaser and Konig, 1995). Use of alternative formulations of nephrotoxic drugs, such as lipid-encapsulated formulations of amphotericin B, may prevent drug-induced AKI (Lamiere, Biesen, and Vanholder, 2005). Drugs that decrease regulation of renal blood flow, such as NSAIDs, ACE inhibitors, or angiotensin-II-receptor blockers, should be avoided or used cautiously (Sharfuddin *et al.*, 2012). Aggressive intravascular volume repletion has been reported to prevent ATN in patients with major surgery, trauma, and sepsis (Sever, Vanholde, and Lameire, 2006; Sharfuddin *et al.*, 2012).

Hemodynamic monitoring

Hemodynamic monitoring is an important tool to guide resuscitation. Measures such as central venous monitoring, pulmonary arterial catheter monitoring, or devices that measure stroke volume and pulse pressure variation should be considered. The use of hemodynamic monitoring is to direct intravascular volume repletion to achieve adequate mean arterial pressure and cardiac output (Bagshaw *et al.*, 2010). See Chapter 5 for further discussion on hemodynamic monitoring.

Volume expansion

Volume expansion is needed to prevent or treat hypovolemia or renal hypoperfusion caused by vasodilation and decreased intravascular resistance. The choice of colloid versus crystalloids for volume resuscitation remains controversial. Fluid resuscitation with saline with or without albumin have similar results in critically ill patients (Finfer *et al.*, 2004). If the patient's hemoglobin is low, blood transfusion may be considered. Close monitoring of hemodynamics is essential to prevent fluid overload from overly aggressive volume resuscitation. A foley catheter should be considered to closely monitor urinary output in response to fluid resuscitation. Macedo *et al.* (2011) found that oliguria measured by hourly outputs significantly predicted AKI sooner even in patients without elevated serum creatinine, providing for earlier diagnosis and intervention in the management of critically ill adults. Patients who were oliguric for more than 12 h or had multiple episodes of oliguria had higher mortality in this study (Macedo *et al.*, 2011).

Management of electrolyte and acid–base imbalance

Hyperkalemia is the most serious electrolyte imbalance associated with AKI. Mild hyperkalemia (serum potassium < 5.5 mEq/l) is controlled by dietary restrictions of potassium. Severe hyperkalemia (serum potassium > 5.5 mEq/l) is treated with sodium polystyrene sulfonate, which enhances intestinal potassium losses. Loop diuretics, such as furosemide, can be used in a patient with severe hyperkalemia to excrete potassium if the patient is still diuretic responsive. If ECG changes indicative of hyperkalemia are present, 10–20 units of regular insulin is administered intravenously to increase potassium entry into the cell and decrease serum potassium level. The patient is also given dextrose, 25–50 g IV to prevent hypoglycemia caused by the administration of insulin. Intravenous calcium may also be administered to antagonize the cardiac and neuromuscular effects of hyperkalemia. Intravenous bicarbonate can be given to enhance bicarbonate intake into the cell; however, its effect is not rapid enough to be clinically significant (Sharfuddin *et al.*, 2012).

Clinical Pearls

If dialytic therapy is needed to treat hyperkalemia, hemodialysis is the most efficent modality to remove potassium, and is the preferred method if life-threatening ECG changes are present.

Hyponatremia, accompanied by a corresponding fall in serum osmolality, is treated with water restriction. Hypernatremia is treated with the administration of water or hypotonic IV solutions (Sharfuddin *et al.*, 2012).

Hyperphosphatemia is controlled by restricting dietary phosphate intake and administration of a phophate-binding agent. Common phosphate-binding agents are aluminum hydroxide, calcium salts, sevelamer carbonate, or lanthanum carbonate.

Acidosis is usually not treated unless the serum bicarbonate is ≤15 mEq/l or the blood pH is <7.15–7.20. When metabolic acidois is due to AKI, oral or parenteral bicarbonate may be administered. Administration of bicarbonate requires careful monitoring for undesired effects such as metabolic alkalosis, hypocalcemia, hypokalemia, hypernatremia, and volume overload (Sharfuddin *et al.*, 2012).

Pharmacologic interventions

Furosemide is frequently used during various stages of AKI. A meta-analysis examined the use of furosemide with AKI and found that it did not have a direct affect on mortality or improvement in renal function (Ho and Sheridan, 2006). Furosemide may be useful to decrease fluid retention in patients receiving mechanical ventilation. Patients will respond to furosemide more favorably in mild versus severe AKI (Ho and Power, 2010).

In the past, low-dose dopamine was routinely used as a renal vasodilator to maintain renal perfusion. Multiple studies revealed that it does not reduce mortality or contribute to renal recovery, even when used in combination with furosemide. In light of the current evidence, renal dose dopamine should not be used to prevent AKI (Kellum and Decker, 2001).

The use of *N*-acetylcysteine (NAC) to prevent contrast nephropathy is controversial. Its use is not supported by evidence. NAC may cause a decrease in serum creatinine concentration that does not seem to cause a protective effect on the kidneys (Alonso *et al.*, 2004; Hoffmann *et al.*, 2004).

The management of AKI caused by decomponsated heart failure may include many agents. Furosemide may be used with caution. It may have a favorable response by decreasing vascular congestion, venous congestion, and intravascular volume. Care must be taken by the practitioner to prevent overdiuresis causing renal hypoperfusion. Inotropes and vasodilators may also be needed to improve cardiac output and reduce afterload (Sharfuddin *et al.*, 2012).

Vasoconstrictors are used in the setting of hepatorenal failure. Octreotide and midodrine, used in conjunction with albumin may improve renal perfusion. It is recommended that patients with hepatorenal failure have an expedited referral for livery transplant (Runyon, 2009).

Water-soluble vitamins are administered to patients receiving renal replacement therapy (Sharfuddin *et al.*, 2012). Calcium carbonate is administered as needed for hypocalcemia. Doses of medications often need to be adjusted if AKI is present. If the patient is receiving renal replacement therapy, doses need to be adjusted based on the dialytic therapy used. Consultation with the clinical pharmacist is helpful to ensure appropriate medication dosing.

Prevention of radiocontrast nephropathy

Prehydration is effective in reducing radiocontrast-induced nephropathy (Calzavacca, Licari, and Bellomo, 2010) and the use of 0.9% saline has been found to be more effective than 0.45% saline (Mueller, Buerkle, and Buettner, 2002). Intravenous sodium bicarbonate solutions can also be used to prevent radiocontrast nephropathy, although the evidence is conflicting about its efficacy.

Clinical Pearls

The recommended hydration regimen for hospitalized patients is 0.9% NS or sodium bicarbonate solutions infused at 1 ml/kg/h for 12 h before and after the administration of the radiocontrast agent (Sharfuddin et al., 2012). Intravenous hydration is more effective than oral hydration to prevent radiocontrast nephropathy (Calzavacca, Licari, and Bellomo, 2010).

Nutrition

Considerations when assessing nutritional needs of patients with AKI include severity of AKI, other comobidities present, and whether or not renal replacement therapies are being used (Yaklin, 2011). Patients with AKI should have a complete nutritional assessment and an individualized nutrition plan established. Protein intake should be based on catabolic rate, renal function, and dialysis losses. Electrolyte intake is adjusted based on serial monitoring of serum electrolyte concentrations. If the patient is nil per os (NPO) or cannot take oral nutrition, enteral feeds should be initiated (Brown, Compher, and Directors, 2010).

Renal replacement therapy

Timing and dosing of renal replacement therapy (RRT) remains controversial. Little evidence is available to support a standardized dose and timing for initiation of RRT to optimize patient outcomes (Bouchard, Macedo, and Mehta, 2010). Intermittent hemodialysis (IHD), continuous renal replacement therapies (CRRT), sustained low-efficiency dialysis (SLED), extended daily dialysis (EDD), and peritoneal dialysis (PD) are dialytic therapies currently being used in the critical care unit. IHD, CRRT, and PD are the most common modalities of RRTs used in the critical care unit (Carlson, 2009).

Intermittent hemodialysis

IHD is the most effective method to remove fluid and electrolytes in a short period of time. The patient's blood is pumped through a filter with a semipermeable membrane where the transfer of fluids, electrolytes, waste products, and other solutes takes place. A counterflow of dialysate through the filter, outside of the blood compartment, enhances the removal of solutes by diffusion. IHD is the most efficient modality of RRT, and is the treatment of choice for severe hyperkalemia. Typically, treatments last 3–4 h. The frequency of treatments is based on individual patient need and usually ranges from daily to three times per week. Rapid fluid shifts can decrease cardiac output, decrease renal perfusion, and delay healing of the injured kidneys. Anticoagulation is necessary to maintain the high blood flow required for this therapy to be efficient. SLED and EDD are hybrid therapies of IHD. A conventional hemodialysis machine is used but operated at a slower rate, and it is better tolerated in hemodynamically unstable patients.

Continuous renal replacement therapies

The use of CRRT results in a more gradual dialysis that is better tolerated by the hemodynamically unstable patient. Fluids, electrolytes, waste products, and small to medium-sized solutes are removed. Arteriovenous or venovenous vascular access is used based on the therapy being performed. Venovenous access tends to be less problematic because blood is pumped through the blood circuit using a blood pump while arteriovenous therapies rely on the patient's blood pressure to circulate the blood. Arteriovenous therapies require a single lumen catheter in a large artery, such as the femoral artery, and a single lumen dialysis catheter in a large vein, such as the femoral or internal jugular vein. Venovenous therapies use a dual

Table 7.10 Modalities of CRRT.

	Catheter access	Method of fluid and solute removal	Fluids used
Slow continuous ultrafiltration (SCUF)	Arteriovenous Venovenous	Ultrafiltration	None
Continuous arteriovenous hemofiltration (CAVH)	Arteriovenous	Ultrafiltration Convection Adsorption	Replacement
Continuous arteriovenous hemodialysis (CAVHD)	Arteriovenous	Ultrafiltration Diffusion Adsorption	Dialysate
Continuous arteriovenous hemodialfiltration (CAVHDF)	Arteriovenous	Ultrafiltration Convection Diffusion Adsorption	Replacement Dialysate
Continuous venovenous hemofiltration (CVVH)	Venovenous	Ultrafiltration Convection Adsorption	Replacement
Continuous venovenous hemodialysis (CVVHD)	Venovenous	Ultrafiltration Diffusion Adsorption	Dialysate
Continuous venovenous diafiltration (CVVHDF)	Venovenous	Ultrafiltration Convection Diffusion Adsorption	Replacement Dialysate

Ultrafiltration – the movement of fluid through a semi-permeable membrane
Diffusion – the movement of solutes from an area of higher concentration to an area of lower concentration
Convection – movement of solutes with fluid through a semi-permeable membrane
Adsorption – binding of solutes to a semi-permeable membrane

lumen dialysis catheter placed in a large vein, such as the femoral or internal jugular veins. Venovenous therapies are used more frequently than arteriovenous therapies. Table 7.10 summarizes available CRRTs. Blood is circulated through a filter containing a semipermeable membrane. Depending on the modality used, dialysate and replacement fluids may be used to enhance solute clearance. Dialysate is infused into the outer compartment of the filter and does not make contact with blood. Replacement fluid is infused directly into the blood circuit and mixes with the blood. Replacement fluids enhance convective clearance. Because CRRT is a continuous therapy, rapid fluid and electrolyte shifts are avoided, giving the injured kidney a better chance to heal.

Peritoneal dialysis

PD uses the peritoneal membrane as a semi-permeable membrane. PD is not as efficient as IHD or CRRT because fluid and solute removal is less predictable. Dialysate is infused through a catheter into the peritoneal space. The fluid and solutes are exchanged through the peritoneal membrane using diffusion, osmosis, and filtration. PD is not the first choice of RRT for the critically ill patient because its effects are slow to occur and abdominal surgery or interventions preclude the use of PD. Fluid management can become problematic when PD is used for the patient with ascites. The risk of infection is greater due to catheter placement in the peritoneal space. Table 7.11 compares IHD, CRRT, and PD.

Prevention and treatment of AKI presents many challenges to the advanced practice nurse. Identification of patients at risk is essential to develop interventions to prevent or minimize AKI. Interdisciplinary collaboration is key to ensure safe, proactive patient care. Many controversies about the care of the patient with AKI continue to exist and more research is needed to resolve them. Identification of patients at risk is essential to develop interventions to prevent or minimize AKI.

Table 7.11 Comparison of renal replacement therapies.

	Advantages	Disadvantages	Potential complications
IHD	Efficient removal of fluids and solutes	Requires specialized equipment and specialized staff	Hemodynamic instability
	Fluid and electrolyte balance can be rapidly altered	Hemodynamic instability from rapid fluid shifts	Dialysis disequilibrium syndrome
	Treatment is short and intermittent	Often requires heparinization	Electrolyte imbalance
		Difficulties in maintaining adequate vascular access	Fluctuations of acid–base balance
		Biocompatibility issues related to hemodialyzers	Inadequate nutrition
			Central line–associated bloodstream infection
			Bleeding due to anticoagulation
			Air embolism
CRRT	Large amounts of fluids can be infused without fluid overload	Less efficient solute removal than hemodialysis	Hemodynamic instability
	Can be used with hemodynamic instability	Potential for electrolyte imbalance	Electrolyte imbalance
	Continuous, gradual fluid and solute removal	Increased responsibility for critical care nurse	Central line–associated bloodstream infection
	More precise fluid management	Does not quickly remove potassium	Bleeding due to anticoagulation
	Performed by critical care nurse	Requires vascular access	Hypothermia
		May require anticoagulation	Air embolism
		Clotting of the circuit may occur	Clotting of circuit
		May induce hypothermia	
		Access complications can occur (clotting, bleeding, infection)	
PD	Simple equipment	High risk of infection (peritonitis, catheter site infection)	Protein loss
	Requires less technical support	Desired effects slower to occur, inefficient in an emergency	Hyperglycemia
	Rapid initiation of treatment	Possible patient discomfort	Infection/peritonitis
	No anticoagulation needed	Possible pulmonary compromise (due to reduced diaphragmatic compliance, decreased ventilation)	Hypoglycemia
	Vascular access not required	Less predictable for fluid removal	Constipation
	Lower risk of hypotension, rapid fluid and electrolyte shifts	Risk for hyperglycemia and hyperosmolarity (due to glucose in dialysate)	
		May be contradicted by abdominal surgery, adhesions, abdominal drains, abdominal wounds, or peritonitis	

References

Acute Kidney Injury Work Group (2012) KDIGO Clinical practice guideline for acute kidney injury. *Kidney International Supplement*, **2**, 1–138.

Alonso, A., Lau, J., Jaber, B. *et al.* (2004) Prevention of radiocontrast nephropathy with N-acetylcysteine in patients with chronic kidney disease: a meta-analysis of randomized, controlled trials. *American Journal of Kidney Diseases*, **43** (1), 1–9.

Appel, G. (1990) Aminoglycoside nephrotoxicity. *American Journal of Medicine*, **88** (3 Suppl), 16S–20S.

Bagshaw, S., Bellomo, R., Devarajan, P. *et al.* (2010) Review article: acute kidney injury in critical illness. *Canadian Journal of Anesthesia*, **57** (11), 985–998.

Bellomo, R., Ronco, C., Kellum, J.A. *et al.* (2004) Acute renal failure – definition, outcome measures, animal models, fluid therapy, and information technology needs: the Second International Consensus Conference of the Acute Dialysis Quality Initiative (ADQI) Workgroup. *Critical Care*, **8** (4), R204–R212.

Bentley, M. (2011) Acute kidney insufficiency in the critically ill. *Journal of Pharmacy Practice*, **24** (1), 61–69.

Bentley, M., Corwin, H., and Dasta, J. (2010) Drug-induced acute kidney injury in the critically ill adult: recognition and prevention strategies. *Critical Care Medicine*, **38**, S169–S174.

Blaser, J. and Konig, C. (1995) Once-daily dosing of aminoglycosides. *European Journal of Microbiology and Infectious Disease*, **14** (12), 1029–1038.

Bouchard, J., Macedo, E., and Mehta, R. (2010) Dosing of renal replacement therapy in acute kidney injury: lessons learned from clinical trials. *American Journal of Kidney Diseases*, **55** (3), 570–579.

Brown, R., Compher, C., and Directors, A. S. (2010) A.S.P.E.N. Clinical guidelines: nutrition support in adult acute and chronic renal failure. *Journal of Parenteral and Enteral Nutrition*, **4** (4), 366–376.

Calzavacca, P., Licari, E., and Bellomo, R. (2010) Acute kidney injury, in *Surgical Intensive Care*, 2nd edn (eds J. O'Donnell and F. Nacul), Springer, New York, pp. 421–430.

Carlson, K. (ed.) (2009) *Advanced Critical Care Nursing*. Saunders, St. Louis.

Coca, S. (2010) Acute kidney injury in elderly persons. *American Journal of Kidney Diseases*, **56** (1), 122–131.

Dennen, P., Douglas, I., and Anderson, R. (2010) Acute kidney injury in the intensive care unit: an update and primer for the intensivist. *Critical Care Medicine*, **38** (1), 261–275.

Devarajan, P. (2011) Bimarkers for the early detection of acute injury. *Current Opinions in Pediatrics*, **23** (2), 194–200.

Dirkes, S. (2011) Acute kidney injury: Not just acute renal failure anymore. *Critical Care Nurse*, **31** (1), 37–49.

Finfer, S., Bellomo, R., Boyce, N. *et al.* (2004) A comparison of albumin and saline for fluid resuscitation in the intensive care unit. *New England Journal of Medicine*, **350** (22), 2247–2256.

Hall, I., Yarlagadda, S., Coca, S. *et al.* (2010) IL-18 and urinary NGAL predict dialysis and graft recovery after kidney transplantation. *Journal of the American Society of Nephrology*, **21** (1), 189–197.

Hall, J. (2011) *Guyton and Hall Texbook of Medical Physiology*. Saunders, Philadephia, PA.

Hassse-Fielitz, A., Bellomo, R., Devarajan, P. *et al.* (2009) Accuracy of neutrophil gelatinase-associated lipocalin (NGAL) in diagnosis and prognosis in acute kidney injury: a systematic review and meta-analysis. *American Journal of Kidney Diseases*, **54** (6), 1012–1024.

Herget-Rosenthal, S., Marggraf, F., Husing, J. *et al.* (2004) Early detection of acute renal failure by serum cyctatin C. *Kidney International*, **66** (3), 1115–1122.

Ho, J. and Power, B. (2010) Anaesthesia. *Benefits and Risks of Furosemide in Acute Kidney Injury*, **65** (3), 283–293.

Ho, K.M. and Sheridan, D.J. (2006) Meta-analysis of furosemide to prevent or treat acute renal failure. *British Medical Journal*, **333**, 1–6.

Hoffmann, U., Fischereder, M., Kurger, B. *et al.* (2004) The value of *N*-acetylcysteine in the prevention of radiocontrast agent-induced nephropathy seems questionable. *Journal of the American Society of Nephrology*, **15** (2), 407–410.

James, M., Bouchard, J., Ho, J. *et al.* (2013) Canadian society of nephrology commentary on the 2012 KDIGO clinical practice guidelines for acute kidney injury. *American Journal of Kidney Disease*, **61** (5), 673–685.

Kellum, J. and Decker, M. (2001) Use of dopamine in acute renal failure: a meta-analysis. *Critical Care Medicine*, **29** (8), 1526–1531.

Lamiere, N. Biesen, N., and Vanholder, R. (2005) Acute renal failure. *Lancet*, **365**, 417–430.

Liangos, O., Perianayagam, M., Vaidya, V. *et al.* (2007) Urinary *N*-acetyl-beta-(D) glucosaminidase activity and kidney injury molecule-1 level are associated with adverse outcomes in acute renal failure. *Journal of the American Society of Nephrology*, **18** (3), 904–912.

Lippincott Manual of Nursing Practice Series: Diagnostic Tests, 1st edn. (2007), Lippincott, Williams & Wilkins, Philadelphia, pp. 1834–1838.

Longo, D., Fauci, A., Kasper, D. *et al.* (eds) (2012) *Harrison's Priniciples of Internal Medicine*, 18th edn, McGraw-Hill, New York.

Macedo, E., Malhotra, R., Bouchard, J. *et al.* (2011) Oliguria is an early predictor of higher mortality in critically ill patients. *Kidney International*, **80**, 760–767.

Mehran, R., Aymong, E., Nikolsky, E. *et al.* (2004) A simple risk score for prediction of contrast induced nephropathy after percutaneous coronary intervention. *Journal of the American College of Cardiology*, **44** (7), 1393–1399.

Mehta, R., Kellum, J., Shah, S. *et al.* (2007) Acute kidney injury network: report of an initiative to improve outcomes of acute kidney injury. *Critical Care*, **11** (2), R31.

Molitoris, B., Levin, A., Warnock, D.J. *et al.* (2007) Improving outcome of acute kidney injury: report of an initiative. *Nature Clinical Practice of Nephology*, **3** (8), 439–442.

Mueller, C., Buerkle, G., and Buettner, H. (2002) Prevention of contrast media-associated nephropathy: randomized comparison of 2 hydration regimens in 1620 patients undergoing coronary angioplasty. *Archives of Internal Medicine*, **162** (3), 329–336.

Naughton, C. (2008) Drug-induced nephrotoxicity. *American Family Physician*, **78** (6), 743–750.

Nickolas, T., O'Rourke, M., Yang, J. *et al.* (2008) Sensitivity and specificity of a single emergency department measurement of urinary neutrophil gelatinase–associated lipocalin for diagnosing acute kidney injury. *Annals of Internal Medicine*, **148** (11), 810–819.

Palevsky, P., Liu, K., Brophy, P. *et al.* (2013) KDOQI US commentary on the 2012 KDIGO clinical practice guideline for acute kidney injury. *American Journal of Kidney Disease*, **61** (5), 649–672.

Parikh, C. and Devarjan, P. (2008) New biomarkers for acute kidney injury. *Critical Care Medicine*, **36** (4 Suppl), S159–S165.

Parikh, C., Abraham, E., Ancukiewicz, M. *et al.* (2005) Urine IL-18 is an early diagnostic marker for acute kidney injury and predicts mortality in the intensive care unit. *Journal of the American Society of Nephrology*, **16** (10), 3046–3052.

Runyon, B. (2009) Management of adult patients with ascites due to cirrhosis: an update. *Hepatology*, **49** (6), 2087–2107.

Sever, M., Vanholde, R.R., and Lameire, N. (2006) Management of crush-related injuries. *New England Jouranl of Medicine*, **354** (14), 1052–1063.

Sharfuddin, A., Weisbord, S., Palevsky, P. *et al.* (2012) Acute kidney inury, in *Brenner & Rector's The Kidney*, 9th edn, Vol. I (eds M. Taal, G. Chertow, P. Marsden, *et al.*), W.B. Saunders, Philadelphia, PA, pp. 1049–1099.

Thakar, C., Arrigain, C., Worley, S. *et al.* (2005) A clinical score to predict acute renal failure after cardiac surgery. *Journal of the American Society of Nephrology*, **16** (1), 162–168.

Thakar, C., Christianson, A., Freybery, R. *et al.* (2009) Incidence and outcomes of acute kidney injury in the intensive care units: a veterans administration study. *Critical Care Medicine*, **37** (9), 2552–2558.

Uchino, S., Kellum, J., Bellomo, R. *et al.* (2005) Acute renal failure in critically ill patients: a multinational, multicenter study. *JAMA*, **294** (7), 813–818.

Vincenti, F. and Amend, J.W. (2008) Diagnosis of medical renal diseases, in *Smith's General Urology*, 17th edn (eds E. Tanagho and J. McAninch), McGraw-Hill, New York.

Yaklin, M. (2011) Acute kidney injury: an overview of pathophysiology and treatments. *Nephrology Nursing Journal*, **38** (1), 13–18, 30.

Yaqub, M. and Molitoris, B. (2009) Acute kidney injury, in *Current Diagnosis & Treatment: Nephrology & Hypertension* (eds E. Lerma and J.A. Berns), McGraw-Hill, New York, pp. 89–98, http://www.accessmedicine.com/content.aspx?aID=6343318 (accessed July 24, 2014).

CHAPTER 8

Monitoring for blood glucose dysfunction in the intensive care unit

Laura Kierol Andrews

Yale School of Nursing, Orange, CT., USA

Diabetes management in the ICU

Hyperglycemia in critical care patients is common, linked to poor outcomes, and can occur in both diabetic and nondiabetic patients (Finfer *et al.*, 2012; Merrill and Jones, 2011; Moghissi *et al.*, 2009). In nondiabetic patients, this is called critical illness or stress-induced hyperglycemia and is an adaptive reaction to provide the brain and central nervous system with a steady source of energy. Increased production of catacholamines, cortisol, glucagon, growth hormone, and cytokines, along with the production of glucose from glycogenolysis and glyconeogenesis, contribute to hyperglycemia in critically ill patients as part of the stress response; this may also be enhanced in patients with sleep disorders (Taub and Redeker, 2008). Treatment of sleep-disorded breathing in patients with diabetes improves quality of life and physiologic status (ADA, 2013). Additionally, insulin resistance, in both hepatic and skeletal muscles of the critically ill, exacerbates hyperglycemia (see Fig. 8.1).

In the critical care unit, risk factors for hyperglycemia also include preexisting or undiagnosed diabetes, infection, sepsis, trauma, shock, hyperalimentation, older age, and the use of glycogenic drugs such as epinephrine, steroids, and immunosuppressive agents. The effects of hyperglycemia, including delayed wound healing, infection, and end-organ damage are thought to be related to alterations in neutrophil and lymphocyte function that impair immunity and inflammatory processes, and an increase in the release of fatty acids from lipolysis and oxidative damage and protein degradation (ADA, 2013; Clement *et al.*, 2004).

Effects of hyperglycemia

Hyperglycemia is associated with poor outcomes (including increased morbidity and mortality) in cardiovascular, neurologic, and trauma patients. Landmark studies in surgical and medical intensive care unit (ICU) patients examined the effects of intensive insulin therapy (IIT) (glucose = 80–110 mg/dl) versus usual insulin therapy (glucose levels up to 215 mg/dl) (Van den Berghe *et al.*, 2001, 2006). Decreased mortality was seen in both studies with the use of IIT, but administration of parenteral nutrition and administration of IV glucose (200–300 g/day) to study subjects clouded the applicability of the findings. Current studies have shown that IIT increased mortality and patients had significantly higher numbers of severe hypoglycemic events (glucose < 40 mg/dl) (Finfer *et al.*, 2009; Griesdale *et al.*, 2009; Wiener, Wiener, and Larson, 2008). Krinsley and Grover (2007) found that a single episode of hypoglycemia increased mortality by 16.4% compared to patients without any episodes of hypoglycemia. In the Normoglycemia in Intensive Care Evaluation and Surviving Using Glucose Algorithm Regulation (NICE–SUGAR) study (Finfer *et al.*, 2012), investigators demonstrated that using tight versus IIT glucose targets (140–180 versus 80–110 mg/dl) resulted in fewer hypoglycemic episodes and lower 90-day mortality in the tight target group. The latest American Diabetes Association (ADA)

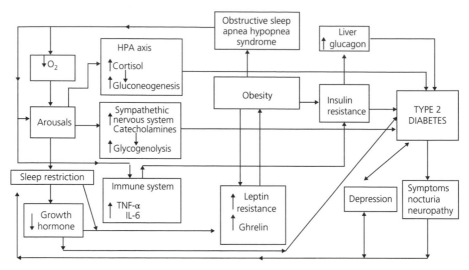

Figure 8.1 Potential pathophysiological associations between sleep disorders and diabetes. Reprinted with permission of Sage Publications.

guidelines recommend target glucose levels of 140–180 mg/dl and suggest that the lower end of the range is potentially associated with less patient risk (ADA, 2013).

Hyperglycemia management recommendations

National organizations have published recommendations that target glucose control levels to be between 140 and 180 mg/dl in most ICU patients (AACE and ADA, 2009; ADA, 2012). Additional recommendations by the ADA (2013) include intravenous (IV) administration of insulin using protocols and management plans to minimize and treat hypoglycemic events in critically ill patients. Noncritically ill patients should have premeal glucose targets less than 140 mg/dl. In nondiabetic patients, glucose monitoring should be considered for high-risk patients and treatment based on severity of illness (critical versus noncritical) (ADA, 2013).

Glucose monitoring

The use of insulin therapy to treat hyperglycemia requires point-of-care (POC) testing systems that are fast and accurate. POC glucose monitors conduct whole blood testing, which is less accurate than laboratory

plasma glucose tests by 11%. In anemic patients, falsely elevated glucose levels from POC testing can lead to overtreatment. Oxygen tension levels in the blood can also affect glucose readings if the POC monitor uses a glucose oxidase method, with hypoxemia ($_pO_2 < 44$ mmHg) falsely elevating readings and hyperoxygenated samples ($_pO_2 > 100$ mmHg) falsely lowering readings (Egi, Finfer, and Bellomo, 2011). Shearer et al. (2009) found that blood glucose samples from finger sticks and central venous catheters differed significantly from laboratory plasma levels, but not from each other. Although POC testing is faster and less expensive, caution is warranted when using it solely as a means to titrate insulin therapy in critically ill patients. A frequent comparison to laboratory plasma glucose samples is necessary until the technology improves.

Carbohydrate administration

Sources of glucose administration must be assessed when initiating and maintaining insulin therapy. Common sources, such as maintenance of IV fluids with dextrose, IV drips mixed in dextrose, and nutritional supports such as enteral and parenteral feeds, if not monitored carefully, can contribute to hyperglycemia. An example demonstrating this point is that administering D_5NS at 100 cc/h IV results in 120 g of dextrose per day, but only 60 g if the IV rate is decreased to 50 cc/h. Use of IV solutions with dextrose may require adjustments in insulin doses. Additional sources such as peritoneal dialysis fluid, in which 75% of the dextrose is absorbed, should also be included in carbohydrate calculations. Careful consideration must also be given to initiating glycogenic medications such as epinephrine and steroids when assessing hyperglycemia, and when weaning these medications, adjustments to insulin dosing can be anticipated.

Insulin therapy

It is recommended that IV regular insulin infusions be used in critically ill patients to guarantee full absorption of doses. ICU patients, especially those in shock states or with anasarca, will have erratic absorption from subcutaneous administration of insulin. The onset of IV insulin is immediate and its half-life is 5–17 min, allowing for POC testing in unstable patients at least every hour. The use of nurse-driven protocols has shown promising results in the literature (Holzinger et al., 2008; Krinsley, 2004; Shearer et al., 2009). Many institutions have adapted tight glucose control targets and currently utilize protocols that allow nurses to manage hyperglycemia (see Fig. 8.2).

For patients on oral or tube-feeding nutrition, insulin protocols include testing frequency and administration of insulin coverage (Fig. 8.3). In addition, as patients stabilize, conversion to less restrictive insulin-testing protocols is made. Generally, guidelines for fingerstick glucose (FSG) testing in patients with tube feedings will be guided by testing every 6 h and for those who can eat, testing is generally done prior to meals and at bedtime.

See Table 8.1 for a guide used at the author's hospital which also contains protocol options for hypoglycemic management based on the POC testing value and the patient's mental status.

Once a patient is hemodynamically stable, taking in a consistent carbohydrate diet (enteral or parenteral), and is able to predictably absorb subcutaneous insulin, he or she can be transitioned to subcutaneous insulin. When transitioning from IV insulin to oral intake, conduct the following procedures:

- Calculate the total amount of IV insulin given in the last 24 h.
- Give half that amount in basal form (glargine or detemir).
- Give the other half as rapid-acting insuline (Glulisine, lispro, or aspart) in three divided premeal doses.
- Supplement with rapid-acting insulin sliding scale as needed (based on premeal glucose levels).

Discontinue IV insulin 2 h after basal dose is given.

Hypoglycemia management

Prevention and treatment of hypoglycemic episodes is very important and nurses must be clear on adopted protocols for monitoring and treatment. Finer et al. (2012) summarized the increased risk of death associated with hypoglycemia in ICU settings. Table 8.2 demonstrates an adopted hypoglycemia protocol used at the author's institution in Connnecticut. The use of guidelines and nurse driven protocols are increasingly recognized by the national guidelines (ADA, 2013; Moghissi et al., 2009).

Conclusion

Research continues on the most effective management and safety protocols to treat critically ill patients with blood glucose dysfunction. Recent analyses by Mackenzie, Whitehouse, and Nightingale (2011) may influence and change the way clinicians think about glycemic control in critically ill patients. In an examination of glucose control metrics that were linked to mortality in critically ill patients, Mackenzie, Whitehouse, and Nightingale (2011) found a number of patient values that were linked to negative outcomes in four types of critical care units. The three metrics were variables measuring central tendancy (average glucose, time-averaged glucose, hyperglycaemic

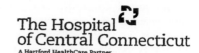

The Hospital
of Central Connecticut
A Hartford HealthCare Partner
Critical Care/Intensive Care Insulin Infusion
Physician Order

ALLERGY STICKER

DO NOT USE ABBREVIATIONS: µ, mcg, u, iu, QD, QID, QOD, B.I.W., T.I.W., MgS04, MS04, MS, HISS, RISS, AD, AU, AS

Please check box to activate the order.

Initiation:
1.   If glucose is greater than 250mg/dL, discontinue all IV glucose infusions.
2.   When the patient's glucose is ≤ 250 mg/dL add dextrose to IV's or ensure patient is receiving enteral feeds.
3.   **INITIATION TABLE**

Glucose (mg/dL)	Infusion rate (units/hour)	Infusion rate (mL/hour)
181 - 210	1	1
211 - 240	1.5	1.5
241 - 270	2	2
>270	3	3

4.   Check glucose q 1 x 4 hours, then q 2 hours.
     Calculate % changes for EACH new glucose and follow steps 4A-D.

     A.   Use *Maintenance Infusion Table* if
          i.   Glucose < 120, regardless of % change
          ii.   Gluscose fails to fall by 10%
     B.   If glucose falls **between 10-25%** and glucose > or = 120, leave infusion the same.
     C.   If glucose falls **more than 25%** and glucose > or = 120, decrease infusion by half.
     D.   If glucose remains within 120-180 mg/dL range for 8 hours, change glucose checks to q 4 hours.

5.   **MAINTENANCE INFUSION TABLE**

Glucose (mg/dL)	Insulin infusion (units/hour)
<80	D/C insulin infusion. Inform MD/APRN/PA. Administer 12.5 grams glucose (1/2 amp D50)IVP. Recheck glucose q 30 min x 2, then in 1 hour. If glucose > 180 after 2 hours, resume insulin infusion using Initiation Table.
80 – 119	D/C insulin infusion. Recheck glucose in 1 hour. If > 120, restart infusion at 1/2 previous rate. If < 120, continue to follow maintenance table.
120 – 180	No change
181 – 210	Increase by 0.5 units/hour (+ 0.5 mL/hour)
211 – 240	Increase by 1.0 units/hour (+ 1 mL/hour)
241 – 270	Increase by 1.5 units/hour (+ 1.5 mL/hour)
271 – 300	Increase by 2 units/hour (+ 2 mL/hour)
>300	Increase by 3 units/hour (+ 3 mL/hour)

6.   If tube feedings are discontinued for **any** reason, while patient is on maintenance insulin infusion, obtain an order for IVFs with Dextrose 5% at a maintenance rate and continue protocol using step 4 above and *hourly* glucose checks for the *next 4 hours.*

     NOTE: This protocol is not designed for the initial treatment of the DKA patient.*

Physician Signature: _____ Beeper #: _____ Date: _____ Time: _____

HCC Form # 1307 Revised 8-11   Critical Care/Intensive Care Insulin Infusion Physician Order

Figure 8.2 Critical care insulin infusion protocol (Hospital of Central Connecticut).

ALLERGY STICKER

Insulin Dose calculations on Reverse Side (Print) /Next Page (Alnet)

TARGET BLOOD GLUCOSE RANGES	**GLUCOSE MONITORING**
• Target Goal: 100 to 150 mg/dL • Random: < 180 mg/dL	☐ HbA1C on admission *(if not obtained within 30 days)* • Call Provider for FSG < 70 mg/dL (refer to <u>HYPOGLYCEMIA</u> <u>MANAGEMENT</u>) or > 400 mg/dL

SCHEDULED BASAL AND BOLUS INSULIN ORDERS
Check Only One Tube Feed Option And The Related Boxes

☐ **If transitioning from IV to SC Insulin Protocol, D/C the insulin infusion 2 hours after the initial SC glargine (Lantus) dose.**

☐ **PATIENT RECEIVING TUBE FEED SUPPLEMENT IN PM WITH MEALS DURING THE DAY** *[glulisine (Apidra®) & NPH insulin]*

☐ Check FSG 3 times daily before meals & every 6 hour <u>once tube feed starts</u>	☐ _____units SC glulisine **(Apidra)** Insulin <u>pre-meal</u> ☐ _____units SC **NPH Insulin** 30 minutes prior to start of <u>tube feed</u> every night ☐ **GLULISINE (APIDRA) INSULIN** dosed per **CORRECTION DOSE** orders below

☐ **FOR PATIENT RECEIVING BOLUS TUBE FEEDS ONLY** *[glulisine (Apidra®)& glargine (Lantus®) insulin]*

☐ Check FSG ___ times daily before boluses	☐ _____units **glargine (Lantus)** SC every 24 hours ☐ _____units **glulisine (Apidra)** Insulin SC _____ times daily before boluses ☐ **GLULISINE (APIDRA) INSULIN** dosed per **CORRECTION DOSE** orders below

☐ **FOR PATIENTS ON CONTINUOUS TUBE FEEDS** *[regular & glargine (Lantus®) insulin]*

☐ Check FSG Every 6 hours	☐ _____units **glargine (Lantus)** SC every 24 hours ☐ **REGULAR INSULIN** every 6 hours dosed per **CORRECTION DOSE** orders below

CHECK ONE *INSULIN* CORRECTION DOSE

☐ **SENSITIVE**		☐ **USUAL**		☐ **RESISTANT**	
Blood Glucose	Dose (SC)	Blood Glucose	Dose (SC)	Blood Glucose	Dose (SC)
151 – 200 mg/dL	1 units	151 – 200 mg/dL	3 units	151 – 200 mg/dL	6 units
201 – 250 mg/dL	2 units	201 – 250 mg/dL	4 units	201 – 250 mg/dL	8 units
251 – 300 mg/dL	3 units	251 – 300 mg/dL	5 units	251 – 300 mg/dL	10 units
301 – 350 mg/dL	4 units	301 – 350 mg/dL	7 units	301 – 350 mg/dL	12 units
351 – 400 mg/dL	5 units	351 – 400 mg/dL	8 units	351 – 400 mg/dL	14 units
> 400mg/dL	6 units	> 400mg/dL	10 units	> 400mg/dL	16 units

HYPOGLYCEMIA MANAGEMENT AND ORDERS

☐ **HYPOGLYCEMIA MANAGEMENT**
*Checking above box denotes activation of **HYPOGLYCEMIA ORDERS** on Right Side based on instructions below.*
  • If initial FSG <70mg/dL, follow **HYPOGLYCEMIA ORDERS** <u>OPTIONS 1 , 2, 3, or 4</u> and repeat FSG in 15 minutes
 	
  • If repeat FSG <100mg/dL, follow **HYPOGLYCEMIA ORDERS** <u>OPTIONS 1 , 2, 3, or 4</u> and recheck FSG every 15 minutes until FSG >100mg/dL
 	
  • When FSG reaches >100mg/dL, no further treatment needed.
	OPTIONS based on Mental Status
	Only applies if Hypoglycemia Management checked on Left Side
	♦ **OPTION 1: ALERT AND TOLERATES ORAL INTAKE**
	  Give 15 grams of fast acting carbohydrate (4 oz.
	  Cranberry Juice or 5-6 oz. regular soda or 6 saltine
	  crackers) & recheck FSG glucose in 15 min
	
	♦ **OPTION 2: ALERT, NO ORAL INTAKE WITH IV ACCESS**
	  Half ampule (25mL) of Dextrose 50% IV push x1
	
	♦ **OPTION 3: NOT ALERT WITH IV ACCESS**
	  1 ampule (50 mL) of Dextrose 50% IV push x 1
	
	♦ **OPTION 4: NOT ALERT WITHOUT IV ACCESS**
	  Glucagon 1mg IM/SC X 1

Physician Signature: _____ Beeper #: _____ Date: _____ Time: _____

HCC Form # 1547 Revised 3-12   Tube Feed Subcutaneous Insulin Protocol Physician Order

Figure 8.3 Subcutaneous insulin correction scales for patients on tube-feeding diets.

index, and median glucose), metrics of variability (e.g., standard deviation, glycemic lability index, maximum glucose, coefficient of variation), and a single metric of hypoglycemia (minimum glucose). Makenzie *et al.* (2011) found an independent association of each category with mortality and recommend that these categories be studied further to better define the actual metrics accountable for the variation in outcomes for critically ill patients.

Table 8.1 Management options for insulin coverage of fingerstick glucose (FSG) testing before meals and at bedtime (Hospital of Central Connecticut).

Check one	Sensitive	Usual	Resistant
FSG	Dose (SC)	Dose (SC)	Dose (SC)
Premeal < 70 mg/dl or bedtime < 100 mg/dl	Notify HO and initiate hypoglycemia treatment	Notify HO and initiate hypoglycemia treatment	Notify HO and initiate hypoglycemia treatment
151–200 mg/dl	1 unit	2 units	4 units
201–250 mg/dl	2 units	4 units	6 units
251–300 mg/dl	3 units	6 units	8 units
301–350 mg/dl	4 units	8 units	10 units
351–400 mg/dl	5 units	10 units	12 units
>401 mg/dl	Notify HO	Notify HO	Notify HO

- **Patients on oral diets: FSG testing is before meals and at bedtime**
  - Coverage is with Glulisine (Apidra ©)
- **Patients on continuous tube feedings: FSG testing is every 6 h**
  - Coverage is with regular insulin

HO, house officer; SC, subcutaneous.

Table 8.2 Hypoglycemia protocol: options based on mental status.

Alert and tolerates oral intake
Give 4 oz. cranberry juice or 6 oz. of regular sodium
Recheck FSG in 15 min
Alert, no oral intake with IV access
25 ml of Dextrose 50% IV push X 1 (1/2 bristojet of 50% Dextrose)
Not alert with IV access
50 ml of Dextrose 50% IV push X 1 (whole bristojet of 50% Dextrose)
Recheck FSG in 15 min
Not alert without IV access
Glucagon 1 mg IM/SC X 1
Recheck FSG in 15 min

References

American Association of Clinical Endocrinologists (AACE) and American Diabetes Association (2009) American Association of Clinical Endocrinologists and American Diabetes Association consensus statement on inpatient glycemic control. *Endocrine Practice*, **15** (4), 353–369.

American Diabetes Association (ADA) (2013) Standards of medical care in diabetes—2013. *Diabetes Care*, **36**, S11–S66.

Clement, S., Braithwaite, S.S., Magee, M.F. *et al.* (2004) Management of diabetes and hyperglycemia in hospitals. *Diabetes Care*, **27** (2), 553–591.

Egi, M., Finer, S., and Bellomo, R. (2001) Glycemic control in the ICU. *Chest*, **140** (1), 212–220.

Finfer, S., Chittock, D.R., Su, S.Y. *et al.* (2009) Intensive versus conventional glucose control in critically ill patients. *New England Journal of Medicine*, **360** (36), 1283–1297.

Finfer, S., Liu, B., Chittock, D.R. *et al.* (2012) Hypoglycermia and risk of death in critically ill patients. *New England Journal of Medicine*, **357**, 1108–1118.

Griesdale, D.E., de Souza, R.J., van Dam, R.M. *et al.* (2009) Intensive insulin therapy and mortality among critically ill patients: a meta-analysis including NICE-SUGAR study data. *Canadian Medical Association Journal*, **180** (8), 821–827.

Holzinger, U., Feldbacher, M., Bachlechner, A. *et al.* (2008) Improvement of glucose control in the intensive care unit: an interdisciplinary collaboration study. *American Journal of Critical Care*, **17** (2), 150–158.

Krinsley, J.S. (2004) Effect of an intensive glucose management protocol on the mortality of critically ill adult patients. *Mayo Clinic Proceedings*, **79**, 992–1000.

Krinsley, J.S. and Grover, A. (2007) Severe hypoglycemia in critically ill patients: risk factors and outcomes. *Critical Care Medicine*, **35**, 2262–2267.

Mackenzie, I.M.J., Whitehouse, T., and Nightingale, P.G. (2011) The metrics of glycaemic control in critical care. *Intensive Care Medicine*, **37**, 435–443.

Merrill, A. and Jones, S. (2011) Effectiveness of tight glycemic control in the medical Intensive Care Unit: a systematic review. *JBI Library of Systematic Reviews*, **9**, 417–436.

Moghissi, E.S., Korytkowski, M.T., DiNardo, M. *et al.* (2009) American Association of Clinical Endocrinologists and American Diabetes Association consensus statement on inpatient glycemic control. *Diabetes Care*, **32**, 1119–1131.

Shearer, A., Boehmer, M., Closs, M. *et al.* (2009) Comparison of glucose point-of-care values with laboratory values in critically ill patients. *American Journal of Critical Care*, **18**, 224–230.

Taub, L.F.M. and Redeker, N.S. (2008) Sleep disorders, glucose regulation, and type II diabetes. *Biological Research in Nursing*, **9**, 231–243.

Van den Berghe, G., Wouters, P., Weekers, F. *et al.* (2001) Intensive insulin therapy in critically ill patients. *New England Journal of Medicine*, **345** (19), 1359–1367.

Van den Berghe, G., Wouters, P., Hermans, G. *et al.* (2006) Intensive insulin therapy in the medical ICU. *New England Journal of Medicine*, **354** (5), 449–461.

Wiener, R.S., Wiener, D.C., and Larson, R.J. (2008) Benefits and risks of tight glucose control in critically ill adults: a meta-analysis. *JAMA*, **300** (8), 933–944.

CHAPTER 9

Monitoring for hepatic and GI dysfunction

Eleanor R. Fitzpatrick

Surgical Intensive Care & Intermediate Care Units, Thomas Jefferson University Hospital, Philadelphia, USA

Physiologic guidelines

The gastrointestinal (GI) system comprises the alimentary canal, beginning at the mouth; extending through the pharynx, esophagus, stomach, small intestine, colon, rectum, and anal canal; and ending at the anus (Linton, 2012). The GI tract spans approximately 30 ft in length (see Fig. 9.1). It incorporates structures that are auxiliary organs of the GI (or digestive) tract including the liver, pancreas, and gallbladder (Linton, 2012).

The GI system is responsible for essential functions including ingestion and propulsion of food, mechanical and chemical digestion of food, synthesis of nutrients such as vitamin K, absorption of nutrients into the blood stream, and the storage and elimination of nondigestible waste products from the body (Linton, 2012). The liver, the gallbladder and its bile ducts, and the pancreas are called accessory glands in the GI system. Their function is to aid digestion through the delivery of bile and enzymes to the small intestine. The role of the liver is detoxification of chemicals and synthesis and storage of nutrients (Linton, 2012). The pancreas performs the endocrine functions of insulin and glucagon production as well as the exocrine function of digestive enzyme secretion. GI dysfunction can result in acute and critical illness due to a variety of malfunctions within the hollow tube-like structure of the tract or within its auxiliary organs. The GI system is fraught with disorders, potentially requiring intensive assessment and monitoring.

Gastrointestinal dysfunction

GI dysfunction may first be noted in the development of metabolic abnormalities when there is disruption of the normal activities of digestion and absorption. The major function of the GI tract is digestion, converting ingested nutrients into simpler forms carried to the portal circulation for use in metabolic processes (Urden, Stacy, and Lough, 2010). The GI system also has an important role in the detoxification and elimination of bacteria, viruses, chemical toxins, and drugs. Disturbances within the hepatic and GI systems or their hormonal and neural controls can cause critical illness complicated by severe derangement in nutritional status (Urden, Stacy, and Lough, 2010).

GI dysfunction arises from alterations in normal function within the esophagus (esophageal varices), the stomach (ulcers, tumor), as well as small and large intestines (inflammation, ulceration, tumors). The auxiliary organs of the GI tract may also contain the onus of severe disease. Pancreatic function may go awry with the development of pancreatitis or a malignant or benign tumor. Patients may fall victim to abnormalities of the liver with hepatic dysfunction due to end-stage liver disease (ESLD) from cirrhosis or hepatitis or due to acute liver failure (ALF). The numerous functions of the liver cause its dysfunction to result in a multitude of metabolic and synthetic abnormalities. Any significant alteration in any of these functions can result in critical illness. Bleeding from esophageal varices may arise as a liver damaged by alcohol, hepatitis, or other

Critical Care Nursing: Monitoring and Treatment for Advanced Nursing Practice, First Edition. Edited by Kathy J. Booker.
© 2015 John Wiley & Sons, Inc. Published 2015 by John Wiley & Sons, Inc.

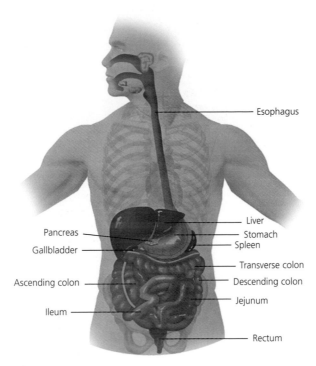

Esophagus

Liver
Stomach
Spleen

Pancreas
Gallbladder

Transverse colon
Descending colon
Jejunum

Ascending colon

Ileum

Rectum

Figure 9.1 Gastrointestinal tract.

cause of cirrhosis becomes fibrotic and portal hypertension ensues. The development of refractory ascites is not fully understood but it seems that it is due, in part, to multifactorial causes of inappropriate sodium and water retention, hypoalbuminemia with reduced intravascular osmotic pressure, portal hypertension, and hyperpermeable capillaries (Smeltzer *et al.*, 2010). Hepatic encephalopathy is another sequelae of ESLD that also has a complex pathophysiology. This phenomenon is thought, in part, to be related to ineffective conversion of ammonia into urea for excretion. Ammonia, which crosses the blood–brain barrier, has sedating neurologic effects. There are four stages of hepatic encephalopathy, the fourth being coma (Smeltzer *et al.*, 2010) (Table 9.1).

Blunt-force trauma due to motor vehicle crash, falls, or contact during sports or penetrating injury due to gunshot wounds or stabbing to the abdomen can injure underlying GI structures. Intraabdominal structures can also be disrupted by gunshot or stab wounds to the chest, anywhere below the fourth intercostal

Table 9.1 Clinical grades of hepatic encephalopathy.

(I) Mild confusion, euphoria, anxiety, or depression
     Shortened attention span
     Slowing of ability to perform mental tasks (addition/ subtraction)
     Reversal of sleep rhythm
(II) Drowsiness, lethargy, gross deficits in ability to perform mental tasks
     Obvious personality changes
     Inappropriate behavior
     Intermittent disorientation of time (and place)
     Lack of sphincter control
(III) Somnolent but rousable
     Persistent disorientation of time and place
     Pronounced confusion
     Unable to perform mental tasks
(IV) Coma with (IVa) or without (IVb) response to painful stimuli

From: Sherlock, S. *Diseases of the Liver and Biliary System, Eleventh Edition*. Published Online: 25 OCT 2007. Wiley Online Library

space anteriorly and seventh intercostal space posteriorly (Wiegand, 2011). These injuries can result in organ disruption with bleeding or spillage of GI contents into the peritoneal space with peritonitis.

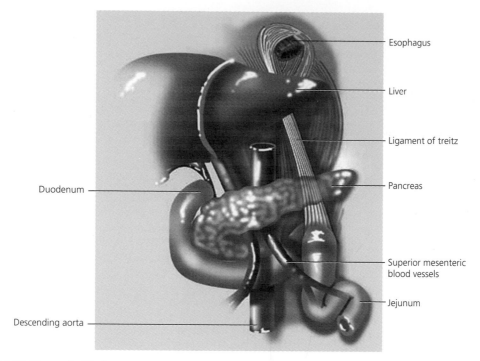

Esophagus

Liver

Ligament of treitz

Pancreas

Duodenum

Superior mesenteric
blood vessels

Jejunum

Descending aorta

Figure 9.2 Ligament of Treitz.

Gastrointestinal bleeding

GI hemorrhage occurs in the critically ill with relative frequency. All critically ill patients should be considered at risk for stress ulcers and therefore GI hemorrhage. This bleeding can arise from upper GI sites (upper GI bleeding) or from lower GI structures (lower GI bleeding). The ligament of Treitz (see Fig. 9.2) is the anatomic site of division between the upper and lower GI tracts.

The most common causes of upper GI bleeding are peptic ulcers (either gastric or duodenal), stress-related mucosal disease, and esophagogastric varices (Urden, Stacy, and Lough, 2010). Lower GI bleeding is most often caused by diverticulosis and arterial–venous malformations.

The assessment of the hepatic and GI systems includes an extensive review of the patient's history as well as a complete physical examination. A complete evaluation of these systems may also include a multitude of laboratory indices and invasive and noninvasive testing (Urden, Stacy, and Lough, 2010; Smeltzer *et al.*, 2010).

Monitoring elements: Nasogastric decompression

In order to monitor the acutely or critically ill patient for signs of abnormalities of the GI system, placing a nasogastric (NG) tube is an important action to determine and to diagnose many abnormal conditions of the GI tract. Placing an NG tube is critical in differentiating upper from lower GI bleeding. NG aspiration with saline lavage is beneficial to detect the presence of intragastric blood, to determine the type of gross bleeding, to clear the gastric field for endoscopic visualization and to prevent aspiration of gastric contents. A grossly bloody aspirate in the absence of a traumatic intubation confirms an upper gastrointestinal bleed (UGIB). Red blood suggests currently active bleeding, whereas the appearance of coffee-ground returns suggests recently active bleeding. A bilious, nonbloody aspirate strongly suggests that bleeding is distal to the ligament of Treitz or stopped many hours before (Cappell and Freidel, 2008b). The patient vomiting blood or with bloody NG drainage is usually bleeding from a source above the duodenojejunal junction because reverse peristalsis is seldom sufficient to cause hematemesis if the bleeding point is below this area (Urden, Stacy, and Lough, 2010). Once an NG tube is placed, the drainage must be closely scrutinized for bleeding or for conditions that could precipitate bleeding. Normal gastric drainage is green or gold bilious in color.

The process of testing gastric contents for blood is an integral assessment criterion when one suspects GI bleeding, but the bleeding is occult. Occult blood is not visible to the naked eye. NG aspirate or vomitus may be tested for occult blood by obtaining a small specimen, placing it on a specialized paper surface (of a commercially available product), and then treating it with a chemical designed to detect the presence of blood through specific color changes identified by the practitioner (Linton, 2012). Additionally, monitoring the stool for the presence of gross or occult blood can also be performed with similar technology. A stool specimen is applied to a commercially available slide. When hydrogen peroxide or another commercially available developer is added to the sample, any blood cells present liberate their hemoglobin and a bluish ring appears on the electrophoretic paper. This reading is made at precisely the 30 s mark after the developer is added (Nettina, 2010). Though this test is often used as a screen for colon cancer in the outpatient setting, such an assessment made in the critical care unit may provide more information about the location of a possible bleeding site and the severity of the bleeding.

Evidence-based treatment guidelines

There are no currently published guidelines for the insertion of an NG tube in the setting of GI hemorrhage or other GI disorders. However, this practice is commonplace and frequently performed. Published guidelines do exist, however, recommending rapid assessment and volume resuscitation of the bleeding patient. These recommendations include the use of crystalloid and colloid infusion and the transfusion of blood products when blood loss is

estimated at 30% or more of circulating intravascular volume. A standardized protocol for resuscitation should exist in facilities that treat patients with GI hemorrhage (Scottish Intercollegiate Guidelines Network [SIGN], 2008). Volume status and hemodynamic stability should dictate the amount of fluid transfused. In hemodynamically unstable patients or patients with large hemorrhage, boluses of 500 ml of normal saline or lactated Ringer solution with continuous reassessment are appropriate. Determining the need for invasive monitoring should be based on the clinical presentation and need for close assessment and management of volume status. Transfusion of blood products is recommended in those patients with hemodynamic instability despite crystalloid resuscitation and in those with continuous bleeding. A patient's age, comorbid conditions, briskness of bleed, baseline hemoglobin, and hematocrit levels, as well as evidence of cardiac, renal, or cerebral hypoperfusion should all be taken into consideration when determining the quantity of blood to transfuse. Coagulopathic patients may require platelets or fresh frozen plasma as appropriate (Kumar and Mills, 2011). To replace coagulation factors, it is recommended that for every four units of packed red blood cells (RBCs) transfused, a patient be given one unit of fresh frozen plasma (Maltz, Siegel, and Carson, 2000). A consensus statement regarding platelet transfusion recommends that patients with platelet counts in the range of 50 000–90 000 mm^3 do not require platelet transfusion, whereas those with counts less than 50 000 mm^3 and active bleeding may require transfusion (Conteras, 1998). Clinical parameters, including age, comorbid conditions, and severity of bleed, should be used to determine whether or not platelets should be administered to thrombocytopenic patients (Kumar and Mills, 2011).

Gastric pH

The pH of gastric contents may be measured frequently to assess for an acidic environment, a risk factor for the development of peptic ulceration, especially in the at-risk critically ill. Though the routine monitoring of gastric pH is controversial, this may be performed to maintain the pH between 3.5 and 4.5 with prophylactic agents such as proton pump inhibitors (PPIs), histamine antagonists, or agents such as sulcrafate, which coat and protect the mucosa. Intragastric pH studies have demonstrated that while a pH of more than 4 may be adequate to prevent stress ulceration (prophylaxis), a pH of more than 6 may be necessary to maintain clotting in patients at risk of rebleeding from peptic ulcer. Some studies have indicated that although histamine 2 receptor antagonists and PPIs effectively raise the pH of intragastric fluids to more than 4, PPIs are more likely to maintain a pH of more than 6, a factor to consider for patients in the intensive care unit (ICU) who are at risk for rebleeding from peptic ulcers after hemostasis (Fennerty, 2002; SIGN, 2008). Gastric pH measurements can be made with litmus paper or direct NG tube probes (Urden, Stacy, and Lough, 2010). In performing this assessment, the nurse will also be alert for the presence of obvious bleeding. With the hypoperfusion of the GI tract in shock, sepsis, and other serious conditions, the mucosa may slough and ulcerate, causing bleeding.

Evidence-based treatment guidelines

No published guidelines currently exist regarding the routine testing of pH of intragastric contents. The SIGN guidelines (2008) discuss the controversial issue of medications used to treat

---

Clinical Pearls—Patient Management and Treatment

NG lavage is often performed during an upper GI hemorrhage event. It is used to control active bleeding by decreasing gastric mucosal blood flow and to evacuate blood from the stomach. Gastric lavage is performed by inserting a large-bore NG tube into the stomach and irrigating it with normal saline or water until the returned solution is clear. Room temperature lavage is recommended over cooled or iced lavage fluid as cold fluids shift the oxyhemoglobin dissociation curve to the left, decrease oxygen delivery to the tissues, and prolong bleeding time and prothrombin time (Waterman and Walker, 1973). Iced saline lavage lowers core body temperature, induces shivering, and results in an increased metabolic rate (Andrus, 1987). Iced fluid lavage may also further aggravate bleeding (Gilbert and Saunders, 1981; Ponsky, Hoffman, and Swayngim, 1980; Urden, Stacy, and Lough, 2010).

---

and to prevent UGIB. The SIGN guidelines, however, do recommend that, in the patient at high risk for a rebleeding episode due to peptic ulcer disease, PPIs be used. This class of drugs is more likely to maintain intragastric pH at a level of 6 or over to prevent recurrent bleeding (Ali and Harty, 2009; SIGN, 2008).

Monitoring elements: Laboratory tests for GI bleeding

Laboratory tests may not provide an accurate and timely assessment of GI bleeding. RBCs and plasma are lost in equal amounts during a bleeding episode. The hemoglobin and hematocrit may be helpful for monitoring trends during a bleeding episode and should be assessed on a frequent basis.

Evidence-based treatment guidelines

There are no published guidelines recommending the frequency of laboratory data monitoring but the 2008 guidelines published by SIGN (2008) do advise practitioners that blood urea nitrogen (BUN) should be measured frequently in patients with GI bleeding as a marker of bleeding extent, with breakdown of RBCs within the GI tract raising the BUN level (SIGN, 2008).

Endoscopic procedures

Endoscopic procedures incorporate a flexible tube (the fiber-optic endoscope) to visualize the GI tract and to perform certain diagnostic and therapeutic procedures. Images are produced through a video screen or telescopic eyepiece. The tip of the endoscope moves in four directions, allowing for wide visualization. The endoscope can be inserted via the mouth or the rectum, depending on which portion of the GI tract is to be viewed. Capsule endoscopy utilizes an ingestible camera device rather than an endoscope (Nettina, 2010). The capsule endoscopy's current utilization is in the ambulatory, outpatient setting, for the most part, but could gain applicability in the acute care setting in the future. The scopic procedure of endoscopic esophagogastroduodenoscopy (EGD) is the principal diagnostic procedure to identify the presence of upper or lower GI bleeding. EGD can accurately identify the site of bleeding, provide prognostic information about rebleeding risk, and offer therapeutic potential (Ali and Harty, 2009). To isolate the source of bleeding in a patient with an acute bleeding episode, an urgent fiber-optic endoscopy should be performed. When performed within 12h of the bleeding episode, endoscopy has a 90–95% accuracy rate (Urden, Stacy, and Lough, 2010). EGD provides direct visualization of the upper GI tract including the esophagus, stomach, and duodenum. It has several diagnostic indications including the evaluation of dysphagia, gastroesophageal reflux disease (GERD), epigastric pain, and GI bleeding (Ali and Harty, 2009; Stonesifer, 2004). The stomach must be prepared adequately for the endoscopy to be as accurate as possible. An NG tube should be lavaged with room temperature saline to evacuate blood and clots prior to the test being performed. Room temperature lavage is preferred to ice lavage since cold temperatures may potentiate vasoconstriction and suppressed blood supply to an already potentially ischemic mucosa.

In the case of a nondiagnostic endoscopic test, there are other radiologic diagnostic interventions that can be made. Namely, a tagged RBC radionucleotide study can be performed to identify an obscure but dangerous site of bleeding. Angiography may also be performed in the setting of a nondiagnostic EGD. In patients who are actively bleeding at a site of at least 0.5ml/min this test may accurately identify a site of bleeding. A bleeding rate of less than 0.5ml/min precludes its identification by this diagnostic method (Urden, Stacy, and Lough, 2010). Therapeutic interventions may also be performed via endoscopy or angiography. These strategies may include treatment of esophageal varices or bleeding ulcers, biopsy, or dilatation. Endoscopic treatments also include thermal coagulation, injection therapy, hemostatic clips, argon plasma coagulation, and combination therapy. During these diagnostic and at times therapeutic interventions, the patient is sedated. It is important to ensure safe management of the patient undergoing these procedures and avoid oversedation. This is accomplished by adhering strictly to institutional standards for the management of moderate sedation.

Evaluation of the lower GI tract also incorporates a scopic procedure for complete assessment of the GI tract below the ligament of Treitz. Colonoscopy assesses the mucosa of the entire colon and frequently the distal terminal ileum via a flexible, fiber-optic scope. These scopes have the same capabilities as those used for EGD but are larger in diameter and longer. Still and video recordings can be used to document the procedure and relative findings (Smeltzer et al., 2010). Through this procedure, bleeding, masses, strictures, polyps, and other pathology may be identified and treated as noted with EGD: with lasers, heat, or uni- or bipolar coagulation (see Table 9.2).

If colonoscopy does not yield a diagnostic or therapeutic result, angiography may be used to identify the bleeding site (if there is still active bleeding of 0.5ml/min) and to correct via embolization with fat, coils, gelfoam, or other commercial products. The colon must be adequately prepared with the use of laxatives or enemas prior to the patient undergoing the study. The use of moderate sedation by trained nursing or anesthesia personnel affords the patient needed comfort during the procedure and avoidance of oversedation. See Table 9.3 for other monitoring priorities for intra- and postendoscopic therapy.

Evidence-based treatment guidelines

Currently published guidelines for the evaluation and treatment of upper or lower GI hemorrhage include treatment of patients in a critical care unit (with at least hourly monitoring of vital signs) and prompt and aggressive stabilization with volume resuscitation. All nonsteroidal anti-inflammatory drugs (NSAIDs) and aspirin should be discontinued. Early EGD or colonoscopy (within 24h of initial presentation) is also recommended for diagnosis and therapeutic interventions. It is also recommended that patients experiencing an upper GI bleeding episode be evaluated for the presence of *Helicobacter pylori* either during EGD biopsy or with a urea breath test. Patients who test positive for *H. pylori* should receive a course of antibiotic therapy. Patients with GI

Table 9.2 Indications for endoscopic and angiographic therapy in acute upper and lower GI bleeding.

Bleeding source	Injection	Ablative	Mechanical	Angiographic
Duodenal ulcer	X	X	X	X
Gastric ulcer	X	X	X	X
Esophageal varices	X		X	
Mallory–Weiss tears	X	X	X	
Angiodysplasia of the upper or lower GI tract	X	X		X
Colonic ulcer	X	X	X	X

Esophagogastroduodenoscopy is the procedure of choice for the diagnosis and therapy of upper gastrointestinal bleeding lesions. Endoscopic therapy is indicated for lesions with high-risk stigmata of recent hemorrhage, including active bleeding, oozing, a visible vessel, and possibly an adherent clot. Use of these therapies is dictated by personal experience, training, preference, cost, and availability (Cappell and Friedel, 2008b).

Colonoscopy and angiography are diagnostic and therapeutic interventions. Injections, as well as ablative and mechanical interventions, are performed via scopic guidance. Once bleeding sites are identified angiographically, vessels may be embolized with coils, fat, gelfoam, or other commercially available products. Potent vasoconstrictors such as vasopressin may also be administered to coalesce vessels and eradicate bleeding.

Injection therapy may include use of epinephrine or commercially available sclerosants such as sodium tetradecyl sulfate, polidocanol, or ethanol.

Ablative therapy may include electrocautery, heater probe, or argon plasma coagulation.

Mechanical therapy may include endoclips or banding (EVL endoscopic band ligation).

All three therapies are effective as monotherapies, but combined therapies may increase the efficacy.

Table 9.3 Monitoring priorities for intra- and postendoscopic therapy.

Provide patient and family education regarding the procedure, intra- and postprocedure care. Ensure proper consents have been obtained.

Elevate head of bed, monitor for aspiration in patients at risk due to moderate sedation.

Monitor for respiratory depression with use of moderate sedation.

Ensure patency of venous access. Monitor for signs of overt and obscure bleeding, continue volume resuscitation as needed.

Close monitoring of vital signs, cardiac rhythm, and pulse oximetry. Monitor for bradydysrhythmias during passage of the endoscope.

bleeding due to peptic ulcer disease should receive pharmacotherapy in the form of PPIs (Adler, 2004; SIGN, 2008). Intestinal resection or subtotal colectomy is recommended for the management of colonic hemorrhage uncontrolled by scopic interventions (SIGN, 2008).

Evidence-based treatment guidelines for stress ulcers

The published guidelines of the Eastern Association for the Surgery of Trauma for stress ulcer prophylaxis mirror other organizations' recommendations for this effort, especially in the realm of critical care where patients are at greatest risk for the development of stress-related GI bleeding (Guillamondegui et al., 2008). These recommendations state that all critically ill patients with associated risk factors should receive chemical prophylaxis for stress

Clinical Pearls—Patient Management and Treatment

It is critical in the postprocedure phase of patient care to evaluate the patient for the development of a GI perforation, a possible complication of any scopic procedure. A perforation is a break in the wall of the stomach, duodenum, or colon that permits digestive fluids or stool to leak into the peritoneal cavity, causing inflammation of the peritoneum (peritonitis) (Linton, 2012). Monitoring of the patient's vital signs and a thorough assessment for the development of sudden, sharp epigastric or abdominal pain, guarding, rigidity, point and/or rebound tenderness provides the practitioner with a raised index of suspicion for the onset of a GI perforation (stomach, duodenum, colon, etc.). Perforation of the GI tract may also result in other symptoms. The rapid evaluation with an abdominal radiograph will aid the practitioner with this diagnosis and allow for rapid scopic or surgical intervention. The practitioner's initial management initiative is to use gastric decompression, intravenous fluids, and antibiotic agents. A small perforation may seal spontaneously (Linton, 2012).

ulceration. All agents (with the exception of antacids) appear equally adequate for prophylaxis against stress ulceration. The agent of choice is an individual hospital decision. The duration of treatment is ill-defined but should be maintained while risk factors are present. There is insufficient evidence to warrant cessation of prophylaxis in the setting of enteral nutrition (Guillamondegui *et al.*, 2008).

Monitoring elements: Gastric tonometry and capnometry

Blood supply and tissue oxygenation of the GI tract is provided via the splanchnic circulation. When blood flow is decreased due to many disorders, such as in the shock state, the gut may be utilized to provide needed information in assessing for early and accurate warning of tissue hypoperfusion. Oxygenation of the GI (or splanchnic) organs can be quantified using gastric tonometry, which is based upon the knowledge that when oxygen supply to the stomach decreases, anaerobic metabolism in gastric cells produces the by-products of excess hydrogen ions, lactate, and carbon dioxide. As gastric carbon dioxide (CO_2) levels increase, hypoperfusion is likely occurring. Gastric tonometry is a monitor of gastric mucosal hypoperfusion and resultant hypoxia. Measurement of the adequacy of the splanchnic circulation may be particularly important in the critically ill or injured patient. Splanchnic hypoperfusion occurs early in shock, and may occur before the usual indicators of shock such as hypotension or lactic acidosis are present (Marik, 2001). Currently available methods of monitoring gastric CO_2 include gastric tonometry and sublingual capnometry. Gastric tonometry (see Fig. 9.3) is useful for monitoriing the difference between gastric and arterial CO_2. A widening gap indicates compromised blood flow to the splanchnic bed, acidosis, and impaired cellular function (Johnson, 2005). In gastric tonometry, the practitioner withdraws samples of saline placed in the balloon of a specially designed NG tube and sends the saline and an arterial blood gas to the laboratory for analysis of CO_2 and bicarbonate (HCO_3) concentrations. These results are used in the Henderson–Hasselbach equation to determine intramucosal pH (pHi) (Carlesso, Taccone, and Gattinoni, 2006; Marshall and West, 2004; Urden, Stacy, and Lough, 2010). Newer technology known as air tonometry allows for automatic specimen withdrawal (of air within the balloon, not saline) and analysis of pHi (Carlesso, Taccone, and Gattinoni, 2006; Marshall and West, 2004; Urden, Stacy, and Lough, 2010).

Another assessment tool for the GI tract that evaluates regional perfusion and oxygenation has been developed utilizing gastric tonometry principles. Researchers have demonstrated that the very proximal GI tract, namely, the tongue and/or sublingual mucosa, may serve as appropriate sites for measurement of tissue CO_2. Sublingual capnometry or capnography was developed to overcome some of the limitations of gastric tonometry. This noninvasive and portable testing measure provides data that correlates well with gastric oxygen (O_2) levels (Johnson, 2005). Sublingual capnometry is a measurement of the CO_2 level in the vascular bed underlying the tongue, measured in a manner similar to an oral temperature. $SlCO_2$ has been demonstrated to be a sensitive marker of splanchnic perfusion (an early indicator of hypoperfusion) and gut ischemia. Researchers have demonstrated an increase in sublingual PCO_2 ($PslCO_2$) that was closely related to decreases in arterial pressure and cardiac index during circulatory shock produced by hemorrhage and sepsis (Marik, 2001). Studies in trauma and nontrauma patients have indicated that $SlCO_2$ may be a predictor of organ dysfunction, injury severity, and mortality (Strehlow, 2010).

Widespread adoption of sublingual capnometry monitoring in areas such as Emergency Departments has been limited by the requirement for new equipment, difficulties with obtaining accurate, reproducible measurements, and the need for further study (Strehlow, 2010). Though gastric tonometry and sublingual capnometry are not widely used, they should be considered extremely innovative bedside tools for

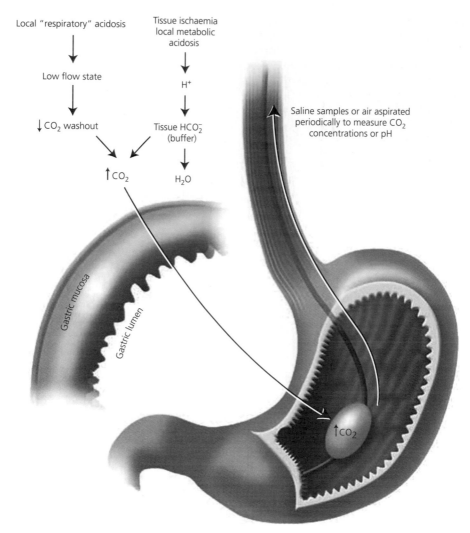

Local "respiratory" acidosis

Low flow state

↓ CO_2 washout

Tissue ischaemia
local metabolic
acidosis

H^+

Tissue HCO_2^-
(buffer)

↑CO_2

H_2O

Saline samples or air aspirated
periodically to measure CO_2
concentrations or pH

Gastric mucosa

Gastric lumen

↑CO_2

Figure 9.3 Gastric tonometry.

assessing for decreased tissue perfusion. Their use may also be of advantage in assessing patient response to therapy such as volume resuscitation with crystalloid but further investigation is needed to determine the role of these technologies.

Evidence-based treatment guidelines

No evidence-based treatment guidelines have been established to date for the use of routine gastric tonometry and sublingual capnometry.

Radiographic diagnostics

Plain radiographic films play an important role in evaluating the critically ill patient for GI abnormalities. A likely application for this testing is in the patient with abdominal pain. Optimally two views of the abdomen should be obtained for the most thorough evaluation. Air–fluid levels may be assessed as well as an evaluation for the presence of free air, indicating perhaps a perforated viscus. Other disease states may be evaluated by plain radiographic films including small or large bowel obstruction or paralytic ileus, all resulting in distended loops of bowel evident on the exam. The addition of contrast to the study allows for assessment of filling defects and mucosal abnormalities along the entire GI tract (Stonesifer, 2004).

Evidence-based treatment guidelines

Many experts dispute the use of the plain abdominal radiograph in the diagnosis of GI disorders, particularly in vascular emergencies of the GI tract. However, the general consensus has been and will continue to be (at least for the foreseeable future) that this is an easily and rapidly performed test, which is advantageous in identifying the presence of a perforated viscus or intestinal obstruction. It can be completed without prolonging time to the operating room for definitive treatment of intestinal infarction and other conditions (Cappell and Batke, 2008; Shanley and Weinberger, 2008). The Royal College of Radiologists (RCR) recommends the use of plain abdominal radiography in many acute conditions of the abdomen including acute abdominal pain, large or small bowel obstruction, pancreatitis, foreign body ingestion, and blunt or stab wound injury to the abdomen (Smith and Hall, 2009).

Ultrasonography

Abdominal ultrasound and, in particular, focused abdominal sonography in trauma (FAST) are important tools in critical care and gastroenterology. They allow for the evaluation of liver size and texture, important factors associated with cirrhosis or fatty liver infiltration. They may also detect masses and ascites as well as abnormalities indicative of cholecystitis. FAST is the mainstay of diagnosis in patients sustaining blunt abdominal trauma. It allows for rapid, noninvasive detection of free fluid within the abdominal cavity and, if found, is an indication for surgical intervention. FAST may also identify solid organ injuries but its sensitivity for this assessment is less than that

for fluid. If FAST results are inconclusive for injury, computed tomography (CT) of the abdomen may be performed (Stonesifer, 2004).

Evidence-based treatment guidelines

The American Institute of Ultrasound in Medicine (AIUM) and the American College of Emergency Physicians (ACEP) state that the FAST examination is a proven and useful procedure for the evaluation of the injured patient immediately during resuscitation to detect large abnormal fluid collections, which require immediate treatment. The FAST guideline includes indications for performing the examination, qualifications of the performing practitioner, specifications for individual examinations, documentation requirements, quality control, and patient safety standards (Bahner, 2008). Table 9.4 provides a summary of the FAST guideline.

Intraabdominal pressure management

In the patient who has sustained abdominal trauma or other abdominal visceral catastrophe such as mesenteric ischemia or severe acute pancreatitis, intraabdominal hypertension (IAH) and abdominal compartment syndrome (ACS) may occur. IAH and ACS develop when the abdominal contents expand in excess of the capacity of the abdominal cavity, potentially suppressing organ perfusion and causing organ dysfunction or failure and increased morbidity and mortality (Stonesifer, 2004; Wiegand, 2011). Increased pressure within the abdominal compartment can be caused by bleeding, ileus, visceral edema, or a noncompliant abdominal wall. Increased abdominal pressure can impinge on diaphragmatic excursion and affect ventilation, often identified by increasing peak inspiratory pressures when patients are mechanically ventilated. Additional clinical manifestations of ACS include decreased cardiac output, decreased urine output, and hypoxia (Urden, Stacy, and Lough, 2010). Measurement of bladder pressure and, thus, indirectly intraabdominal pressure (IAP), is a useful way to detect IAH as well as the progression to ACS. Both conditions are associated

Table 9.4 FAST guideline summary for abdominal ultrasonography.

Indications/contraindications	Patient safety standards
Indications for an ultrasound examination of the abdomen and/or retroperitoneum include but are not limited to the following:	
Abdominal trauma	The request for the examination must be originated by a physician or other appropriately licensed health-care provider or under their direction.
Abdominal, flank, and/or back pain	The accompanying clinical information should be provided by a physician or other appropriate health-care provider familiar with the patient's clinical situation and should be consistent with the relevant legal and local health-care facility requirements.
Search for the presence of free or loculated peritoneal and/or retroperitoneal fluid	For evaluating peritoneal spaces for bleeding after traumatic injury, particularly blunt trauma, the examination known as focused abdominal sonography for trauma (or focused assessment with sonography for trauma) may be performed.
Follow-up of known or suspected abnormalities in the abdomen and/or retroperitoneum	The objective of the examination is to analyze the abdomen for free fluid. Images should be obtained in the right upper quadrant through the area of the liver with attention to fluid collections peripheral to the liver and in the subhepatic space.
	Images should be obtained in the left upper quadrant through the area of the spleen, with attention to fluid collections peripheral to the spleen.
	Images should be obtained at the periphery of the left and right abdomen in the areas of the left and right paracolic gutters for evidence of free fluid.
	Images of the pelvis are obtained to evaluate free pelvic fluid.
	Analysis through a fluid-filled bladder (which if necessary can be filled through a Foley catheter when possible) may help in the evaluation of the pelvis.
All ultrasound studies of the abdomen	Adequate documentation is essential. There should be a permanent record of the ultrasound examination and its interpretation. Images of all appropriate areas should be recorded. Variations from normal size should be accompanied by measurements. Images should be labeled with the patient identification, facility identification, examination date, and side (right or left) of the anatomic site imaged. An official interpretation (final report) of the ultrasound findings should be included in the patient's medical record.
	Diagnostic information should be optimized while keeping total ultrasound exposure as low as reasonably achievable.
	Equipment performance monitoring should be in accordance with the *AIUM Standards and Guidelines for the Accreditation of Ultrasound Practices*.

Source: Bahner (2008).

with traumatic injury as well as with other conditions such as intraabdominal infection and peritonitis, abdominal surgery, ascites, pancreatitis, and aggressive volume resuscitation for the management of shock or cardiopulmonary arrest.

Intraabdominal pressure measurement

There are many approaches to measuring IAP. The measurement of this pressure via an indwelling urinary catheter is a reliable method (Stonesifer, 2004). The measurement of IAP can be made with equipment readily available in the critical care setting but commercially prepared kits designed for this measurement are also available. Should elevated IAP (20–25 mmHg or greater) accompany clinical manifestations of ACS, a surgical decompressive laparotomy may be performed. Surgical decompression incorporates opening of the abdomen followed by a temporizing coverage of the viscera after the procedure. There are many options for management of the open abdomen after decompressive laparotomy. Coverage with clear sterile dressing with some absorptive material and/or drains, and use of a vacuum-assisted technique are just a few of the options for management of the open abdomen. The wound is then closed by a delayed primary closure once the cause of the ACS has resolved or the wound is allowed to heal by secondary intention and eventual skin grafting (Urden, Stacy, and Lough, 2010).

Care of the patient after decompressive laparotomy poses many challenges including ongoing assessment of the status of the viscera for viability and close monitoring for bleeding. Aggressive volume resuscitation and assessment of patient response is most often indicated. A clear, sterile covering of the dressing affords the practitioner the ability to visualize the viscera under the dressing to ascertain its color, an indicator of viability. Large amounts of intraadominal fluid may drain from the dressing and depending on the type of wound management system used, the fluid may be collected in canisters to allow for accurate assessment of fluid losses. These fluid losses may be replaced once quantified via intravenous fluid administration. Of critical importance is continuing to monitor the IAP so that rapid identification of the recurrence of IAH can be made. Should this result from excess compressive forces of the dressing or other complicating factors, the patient would require an urgent removal and reapplication of the dressing.

Assessment of intravascular volume status and patient response to therapy is an important part of the management strategy of the patient post decompressive laparotomy. Several types of monitoring tools exist to accomplish this task. Central venous pressure may be monitored on an hourly basis providing generalized data on overall fluid balance and providing a line for delivering large volumes of fluid (Urden, Stacy, and Lough, 2010). Monitoring heart rate and blood pressure response and hemodynamics can aid in the assessment but new technology provides the practitioner with added information (see Chapter 5). Minimally invasive cardiac output measurement via pulse contour waveform (derived from an arterial catheter) or fluid therapy guided by esophageal ultrasound analysis calculates stroke volume and/or cardiac output and contractility. Variability in stroke volume and cardiac output are useful assessment tools in establishing patient response to therapy using this technology (Urden, Stacy, and Lough, 2010). See Chapter 5: Hemodynamic monitoring for additional guidelines.

Treatment of abdominal compartment syndrome

When using a urinary catheter to measure IAP, the practitioner should instill only 25 cc of saline to distend the bladder prior to clamping and pressure measurement. Higher amounts of fluid injection have been shown to falsely elevate the IAP recording (Cheatham *et al.*, 2007, Malbrain and Deeren, 2006; Malbrain, Delaet, and Cheatham, 2007; Tiwari, 2006; Wiegand, 2011). The World Society of the Abdominal Compartment Syndrome (WSACS) has published extensive guidelines and recommendations including a comprehensive evidence-based medicine approach to the diagnosis, management, and prevention of IAH/ACS (Malbrain and Deeren, 2006). This group has also published consensus definitions for IAP, IAH, and ACS which up until the point of the Society's meeting in 2006 had never been determined (Malbrain and Deeren, 2006). Effective management strategies as described earlier have been implemented in many institutions based on the education and research activities provided by the WSACS in an effort to improve the survival of patients with IAH and ACS (Malbrain and Deeren, 2006).

Diagnostics for liver function

In the assessment and management of the patient with ESLD or ALF, there is an armamentarium of tools and techniques. Laboratory evaluation of hepatic function is performed by measuring liver function tests. More than 70% of the parenchyma of the liver may be damaged before these tests

Clinical Pearls—Patient Management and Treatment

IAP should be measured with the patient in the supine position with the transducer leveled and zeroed at the iliac crest in the midaxillary line (Wiegand, 2011) (see Fig. 9.4). The sequelae of liver disease often result in the need for patients to be admitted to the critical care environment and to undergo a multitude of intensive diagnostic and therapeutic interventions.

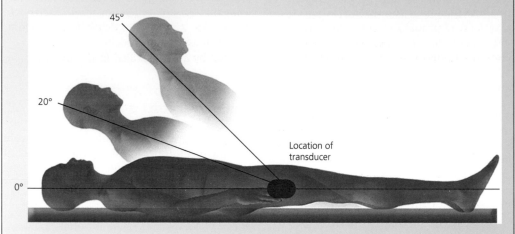

Figure 9.4 Patient positioning for intraabdominal pressure measurement.

become abnormal. Liver function is measured in terms of serum enzyme activity, protein levels, bilirubin, ammonia, clotting factors, and lipids (Smeltzer *et al.*, 2010). Ultrasound, CT, and magnetic resonance imaging (MRI) are also used to identify normal structures of the liver and biliary tree. A radioisotope liver scan may be performed to assess liver size and hepatic blood flow and obstruction (Smeltzer *et al.*, 2010). However, the evaluation of the patient with ESLD is most often guided by the results obtained from the performance of a liver biopsy.

Evidence-based treatment guidelines

Histological assessment of the liver via a liver biopsy is a cornerstone in the evaluation and management of patients with liver disease (Rockey *et al.*, 2009). A liver biopsy is the removal of a small amount of liver tissue usually through needle aspiration to examine liver cells. The most common indication is to evaluate disorders of the parenchyma. Therefore, liver biopsy is currently recommended for three major roles: (1) diagnosis,

(2) assessment of prognosis (disease staging), and/or (3) therapeutic management decisions (Rockey *et al.*, 2009). The practitioner must monitor for the development of intra- and postprocedure bleeding and bile peritonitis as potential serious complications after liver biopsy as well as for the occurrence of pain. Liver biopsy can be performed percutaneously with ultrasound guidance or transvenously via the right internal jugular vein to right hepatic vein under fluoroscopic guidance. Due to the risk of bleeding, the evidenced-based recommendation of the American Association for the Study of Liver Disease (AASLD) is that platelet transfusion be considered when platelet levels are less than 50 000–60 000/ml (Rockey *et al.*, 2009).

Liver support devices

Encephalopathy, coagulopathy, and hemodynamic instability may arise in patients with chronic liver failure or ALF. For the patient with ALF, however, these disorders can be even more life-threatening. As these patients are treated in the ICU and often await liver transplantation, they may require the additional support of liver dialysis to remove toxins the damaged liver can no longer metabolize and excrete. Artificial liver support systems are designed to purify blood by removing protein-bound and water-soluble toxins without providing liver synthetic functions. Currently available systems are based on albumin dialysis of plasma separation and filtration. Bioartificial liver support (BAL) refers to systems that use viable hepatocytes as components of an extracorporeal device connected to the patient's circulation, and thus have the potential to provide liver function. They consist of a bioreactor containing hepatocytes with or without a blood purification device. Studies examining the role of extracorporeal liver support systems have consistently demonstrated an improvement in hepatic encephalopathy (Sundarum and Shaikh, 2009) and other end-stage phenomenon of liver disease.

Liver support devices are used in many specialized facilities and units that manage liver failure in its chronic and acute (or fulminant) form. These devices seek to detoxify substances, and metabolize and synthesize materials when the liver no longer functions, in particular, in the patient with ALF. A variety of systems are available and/or under study such as sorbent systems that detoxify but have no hepatocyte replacement. These systems use charcoal or other adherent particles in an extracorporeal circuit. Transient improvement of hepatic encephalopathy may be observed but no improvement in hepatic function is seen. Other systems have attempted the use of porcine hepatocytes in a bioartificial liver (Polson and Lee, 2005).

Evidence-based treatment guidelines

The last published guidelines for the management of ALF (Polson and Lee, 2005) did not recommend the use of currently available liver support systems outside of clinical trials. Polson and Lee (2005) also stated that the future use of liver support systems in the management of ALF remains unclear. Since the publication of these guidelines, however, research and development of such systems has continued and, recently, the United States Food and Drug Administration (USFDA) did approve the use of liver support systems for the management of fulminant liver failure resulting from drug overdose, drug toxicity, or other toxic conditions adversely affecting liver function (Camus et al., 2009). This process is undertaken as a bridge to liver transplantation and is performed in an ICU setting, implemented by a team skilled in the management of hepatic disorders.

Guidelines for the management of patients with ALF recommend that these patients be treated in an ICU in a transplant center as the only life-saving measure for these patients is often liver transplantation. These guidelines also recommend that pulmonary artery catheterization (as previously discussed) be considered even in hemodynamically stable patients to ensure that appropriate volume replacement has occurred (Polson and Lee, 2005).

Balloon tamponade therapy

Balloon tamponade therapy is a procedure in which a specialized tube (e.g., Sengstaken–Blakemore, Linton and Minnesota tubes) is inserted into the patient with ESLD who is hemorrhaging from gastric or esophageal varices. The gastric balloon is inflated with 250–300 cc of air. It is then pulled snugly against the gastroesophageal junction. The esophageal balloon is inflated to 20–40 mmHg pressure for tamponade against bleeding esophageal varices. Esophageal balloon tamponade is useful for control of acute bleeding because of the direct, constant pressure that is applied to the varices. Traction on the tubes, which places constant pressure on the varices, is essential for effective tamponading. This may be used for temporary hemorrhage control. Long-term use has been implicated in a higher rate of rebleeding and an increased complication rate. It is recommended that the balloon not be inflated for more than 24 h. Esophageal necrosis, esophageal rupture, and tissue necrosis are some of the adverse effects from tamponade therapy (Baird and Bethel, 2011). Specialized practitioners caring for the patient with liver disease undergoing balloon tamponade therapy monitor the pressures in the esophageal balloon frequently (at least every 4h) and are careful that it does not exceed

40 mmHg, thus contributing to the development of complications. Management of volume resuscitation and blood transfusion are key factors in restoring the hemodynamic stability to an acutely bleeding patient.

As balloon tamponade therapy is a temporizing measure, plans should be made for patients to have a more definitive procedure to decrease portal pressure and the risk of bleeding. Transjugular intrahepatic portosystemic shunts (TIPS) are placed under radiologic guidance to create egress for portal blood flow through a balloon expandable stent to the systemic circulation. This procedure is successful in reducing portal hypertension and decompressing varices to control bleeding (Urden, Stacy, and Lough, 2010).

Evidence-based treatment guidelines

Guidelines have been published by the AASLD regarding the use of balloon tamponade therapy (Garcia-Tsao *et al.*, 2007). These guidelines describe this treatment as very effective in controlling bleeding temporarily with immediate control in the majority of patients. The use of a balloon tamponade, however, is associated with potentially lethal complications such as aspiration, migration, and necrosis/perforation of the esophagus with mortality rates as high as 20%. According to the AASLD guidelines (Garcia-Tsao *et al.*, 2007), its use should be restricted to patients with uncontrolled bleeding for whom a more definitive therapy such as a TIPS procedure is planned within 24 h of placement. Airway protection is strongly recommended when balloon tamponade therapy is used (Garcia-Tsao *et al.*, 2007). In the American Association of Critical Care Nurses Procedure Manual for Critical Care, it is recommended that the esophageal balloon port pressure be measured frequently based upon institution standards and be maintained at 25–45 mmHg (Wiegand, 2011).

The AASLD published practice guidelines for prevention and management of varices and variceal hemorrhage in cirrhosis also include the following recommendations (Garcia-Tsao *et al.*, 2007):

1 Use of beta blocker therapy to reduce portal pressure for the prevention of a first variceal hemorrhage in patients with medium to large esophageal varices.

2 Endoscopic variceal ligation (EVL) as an alternative to beta blockers for the prevention of an initial variceal hemorrhage.

3 Acute variceal hemorrhage should be managed with vasoconstrictive pharmacological therapy and variceal ligation. To prevent recurrent bleeding episodes, the use of EVL and pharmacologic agents is recommended.

4 A TIPS procedure or surgically created shunts may be used for those who fail medical therapy.

ICP monitoring in acute liver failure

As previously described, patients with ALF who develop encephalopathy have significant morbidity and mortality. The onset of cerebral edema and intracranial hypertension is not fully understood but these are two of the most serious consequences of ALF and can result in fatal uncal herniation (Polson and Lee, 2005).

The primary purpose of intracranial pressure (ICP) monitoring in this patient population is to detect elevations in ICP and reductions in cerebral perfusion pressure (CPP) so that interventions can be made to prevent herniation while preserving brain perfusion. The ultimate goal of such measures is to maintain neurological integrity and prolong survival while awaiting receipt of a donor organ or recovery of a sufficient functioning hepatocyte mass (Polson and Lee, 2005).

Evidenced-based treatment guidelines

The AASLD recommends the avoidance of sedation in the early stages of encephalopathy (Garcia-Tsao *et al.*, 2007). They also have stated that as patients progress to higher stages of encephalopathy, the head of the bed should be elevated to 30° to decrease ICP. At this stage, patients should be intubated to protect their airway. ICP monitoring and frequent assessment of neurological status is recommended to evaluate and aid in the treatment of intracerebral hemorrhage (ICH). The guidelines further state that ICH should be managed with hyperventilation and short-acting barbiturates may be considered for refractory ICH (Polson and Lee, 2005).

Ascites management

Ascites is another of the life-threatening sequelae of ESLD. Ascites, the accumulation of fluid in the peritoneal cavity, develops as a result of a multitude of contributing factors and the exact pathophysiology is unknown. Some of the complex, contributing factors include portal hypertension, hyperpermeable capillaries with leakage of lymph fluid, and albumin-rich fluid from the diseased liver, low serum albumin levels, and inappropriate sodium and water retention (Linton, 2012). According to the published clinical practice guidelines for the diagnosis of ascites, the initial evaluation of a patient with ascites should include history, physical examination, abdominal ultrasound, and laboratory assessment of liver function, renal function, serum, and urine electrolytes, as well as an analysis of the ascitic fluid. A diagnostic paracentesis should be performed in all patients with new-onset grade 2 (mild) or 3 (moderate) ascites, and in all patients hospitalized for worsening of ascites or any complication of cirrhosis (European Association for the Study of the Liver, 2010).

These guidelines also address recommended management strategies for ascites including those given in Table 9.5.

Measuring the abdominal girth and obtaining daily weights are important elements to monitor for the patient with ascites. Both these are markers of the severity of the fluid accumulation within the abdominal cavity and these data can assist the practitioner in assessing the progression of ascites and its response to treatment (Smeltzer et al., 2010).

Evidence-based treatment guidelines: Paracentesis

Paracentesis is the removal of ascitic fluid from the peritoneal cavity. This procedure is diagnostic and therapeutic. The procedure is indicated when ascites impairs the patient's breathing. Paracentesis removes fluid that impairs full respiratory excursion but it also removes essential proteins and electrolytes and provides a portal of entry for pathogens (Linton, 2012). The procedure may be performed at the patient's bedside or under ultrasound guidance. Paracentesis may result in the removal of 2–31 of fluid or more (Linton, 2012). The removal of up to 61 of fluid is termed total volume paracentesis (TVP) or large volume paracentesis (LVP) and is performed for those patients with refractory ascites whose ascites reaccumulates quickly. These patients are often awaiting liver transplantation. Whenever paracentesis is undertaken, it is performed slowly since rapid removal of fluid can result in circulatory collapse (Linton, 2012). Patients undergoing TVP may require the infusion of albumin during and after their procedure to replete circulating systemic volume and stabilize vital signs (Smeltzer et al., 2010).

According to the AASLD, abdominal paracentesis should be performed and ascitic fluid obtained from patients with clinically apparent new-onset ascites (Garcia-Tsao

Table 9.5 Management strategies for ascites.

Grade 1 mild ascites—only detectable by ultrasound	Moderate ascites—evident by moderate, symmetrical distension of the abdomen	Severe ascites—large or gross ascites with marked abdominal distension	Refractory ascites
No treatment	Restriction of sodium intake and diuretics	Large-volume paracentesis (LVP) followed by restriction of sodium intake and diuretics (unless patients have refractory ascites)	LVP with albumin administration, continuing diuretic therapy (if effective in inducing natriuresis), insertion of transjugular intrahepatic portosystemic shunt (TIPS), and liver transplantation

Source: European Association for the Study of the Liver (EASL) (2010).

et al., 2007). These guidelines do not recommend the routine prophylactic use of fresh frozen plasma or platelets before paracentesis since bleeding is sufficiently uncommon. The initial laboratory studies of ascitic fluid should include a cell count and differential, total protein, and serum-ascites albumin gradient (SAAG) as well as cultures if infection is suspected. Patient management also includes sodium restriction and diuretics. Liver transplantation should be considered in patients with cirrhosis and ascites. Additionally, serial therapeutic paracenteses should be considered a treatment option for those with refractory ascites. For large-volume paracenteses, an albumin infusion of 6–8 g/l of fluid can be considered. Lesser-volume paracenteses may not require this intervention (Runyon, 2009).

Clinical Pearls—Patient Management and Treatment

In order to identify life-threatening hypovolemia practitioners must closely monitor the ESLD patient after paracentesis. Vital signs are closely scrutinized at 15 min intervals until the patient is stable. The puncture site from the paracentesis should also be monitored for the presence of bleeding or hematoma formation. Fluid resuscitation with albumin, blood, coagulation factors, or other colloids may be needed for the unstable, hypotensive, or bleeding patient.

Nutritional assessment and treatment

The patient with liver disease or other GI disease requires an extensive nutritional history and assessment of nutritional parameters. The nutritional assessment includes an evaluation of laboratory data, anthropometric measurements, physical examination, and pertinent health history (Urden, Stacy, and Lough, 2010). The nutrition assessment includes the measurement of acute phase proteins such as albumin and prealbumin and evaluates hematologic values to determine deficiencies (Urden, Stacy, and Lough, 2010).

Evidence-based treatment guidelines

Ensuring adequate protein-calorie nutrition in all stages of liver disease is a highly recommended intervention for patients with liver disease, particularly ESLD (Sundarum and Shaikh, 2009). Guidelines published by the European Society for Clinical Nutrition and Metabolism recommend that patients with cirrhosis have an energy intake of 35–40 kcal/kg/day and a protein intake of 1.2–1.5 g/kg/day. If oral intake is inadequate, additional oral nutritional supplements or tube feeding should be commenced (Plauth *et al.*, 2006). Monitoring of patients as they receive these recommended nutrients includes nutritional intake history and laboratory assessment as described earlier.

Critical monitoring in acute pancreatitis

Many GI illnesses may result in critical illness and the need for intensive care monitoring. Those patients who develop severe acute pancreatitis often require intensive monitoring and care as they have great potential for experiencing any one of a number of systemic and local complications, none the least of which are hypovolemic shock and infected pancreatic necrosis. The two most important markers of severity in acute pancreatitis are organ failure (particularly multisystem organ failure) and pancreatic necrosis (Banks and Freeman, 2006).

Patients with severe acute pancreatitis are monitored closely for the development of respiratory complications while in the critical care unit. The onset of hypovolemic shock, acute lung injury, or sepsis must be identified rapidly and treated aggressively with volume resuscitation, intubation and mechanical ventilation, antibiotic therapy and/or surgery. Additionally, in order to ensure achievement of the goal of adequate volume resuscitation, central venous pressures or pulmonary artery pressures are often monitored in this population. Most recently, less invasive monitoring with cardiac output measurement via pulse contour waveform analysis, which calculates stroke volume and/or cardiac output derived from an arterial catheter (as previously described), has been used for assessment of volume status.

Evidence-based treatment guidelines for acute pancreatitis

Published guidelines in acute pancreatitis include vigorous fluid resuscitation monitored in a variety of ways including a progressive decrease in hematocrit at 12 and 24 h post diagnosis. Bedside oxygen saturation should be monitored at frequent intervals and blood gases should be obtained when clinically indicated, particularly when oxygen saturation is ≤95%. Patients should be monitored in an ICU if there is sustained organ failure or there are other indications that the pancreatitis is severe including oliguria, persistent tachycardia, and labored respiration (Banks and Freeman, 2006). However, no guidelines currently exist for the use of hemodynamic monitoring in the setting of severe acute pancreatitis.

Monitoring elements: pancreatitis

Meeting nutritional needs in acute pancreatitis is a mainstay of treatment. Based upon many randomized, controlled studies, experts recommend the use of enteral feedings, which are believed to stabilize gut barrier function and reduce gut permeability to bacteria and endotoxins. When the goal of optimum nutritional support is achieved, systemic complications may be reduced and morbidity and mortality statistics improved (Banks and Freeman, 2006).

Evidence-based treatment guidelines for acute pancreatitis

As with many GI disorders there are practice guidelines addressing nutrition in patients with acute pancreatitis. Patients who are unlikely to resume oral nutrition within 5 days due to sustained organ failure or other indications require nutritional support. Whenever possible, enteral feeding rather than total parenteral nutrition (TPN) is suggested for patients who require nutritional support (Banks and Freeman, 2006).

Patients who are suspected of harboring gallstones as the mechanism for their pancreatitis and who have signs of severe systemic toxicity should undergo endoscopic retrograde choangiopancreatography with sphincterotomy and stone removal. Regardless of the cause of the acute pancreatitis, patients should not receive prophylactic antibiotics. It is reasonable to administer appropriate antibiotics in necrotizing pancreatitis with signs of infection and/or organ failure while cultures are being obtained. Antibiotics should be discontinued if no source of infection is identified. In the setting of an expected infection of necrotic pancreatic parenchyma, CT-guided percutaneous aspiration with Gram's stain and culture is recommended. The treatment of choice for infected necrosis is surgical debridement if the patient can tolerate it. Other less invasive techniques such as endoscopic and radiologic debridement may be undertaken in centers that have the capabilities to perform these procedures (Banks and Freeman, 2006).

Summary

GI disturbances are a frequent issue in critically ill patient care. In this chapter, monitoring modalities and nursing management priorities have been highlighted. As research advances clinical understanding of GI management and treatment, additional standards of practice will emerge. Currently, overall evidence for monitoring and surveillance is moderate and much further research on effective protocols to enhance patient outcomes is needed.

References

Adler, D.G. (2004) ASGE guideline: the role of endoscopy in acute non-variceal upper GI hemorrhage. *Gastrointestinal Endoscopy*, **60** (4), 300–304.

Ali, T. and Harty, R.F. (2009) Stress-induced ulcer bleeding in critically ill patients. *Gastroenterology Clinics*, **38** (2), 245–265.

Andrus, C.H. (1987) The effects of irrigant temperature in upper gastrointestinal hemorrhage: a requiem for iced saline lavage. *The American Journal of Gastroenterology*, **82** (10), 1062.

Bahner, D. (2008) AIUM practice guidelines for the performance of the focused assessment with sonography for trauma (FAST) examination. *Journal of Ultrasound Medicine*, **27** (2), 313–318.

Baird, M.S. and Bethel, S. (2011) *Manual of Critical Care Nursing: Nursing Interventions & Collaborative Management*, 6th edn, Mosby, St Louis.

Banks, P.A. and Freeman, M.L. (2006) Practice Guidelines in Acute Pancreatitis. *American Journal of Gastroenterology*, **101**, 2379–2400.

Camus, C., Lavoue, S., Gacouin A. *et al.* (2009) Liver transplantation avoided in patients with fulminant hepatic failure who received albumin dialysis with the molecular adsorbent recirculating system while on the waiting list: impact of the duration of therapy. *Therapeutic Apheresis and Dialysis*, **13** (6), 549–555.

Cappell, M.S. and Batke, M. (2008a) Mechanical obstruction of the small bowel and colon. *Medical Clinics of North America*, **92** (3), 575–597.

Cappell, M.S. and Friedel, D. (2008b) Acute nonvariceal upper gastrointestinal bleeding: endoscopic diagnosis and therapy. *Medical Clinics of North America*, **92** (3), 511–550.

Cappell, M.S. and Freidel, D. (2008) Initial management of acute upper gastrointestinal bleeding: from initial evaluation up to gastrointestinal endoscopy. *Medical Clinics of North America*, **92** (3), 491–509.

Carlesso, E., Taccone P., and Gattinoni, L. (2006) Gastric tonometry. *Minerva Anesthesiology*, **72** (6), 529–532.

Cheatham, M.L., Malbrain, M.L., Kirkpatrick, A. *et al.* (2007) Results from the international conference of experts on intra-abdominal hypertension and abdominal compartment syndrome: II: recommendations. *Intensive Care Medicine*, **33** (6), 951–962.

Conteras, M. (1998) Final statement from the consensus conference on platelet transfusion. *Transfusion*, **38** (8), 796–797.

European Association for the Study of the Liver (EASL) (2010) EASL clinical practice guidelines on the management of ascites, spontaneous bacterial peritonitis, and hepatorenal syndrome in cirrhosis. *Journal of Hepatology*, **53** (3), 397–417.

Fennerty, M.B. (2002) Pathophysiology of the upper gastrointestinal tract in the critically ill patient: rationale for the therapeutic benefits of acid suppression *Critical Care Medicine*, **30** (S), 351–352.

Garcia-Tsao, G., Sanyal, A.J., Grace, N.D., and Carey, W. (2007) Prevention and management of gastroesophageal varices and variceal hemorrhage in cirrhosis. *Hepatology*, **46** (3), 922–938.

Gilbert, D.A. and Saunders, D.R. (1981) Iced saline lavage does not slow bleeding from experimental canine ulcers. *Digestive Diseases and Science*, **26** (12), 1065–1068.

Guillamondegui, O.D., Gunter, O.L., Bonadies, J.A. *et al.* (2008) Practice management guidelines for stress ulcer prophylaxis. Eastern Association for the Surgery of Trauma. EAST Practice Management guidelines committee, www.east.org (accessed July 24, 2014).

Johnson, K.L. (2005) Diagnostic measures to evaluate oxygenation in critically ill adults. *AACN Clinical Issues*, **15** (4), 506–524.

Kumar, R. and Mills, A.M. (2011) Gastrointestinal bleeding. *Emergency Medical Clinics of North America*, **29**, 239–252.

Linton, A.D. (2012) *Introduction to Medical-Surgical Nursing*, 5th edn, Elsevier/Saunders, St Louis.

Malbrain, M.L.N.G. and Deeren, D. (2006) Effect of bladder volume on measuring intravesical pressure: a prospective cohort study. *Critical Care Forum*, **10** (4), 1–6.

Malbrain, M.L.N.G., Delaet, I., and Cheatham, M.L. (2007) Consensus conference definition and recommendations on intraabdominal hypertension (IAH) and the abdominal compartment syndrome (ACS). *Acta Clinica Belgica*, **62** (Suppl 1), 44–59.

Maltz, G.S., Siegel, J.E., and Carson, J.L. (2000) Hematologic management of gastrointestinal bleeding. *Gastroenterology Clinics of North America*, **29** (1), 169–187.

Marik, P.E. (2001) Sublingual capnography: a clinical validation study. *Chest*, **120** (3), 923–927.

Marshall, A.P. and West, S.H. (2004) Gastric tonometry and monitoring gastrointestinal perfusion: using research to support nursing practice. *Nursing Critical Care*, **9** (3), 123–133.

Nettina, S.M. (2010) *Lippincott's Manual of Nursing Practice*, 9th edn, Wolters Kluwer Health/Lippincott, Williams, Wilkins, Philadelphia.

Plauth, M., Cabre, E., Riggio, O. *et al.* (2006) ESPEN guidelines on enteral nutrition: liver disease. *Clinical Nutrition*, **25** (2), 285–294.

Polson, J. & Lee, W.M. (2005) American Association for the Study of Liver Disease position paper: the management of acute liver failure. *Hepatology*, **41** (5), 1179–1197.

Ponsky, J.L., Hoffman, M., and Swayngim, D.S. (1980) Gastric bleeding time in dogs is prolonged when iced saline lavage is used. *Journal of Surgical Research*, **28**, 204–205.

Rockey, D.C., Caldwell, S.H., Goodman, Z.D. *et al.* (2009) American Association on the Science of Liver Disease (AASLD) position paper: liver biopsy. *Hepatology*, **49** (3), 1017–1044.

Runyon, B.A. (2009) Management of adult patients with ascites due to cirrhosis: an update (AASLD Practice Guideline). *Hepatology*, **49** (6), 2087–2107.

Scottish Intercollegiate Guidelines Network (SIGN) (2008) *Management of Acute Upper and Lower*

Gastrointestinal Bleeding: A National Clinical Guideline, Scottish Intercollegiate Guideline Network, Edinburgh.

Shanley, C.J. and Weinberger, J.B. (2008) Acute abdominal vascular emergencies. *Medical Clinics of North America*, **92** (3), 627–647.

Smeltzer, S.C., Bare, B.G., Hinkle, J.L., and Cheever, K.H. (eds) (2010) *Brunner & Suddarth's Textbook of Medical-Surgical Nursing*, 12th edn, Wolters Kluwer Health/Lippincott Williams & Wilkins, Philadelphia.

Smith, J.E. and Hall, E.J. (2009) The use of plain abdominal X-rays in the emergency department. *Emergency Medicine Journal*, **26** (3), 160–163.

Stonesifer, E. (2004) Common laboratory and diagnostic testing in patients with gastrointestinal disease. *AACN Clinical Issues*, **15** (4), 580–594.

Strehlow, M.C., (2010) Early identification of shock in critically ill patients. *Emergency Medicine Clinics of North America*, **28**, 57–66.

Sundarum, V. and Shaikh, O.S. (2009) Hepatic encephalopathy: pathophysiology and emerging therapies. *Medical Clinics of North America*, **93** (4), 819–836.

Tiwari, A. (2006) Recognition and management of abdominal compartment syndrome in the United Kingdom. *Intensive Care Medicine*, **32** (6), 906–909.

Urden, L.D., Stacy, K.M., and Lough, M.E. (eds) (2010) *Critical Care Nursing: Diagnosis & Management*, Mosby/Elsevier, St. Louis.

Waterman, N.G. and Walker, J.L. (1973) The effect of gastric cooling on hemostasis. *Surgical Gynecology & Obstetrics*, **137**, 80–82.

Wiegand, D.L.M. (ed.) (2011) *AACN's Procedure Manual for Critical Care*, Elsevier/Saunders, St. Louis.

CHAPTER 10

Traumatic injuries: Special considerations

Catherine L. Bond and Mary Beth Voights

Carle Foundation Hospital, Urbana, IL., USA

Trauma is the leading cause of death for persons less than 44 years of age and the fifth leading cause for all ages (Center for Disease Control [CDC], 2010). Injury results from a transfer of energy to the body tissues. The exact mechanism and patient's tissue resistance to that force will determine the exact injuries. Expected injuries differ based on type and speed of blunt mechanisms (unrestrained driver with side impact, pedestrian struck by motor vehicle, fall from 30 ft landing upright, diving into 4 foot pool, etc.). Weapon, predicted path, velocity, and caliber of the missile, along with distance of the victim from the perpetrator will provide insight into the expected injuries in the patient with penetrating trauma. The reader is directed to more in-depth kinematic references to further develop their knowledge of this concept if desired (McQuillan, Flynn-Makic, and Whelan, 2008).

Primary, secondary, and tertiary surveys

Standardized, sequential evaluations of the trauma patient are the best methods to identify injuries. This evaluation is divided into three distinct surveys with specific assessments, interventions, and goals (see Table 10.1). The American College of Surgeons (ACS) (2008) has developed the primary and secondary surveys to rapidly evaluate and correct life-threatening injury along with a standardized exam to identify most of the significant injuries.

The primary survey takes approximately 90 seconds and should be performed with each first patient encounter as life-threatening conditions can develop as a result of missed injuries, massive fluid resuscitation, or systemic inflammatory response syndrome (SIRS). The secondary survey is a head-to-toe assessment designed to include each body system, identify significant injuries, and prompt appropriate and prioritized intervention. The tertiary survey is a systems-based assessment including a review of diagnostic studies and lab results (Table 10.2). It should be performed each day to identify covert or evolving injuries or complications. This survey is an essential component for advanced practice nurses (APNs) in the postresuscitation phase of care.

Biffl, Harrington, and Cioffi (2003) noted that this survey is especially important in the absence of a full secondary survey. Not surprisingly, their group identified more missed injuries in patients with higher acuity. The more critically injured patients often have an abbreviated secondary survey to accommodate emergency surgical procedures and altered neurologic function, which limits the secondary survey. Inadequate, misinterpreted, or unordered radiologic exams, admission to a nonsurgical service, and low index of suspicion add to the potential for missed injury or unrecognized development of complications (Hollingsworth-Fridlund, 2001). The surveys should be performed by each provider caring for the patient as the multidisciplinary approach will often reveal the most complete set of injuries that require intervention.

Critical Care Nursing: Monitoring and Treatment for Advanced Nursing Practice, First Edition. Edited by Kathy J. Booker.
© 2015 John Wiley & Sons, Inc. Published 2015 by John Wiley & Sons, Inc.

Table 10.1 Primary and secondary survey of the trauma patient.

Primary survey	Life threat/assessment	Intervention
Airway	Airway obstruction	Airway maneuvers Mechanical airways
Breathing	Tension pneumothorax Massive hemothorax Open pneumothorax Flail chest	Needle thoracentesis/chest tube Chest tube/autotransfusion Three-sided dressing/chest tube Pressure support ventilation
Circulation	Cardiac tamponade Hypovolemic shock	Pericardiocentesis Direct pressure to hemorrhaging wounds/fluid bolus/targeted therapy
Disability	Expanding focal hematoma Neurogenic shock	Craniotomy/targeted therapy Fluid bolus followed by pressor agents
Exposure/back	Missed life threat wound	
Secondary survey: head-to-toe exam	**Assessments**	**Interventions to define/manage**
Head		
Scalp/skull injuries	Scalp for laceration, hematomas, evidence of fracture/palpable defects Otorrhea/rhinorrhea	Soft tissue management (cleansing, repair)
Head injury Eye injury	Level of consciousness, GCS, pupils, and presence of eye injury Nerve and bony integrity; malocclusion	If open fracture, IV antibiotics and anticipate surgical intervention CT scan to define neuroinjury Ocular shield/prevent pressure if open globe CT/panorex scan for facial/dental fractures
Face/dental		
Bone/teeth/nerve or soft tissue injuries		
Neck		
Bony, laryngeal, vascular, esophageal injuries	Deformity, pain, tenderness, crepitus, expanding hematoma, bruit	Maintain spinal stabilization/collars; cervical spine CT scan Laryngoscopy Angiography/duplex exam Esophagoscopy
Chest	Chest wall tenderness, crepitus, decreased breath sounds	Chest X-ray or CT; tube thoracostomy if hemo/hemopneumothorax or pneumothorax visible on plain film or respiratory distress (occult pneumothoraces do not require tube thoracostomy)
Rib, pneumo/hemothoraces, pulmonary contusion, tracheobronchial or vascular/cardiac injury	Sub Q emphysema	Pain management
	Unequal arm BP or pulse	Angiography, contrast CT, or transesophageal (TE) echocardiogram
	Severe back pain Muffled heart tones	Pericardiocentesis

(Continued)

Table 10.1 (*Continued*)

Primary survey	Life threat/assessment	Intervention
Abdomen/flank	Distention, tenderness, guarding, rigidity, signs of bleeding (Kehr, Cullen, Gray–Turner)	Gastric decompression
		Ultrasound or diagnostic Peritoneal lavage
Intraabdominal or retroperitoneal injury; abdominal wall injury	Open wounds/potential trajectory	CT scan with contrast
		Exploratory laparotomy
Pelvis/perineum	Hematuria, perineal hematomas	Retrograde urethrogram
Genitourinary injury	Unstable pelvis/wide symphysis	Cystogram
Pelvis fractures	Rectal exam for select patients: tone/frank blood/high riding prostate	Suprapubic catheter if ureteral or bladder disruption
Rectal injury	Vaginal exam for selected patients	Pelvis X-ray or CT with contrast
		Pelvic stabilization (wrap/binder/C clamp)
		Arterial embolization for persistent hypotension without alternate cause
Spine	Pain, tenderness, stepoffs	Spinal stabilization (collars/logroll) until radiologic or clinical clearance
Bony or cord injuries	Motor function	CT scan or plain X-rays
Nerve root injury	Sensory perception	MRI
Extremities	Pain, tenderness, deformity, edema	Immobilization (splint/surgery)
Fractures	Defects, lacerations	Targeted X-rays
Joint instability	Pulse deficits, pallor	Doppler/angiography/interventional embolization
Soft tissue injury	Tense muscle compartments	Compartment pressure measurement/fasciotomy
Vascular injury	Peripheral nerve deficits	
Peripheral nerve injury		
Skin/wounds	Lacerations, hematomas, deep abrasions, burns/frostbite	Cleansing, repair
		Ice packs

Table 10.2 Tertiary survey of the trauma patient.

Tertiary Survey: head-to-toe exam and review of diagnostic exams/plan	Assessments	Goals
Head	Scalp for laceration, hematomas, evidence of fracture	Confirm/rule out vault fractures
	Level of consciousness, GCS, pupils, eye movement, and visual acuity	Evaluate/confirm severity of brain injury based on clinical exams and diagnostic studies
	Review head CT: results/recommended follow-up	Confirm/rule out ocular and cranial nerve injury
		Potential consultants: neurosurgery, ophthalmology, plastics
Face	Facial nerves; bony integrity; malocclusion; CSF leak, hemotympaneum, hearing loss	Evaluate/rule out facial and basilar skull fractures and cranial nerve injury
		Potential consultants: oral maxillofacial, ENT, plastics
Neck/cervical spine	Soft tissue injury, swelling, subcutaneous emphysema	Evaluate/rule out neck, laryngeal, vascular, and spine injury or need for more detailed radiologic exams
	Spine stepoffs/pain/tenderness	Potential consultants: spine, gastroenterology, vascular, interventional radiology
	Review cervical spine clearance (radiographically or clinically)	
Chest	Soft tissue injury, subcutaneous emphysema, tenderness or deformity, paradoxical movement	Pain control; consideration of epidural analgesia or topical patch
	Breath sounds	Chest tube presence/function/output
	Hemodynamic values	Need for ventilatory support
	Review chest X-ray or CT scan	Need for volume replacement, pressor support or diuresis
		Need for follow-up detailed radiologic exams
		Note incidental findings and implications/need for future evaluation
		Potential consultants: cardiovascular surgery, cardiology
Abdomen	Ecchymosis, open wounds, tenderness, guarding, or masses	Wound care/need for antibiotic therapy
	Hemodynamic values	Evaluate/confirm abdominal or renal injury
	Urinary output	Need for follow-up detailed radiologic exams
	Tube/drain outputs (character and volume)	Note incidental findings and implications/need for future evaluation
	Review CT scan	Potential consultants: urology
Pelvis	Palpate for stability	Confirm or rule out pelvis/acetabular fractures
	Hemodynamic values	Need for follow-up detailed radiologic exams
	Review pelvis CT scan or X-ray	Note incidental findings and implications/need for future evaluation
		Potential consultants: orthopedic, interventional radiology

(Continued)

Table 10.1 (*Continued*)

Tertiary Survey: head-to-toe exam and review of diagnostic exams/plan	Assessments	Goals
Back	Inspect entire posterior surface of head/body for soft tissue injury Palpate spine and ribs for deformity/stepoffs/tenderness Review spine X-rays/CT scan/MRI	Confirm or rule out spine injury Need for follow-up detailed radiologic exams Note incidental findings and implications/need for future evaluation Potential consultants: spine
Extremity	Inspect for soft tissue injury Assess circulation Assess motor function Assess sensory integrity Assess joint integrity Palpate for tenderness, crepitus, edema, pain with movement, tense motor compartments Review X-rays	Confirm or rule out extremity injury Identify need for follow-up detailed radiologic exams Note incidental findings and implications/need for future evaluation Potential consultants: orthopedics, vascular, plastics
Skin	Assess for soft tissue injury	Local wound care Possible consultants: wound care, plastics
Lab	Review lab results	Identify need for follow-up detailed exams Initiate surveillance labs

An additional family survey begins in the intensive care phase. This survey, completed by bedside providers, social work, chaplaincy, case management, and rehabilitation coordinator, assesses the strengths and options of the family considering the acuity, impact, and likely disposition of these patients. For some, the task of caring for the acutely injured patient is overwhelming and alternate dispositions (extended care, nursing home, or hospice) must be pursued early versus targeting disposition to rehabilitation or home. Early survey of the expected physical, psychosocial, and emotional outcomes of the patient's injury and factors that will impact their return to functional status should guide the treatment plan beginning in the intensive care unit (ICU) phase of care.

Fluid resuscitation

Controversy exists regarding fluid resuscitation of the trauma patient. Clear guidelines for which fluid to use, when to introduce colloids, and when to end measures of resuscitation are lacking.

Fluid choice
- Crystalloids remain the fluid of choice for the initial replacement of vascular space losses. Lactated ringers solution remains the preferred choice (American College of Surgeons Committee on Trauma, 2008). Recent studies suggest that lactated ringers could be deleterious and normal saline is

preferred (Adewale, 2009). Targeted initial volume replacement is a 1–2 liter bolus for adults and 20 cc/kg for children. Ongoing volume is calculated to produce adequate urine output (>0.5 cc/h for adults; 1 cc/kg/h for children, and 2 cc/kg/h for infants).
- Hypertonic saline shows some promise for hemorrhagic shock replacement with limited postresuscitation lung injury and the added benefit of osmotic diuresis for the head injured population (Adewale, 2009).
- Approximately 25% of the crystalloids will be retained in the vascular space; 75% will extravasate into the interstitial space (Boldt, 2008). Increased fluid volume will sequester in the thoracic region and associated electrolyte imbalances should be anticipated (McQuillan, Flynn-Makic, and Whelan, 2008).
- Blood products are transfused in response to ongoing hemorrhage. Initial replacement, based on time of availability, will include nontyped or cross-matched blood (O-negative for women of childbearing age; O-positive for others), followed by type-specific and fully cross-matched blood. Additional components (fresh frozen plasma, platelets, cryoprecipitate) are added based on ongoing losses and laboratory results.
- Massive transfusion protocols
- Product ratios differ and no single ratio has been determined to yield the best outcomes at this point (Shaz et al., 2010). Table 10.3 contains a copy of the shipment table used in our institution based on current nonmilitary

Table 10.3 Massive transfusion product (MTP) shipment table.

Labs	Shipment	RBC	FFP	Platelets	CRYO
Original panel with MTP protocol activation	1	6 (O-negative) or O-positive if male >16 years	4 (AB) sent as soon as ready	1	
	2	6	4	1	
Coags collected	3	6	4		
	4	6	4	1 if platelet count <50K	10 if fibrinogen <100 mg/dl
Coags collected	5	6	4		
	6	6	4	1 if platelet count <50K	10 if fibrinogen <100 mg/dl
Coags collected	7	6	4		
	8	6	4	1 if platelet count <50K	10 if fibrinogen <100 mg/dl
Coags collected	9	6	4		

literature. The shipments of blood product continue until the active bleeding has been controlled, injury site oozing becomes limited, end points normalize (arterial pH, hemoglobin/hematocrit, fibrinogen, platelets, core temperature), or efforts are recognized as futile.

Clinical Pearls

The key is to have these protocols in place before they are needed. Their development and ongoing success are a collaborative effort of the surgeons, anesthesiologists, intensivists, blood bank, phlebotomy, and nursing.

End points of resuscitation

An extensive review of the literature was undertaken by Tisherman and colleagues (2004) to define optimal end point measurements for trauma resuscitation. Their work has become a guideline in the Eastern Association of Surgery for Trauma (EAST). Tisherman *et al.* (2004) noted that standard clinical parameters (blood pressure, heart rate, urine volume) are inadequate markers of organ perfusion. Multiple other measurements including hemodynamic profiles, acid–base status, gastric tonometry, and regional measures of tissue O_2 and CO_2 levels have been used and studied to determine which, if any, are preferred. This review could not identify a specific parameter that was optimal in monitoring patients to prevent organ failure and death, resulting in a recommendation to utilize any one of these more discrete measurements rather than the standard vital signs and urinary output to measure effectiveness of resuscitation efforts. No studies since the deployment of this guideline have refuted this recommendation. An entire Critical Care Nursing Clinics volume was devoted to ongoing monitoring and hemodynamics and includes more details on each of these modalities (Leeper, 2006). Articles within this edition that are most useful when addressing patients with traumatic injury include transcutaneous CO_2 Monitoring; End Tidal CO_2 Monitoring; Bispectral Index Monitoring during Sedation; and Brain Tissue Oxygen Monitoring.

Intracompartmental monitoring

The brain lives in a closed space with finite limits and little room for anything extra. In an adult, the intracranial volume is 1200–1500 cc. The three components of cerebral volume are cerebral tissue (80%), cerebral blood flow (12%), and cerebrospinal fluid (8%). Any increase in volume in one compartment must be matched by a similar reduction in another compartment or intracranial pressure (ICP) will rise. This is known as the Monroe–Kellie hypothesis. The objective of ICP monitoring is to optimize cerebral perfusion pressure (CPP) and oxygenation and minimize secondary brain injury while allowing time for the brain to heal. CPP is an indirect reflection of cerebral perfusion: mean arterial pressure (MAP) minus ICP. CPP less than 50 is associated with poor outcomes. Continuous monitoring of ICP and blood pressure is the key to managing the changes in the three components of cerebral volume that shift and can cause cerebral hypoperfusion and ultimately herniation (A Joint Project of the Brain Trauma Foundation and American Association of Neurological Surgeons, 2007). These guidelines support ICP monitoring of patients with severe traumatic brain injury and a normal head computed tomography (CT) and who have any two of the following present on admission: age over 40 years, unilateral or bilateral motor posturing, or systolic blood pressure less than 90. Monitoring of ICP in patients with a Glasgow Coma Score of 8 or less with an abnormal CT scan is a supported recommendation from the Brain Trauma Foundation (2007) Guidelines for the Management of Head Injury. Data from monitoring ICP can be used for prognosis, guiding therapies aimed at reducing ICP, increasing MAP, measurement of intraventricular pressure, and guidance of therapeutic drainage of cerebrospinal fluid to decrease cerebral volume. Increasing ICP can be one of the first signs of worsening brain edema or bleeding that may require surgical intervention. See also Chapter 6.

Figure 10.1 using concepts further detailed in Bullock *et al.* (2006), Coplin, 2001, Cushman *et al.* (2010)., and Schirmer *et al.* (2008), illustrates the relationship of elements used in managing head injury patients.

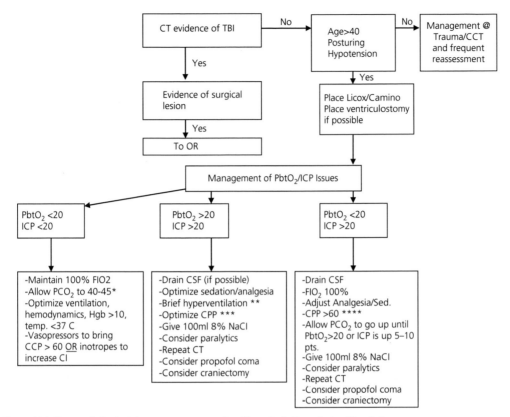

Figure 10.1 Traumatic brain injury management algorithm, Carle Foundation Hospital.
*Unless ICP rises >20.
**Stop if PbtO$_2$ falls <20.
***Vasopressors to bring CPP>60. Inotropes to increase CI.
****If CPP<60, consider inotropes. If CPP<60, consider vasopressors.
NOTE: This protocol provides for all factors that should be considered.

Complications

Caring for trauma patients is not just about knowing how to deal with the injuries, but being able to anticipate and prevent complications. Patients are at risk for some complications simply due to pain and immobility. Other complications are more specific to the mechanism or injury itself. Many times the risks revolve around some alteration in clotting. Many patients are at risk for deep vein thrombosis (DVT) or emboli from areas of vascular injury. Other patients may have prolonged clotting, such as patients who are on chronic anticoagulation or who develop disseminated intravascular coagulation (DIC).

Thromboembolic events

Just as in any bedridden patient, DVT is always a risk. One of the issues in trauma is whether DVT prophylaxis is safe for the patient. Patients with intracranial bleeding, solid organ injury, or major pelvic fractures are at high risk of bleeding, and therefore may need to go without any anticoagulants for 72 h or more. While low–molecular weight heparin or unfractionated heparin may increase risk of expansion of intracranial hemorrhages, Dudley *et al.* (2010)

showed that patients with two consecutive CT scans demonstrating hemorrhagic stability who were started on DVT prophylaxis within 48–72 h had relatively high protection from thromboembolic events and low risk of intracranial hemorrhage. Inferior vena cava (IVC) filters can be used for patients at high risk of DVT who cannot be anticoagulated for many days but IVC filters are not without risk. Other patients can have potential for upper extremity clots either from antecubital peripherally inserted central catheter (PICC) lines or upper extremity vascular injury. Superior vena cava (SVC) filters are difficult to place and come with their own set of potential complications. Patient data from the Trauma Registry of the German Society for Trauma Surgery, including 35,000 trauma patients screened for clinically relevant venous thromboembolic events (VTEs), found that 80.8% of patients with VTE were under chemical or mechanical prophylaxis at the time of the event, and two-thirds of the events occurred within 3 weeks of admission (Paffrath *et al.*, 2010).

Clinical Pearls

Devastating injury from carotid or vertebral artery dissection or flaps causing emboli to travel to the brain resulting in stroke may also arise. Recently, in our trauma center, a 21-year-old patient suffered right-side hemiparesis and expressive aphasia from a clot to the middle cerebral artery following cervical hyperextension in a motor vehicle crash.

Anticoagulation

Many older patients are admitted with some type of anticoagulation. Warfarin and various platelet inhibitors can cause bleeding problems after trauma. Older patients with falls are often admitted with intracranial bleeding related to chronic anticoagulation or antiplatelet drugs. Bleeding risk in solid organ injury or major orthopedic injury also increases with elevated international normalized ratio (INR) or decreased platelet function. Massive transfusion protocols may be utilized for anticoagulated patients who require emergent surgery and develop DIC (see Table 10.3). Older patients requiring reversal of anticoagulation

may require multiple units of fresh frozen plasma and require close monitoring for fluid overload.

Pain management

Many complications are directly related to pain control. In trauma patients, pain control is extremely important to avoid complications associated with immobility and hypoventilation. Patients with chest trauma, including multiple rib fractures and pulmonary contusions, need adequate pain control in order to continue with aggressive pulmonary toilet to prevent pneumonia and lobar collapse. Pneumonia may develop secondary to a combination of factors including hypoventilation, aspiration, inadequate pain management, atelectasis, and pooling of secretions.

Early mobilization

Mobilization is also a key factor in the prevention of complications. While historically the ICU has not been a place where patients spend a lot of time out of bed, new studies support mobilizing even mechanically ventilated patients (Bourdin, 2010; Kress, 2009). This requires a multidisciplinary team effort including nurses, respiratory, physical, and occupational therapies. The improvement in outcomes such as ability of patients to ambulate on discharge and shortened length of stay make the coordination of these interventions essential and worth the effort (Kress, 2009). Bourdin (2010) found that getting the ICU patient into the chair resulted in a decline in heart rate by a mean of 3.5 beats per minute and decreased respiratory rate of 1.4 breaths per minute, while oxygen saturation and arterial blood pressure were not adversely affected. While there can be many barriers to getting trauma patients out of bed, the positive outcomes include improvement in pulmonary status, gut function, and overall endurance.

Thoracic injury management

Rib fractures can easily be underestimated as a major injury. Patients, especially elderly patients, can very quickly decompensate as they take only very shallow inspirations due to pain from multiple rib fractures. The gold standard for pain control in rib fractures is the use of the epidural infusion for analgesia (Simon *et al.*, 2012). However, this can only be used in patients without exposure to anticoagulation and without spinal injury. When an epidural is not possible, scheduled oral medication or patient-controlled analgesia combined with a continuous infusion of narcotic may be warranted. Patients must be carefully monitored for respiratory depression. The balance between adequate pain relief and neurologic and respiratory depression is a key measure for continuous monitoring.

Another risk associated with chest injury is pleural effusion. The patient with rib fractures and/or pulmonary contusion is at risk for effusion 3–5 days post injury. Patients already at risk for respiratory insufficiency may have worsening inspiratory volumes due to the collection of pleural fluid, limiting tidal volume. Drainage with chest tubes or thoracentesis is often required. These patients are followed closely with daily chest X-rays and continuous oxygen saturation monitoring.

Use of narcotics for pain control can contribute to respiratory depression and increasing carbon dioxide levels, not readily apparent in oxygen saturation monitoring. These patients may require alternate modes of both oxygen delivery and ventilation support. Use of bilevel positive airway pressure (BiPAP) for ventilation support or continuous positive airway pressure (CPAP) for oxygenation support may become necessary to prevent progression to respiratory failure (see Chapter 3).

Pneumothorax or hemopneumothorax may occur as the primary injury in blunt chest trauma, or can occur as a possible complication from rib fractures or pulmonary contusion. Chest tube thoracotomy is the treatment of choice. Pain control is again important for these patients and monitoring for adequate oxygenation and ventilation is essential. Not only are rib fractures painful, but the insertion of the chest tube adds to the painful experience. Empyema may develop due to inadequately drained hemothorax, infected parapneumonic effusion, trauma, esophageal perforation, or bronchopleural fistula (Ahmed & Zangan, 2012).

Abdominal trauma

Abdominal trauma can be classified as blunt or penetrating. Complications may include bleeding and infection. Bleeding can occur from inadequate hemostasis or coagulopathy. Hypothermia from administration of multiple blood products, large volumes of room temperature fluids, or prolonged operating room time can also cause coagulopathy. Other complications include intra-abdominal abscess, cholangitis, and biliary fistula. Splenic injuries may result in complications, with the most serious overwhelming post-splenectomy sepsis (OPSS) occurring in 1–2% of patients. OPSS is characterized by an initial "flu-like" syndrome followed by an abrupt onset of fever, chills, nausea, and vomiting. Post-splenectomy patients are prophylactically immunized with pneumococcal (Pneumovax), meningococcal, and *Haemophilus influenzae* vaccines to prevent this. Initial treatment is focused on trying to preserve the spleen, but if watchful waiting is unsuccessful, post-op complications can include bleeding, abscess formation, and pancreatitis.

All trauma patients are at risk for bowel complications. Specific injuries may cause patients to be at higher risk for paralytic ileus. In penetrating trauma, small bowel injury is the most commonly seen (up to 80%) in gun shot wounds (GSWs) and also has a high incidence in general penetrating trauma. Common complications include hemorrhage, suture line disruption, and small bowel malabsorption syndrome. Pelvic fractures, thoracic and lumbar spine injuries, repetitive anesthesia, and abdominal organ injury cause decreased bowel motility and, combined with narcotics for analgesia and immobility, can result in prolonged hospital stays, delay to enteral nutrition, and discomfort to patients (Johnson & Walsh, 2009). See Table 10.4 for differential diagnoses, diagnostic exams, and management strategies.

All patients can benefit from a bowel protocol and timely nutrition. Nutrition can be delayed for days due to a dysfunctional gastrointestinal system. This may necessitate the use of total parenteral nutrition (TPN). Early enteral nutrition (within the first 24 h) is associated with earlier return of bowel function. To encourage bowel function, stool

Table 10.4 Differential diagnosis and management of gastroparesis, small bowel ileus, and colonic ileus.

Condition	Symptoms	Signs	Precipitating factors	Diagnosis	Management
Gastroparesis	Nausea +++ Vomiting +++ Abdominal pain +	Distention Succussion splash	Diabetes Vagal nerve injury (gastric/thoracic surgery) Viral Ideopathic Connective tissue diseases Narcotics Alpha-2-adrenergic agonists (e.g., clonidine) Tricyclic antidepressants Calcium channel blockers Dopamine agonists Muscarinic cholinergic receptor antagonists Octreotide Exenatide and glucagon-like peptide (GLP)-1 agonists Phenothiazines Neurologic disorders Autoimmune disorders Psychiatric disorders	Supine KUB X-ray Gastric emptying study (gastric scintigraphy and electrogastrography)	Nasogastric tube Metoclopramide (Reglan) Erythromycin Limit narcotics Consider jejunal feeding
Small bowel ileus	Nausea ++ Vomiting ++	Bowel sounds: high-pitched or absent Distention No peritoneal signs	Abdominal procedures Abdominal inflammation (appendicitis/abscess/cholecystitis/pancreatitis/abdominal or retroperitoneal hemorrhage) Anticholinergic drugs	Supine KUB X-ray Exclude small bowel obstruction	Nasogastric tube Alvimopan (Entereg) Limit narcotics

	Symptoms	Signs	Causes	Diagnosis	Treatment
	Abdominal pain + "Gasiness"	Dilated loops of bowel, paucity of colonic gas Little or no flatus	Antihistamines Opiates Hypokalemia/hypomagnesemia Sepsis Uremia		
Colonic ileus	Nausea + Vomiting + Abdominal pain +	Bowel sounds: quiet or absent Distention No peritoneal signs Dilated loops of bowel, paucity of colonic gas No flatus	Abdominal procedures Abdominal inflammation (appendicitis/abscess/cholecystitis/pancreatitis/abdominal or retroperitoneal hemorrhage) Anticholinergic drugs Antihistamines Opiates Hypokalemia/hypomagnesemia Sepsis Traumatic injury Uremia	Supine KUB X-ray Exclude colonic obstruction	Neostigmine (Prostigmin) Decompressive colonoscopy Limit narcotics

Adapted from http://www.uptodate.com/contents/etiology-and-diagnosis-of-delayed-gastric-emptying

softeners and laxatives with promotility agents are often added as necessary. A combination of daily laxatives such as milk of magnesia, miralax, and senna/docusate combination is generally effective. In patients with pelvic fractures, thoracic or lumbar spine fractures, or those with abdominal injuries, intravenous metacloprimide (reglan) every 6 h is commonly used and erythromycin may be added intravenously. Constipation is increased by narcotic use and decreased immobility. Close monitoring of patients' bowel movements is essential. This can easily be missed in the face of many other issues in the complex trauma patient. In one study, constipation occurred in 69.9% of ICU patients (Nassar, Queiroz da Silva, and De Cleva, 2009).

Abdominal compartment syndrome

The vital organs of the body are contained within compartments, surrounded by thick walls of fascia, connective tissue, or bone. Increased pressure within a compartment causes decreased blood flow and dysfunction of the organs or tissues contained within. See Table 10.5 for signs and symptoms. Increased pressure in one compartment not only affects the organs within that space, but can cause increased pressure and organ dysfunction in the other compartments of the body.

Abdominal hypertension can cause increased ICP, increased pulmonary pressures causing decreased compliance, as well as bowel ischemia, renal failure, and venous congestion, which can increase risk for DVT and extremity compartment syndromes (Balogh and Butcher, 2010). See Chapter 9 for details of measuring abdominal compartment pressures.

Trauma surgeons have been performing damage control surgery for years. The principle of controlling hemorrhage and keeping the operating time short, leaving the abdominal cavity open to prevent compartment syndrome and facilitate staged procedures has evolved over many years. Open abdominal wounds used to be temporarily closed with towels, Bogota bags, or large wet to dry dressings. Vacuum-assisted wound closure systems have become the standard closure for complex wound management in most trauma centers. By using negative pressure on the wound bed, fluid is removed from the extravascular space, which improves blood supply during the inflammatory phase of healing. Granulation is promoted in the wound bed and dressing changes are generally less painful for patients (Webb, 2002). The time line for the healing process can involve multiple returns to the operating room every 2–3 days for assessment of possible abdominal wound closure. If closure is not possible, then the abdomen may be allowed to granulate followed by a skin graft to close the defect. This process can take 10–14 days. In addition, the patient may have to wait 6–12 months for possible abdominal wall reconstruction to treat ventral hernias (Waibel and Rotondo, 2010). See Figure 10.2 for staging.

Table 10.5 Organ dysfunction caused by increased intracompartmental pressure.

Organ/body part or system	Signs and/or symptoms
Brain	↑ intracranial pressure
Lungs/respiratory	↑ airway pressures, ↓ pulmonary compliance (stiff lungs), hypoxemia, CO_2 retention
Chest/heart/circulation	↑ chamber filling pressures, ↓ cardiac output, ↑ systemic vascular resistance
Gut/intestine	↓ intestinal pH, intolerance of enteral nutrition (↑ residual volumes), bowel edema, ileus, compromised intestinal barrier function
Kidneys/renal	↓ urinary output, ↓ glomerular filtration rate
Lower extremities/venous system	Venous congestion, edema, ↑ deep vein thrombosis risk, extremity compartment syndromes

Adapted from Balogh and Butcher (2010).

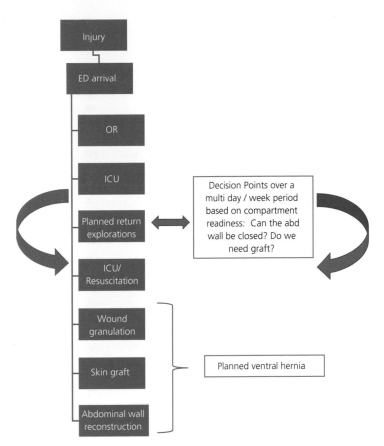

Figure 10.2 Stages of damage control surgery.

Musculoskeletal injuries and management

Musculoskeletal injury is common in the trauma population. While pelvic trauma is the most clinically challenging orthopedic injury to manage, other orthopedic injuries may cause significant lifelong morbidity if they go unrecognized and untreated. The tertiary survey, discussed earlier in this chapter, remains the best offense in injury identification and should be utilized to prevent missed injury.

Assessment for musculoskeletal injury includes inspection for deformity, wounds, ecchymosis, swelling, position abnormality, extremity color; palpation for crepitus, tenderness, discontinuity to palpation of posterior spinous processes, muscle spasm, peripheral pulses; capillary refill time; and motor and sensory assessment. General management strategies for orthopedic injuries include temporary stabilization to prevent blood loss, pain, and nerve damage, followed by long-term stabilization. Timing of operative fixation remains controversial. The current recommendations from EAST favor long bone stabilization within 48 h of injury in polytrauma patients (Dunham *et al.*, 2001). Pelvis stabilization timing is dependent on stability and associated hemorrhage. Early percutaneous fixation provides a minimally invasive option to control hemorrhage and allows for bony stability (Smith and Scalea, 2006). Ongoing monitoring utilizes serial assessments to prevent and identify any complications, including infection, concomitant nerve injury, compartment syndrome, fat

Table 10.6 Prophylactic antibiotic use in open fractures.

Evidence	Recommendation
Level I	Systemic antibiotic coverage directed at gram-positive organisms should be initiated as soon as possible following injury
	Additional gram-negative coverage should be added for grade III fractures
	High-dose penicillin should be added in the presence of fecal or potential clostridial contamination (e.g., farm-related injuries)
	Fluoroquinolones offer no advantage compared with cephalosporin/aminoglycoside regimens and may have a detrimental effect on fracture healing
Level II	Antibiotics should be discontinued 24 h after wound closure for grade I and II fractures
	In grade III fractures, antibiotics should be continued for 72 h following injury or not more than 24 h after soft tissue coverage has been achieved
	Single-dose aminoglycoside dosing is safe and effective for grade II and III fractures

Adapted from Hoff *et al.* (2011).

embolism syndrome, deep vein thrombosis, and ongoing hemorrhage. Preventing infection is paramount given the complications of osteomyelitis and nonunion that are associated with infected bone. Table 10.6 contains the EAST recommendations for prophylaxis and management of open fractures (Hoff *et al.*, 2011).

Concomitant nerve injury is suspected based on injury location and mechanism. Deficits are challenging to identify in the ICU patient who is sedated or has a limited neurologic exam. Serial evaluation of nerve functionality is critical to the surveillance of trauma patients. Table 10.7 demonstrates the best strategy for recognizing deficits.

Compartment syndrome should be suspected with crush injury or significant fracture and is most commonly found in the muscles of the forearm, hand, lower leg, and foot. Fascia is a tough, fibrous sheath that surrounds the skeletal muscle, vessels, and soft tissue. Excessive pressure in the fascial-limiting compartment restricts perfusion to the muscle and neurovascular bundle, which results in tissue ischemia, rebound edema, and tissue necrosis. The presence of open fracture does not preclude compartment syndrome development (McQuillan, Flynn-Makic, & Whelan, 2008). Early signs of this complication, which may be limited in the sedated or neurologically compromised patient, are localized pain out of proportion to the injury and pain with passive stretch of the muscles. Diminished pulses, paresthesia, and paralysis are late signs. Assessing tenseness of the compartment and use of intermittent or continuous compartment pressure measurement devices may be needed to diagnose this complication in the ICU setting. Compartment pressure can be measured by using the Stryker Intracompartmental Pressure Monitor® (Stryker Corporation, Kalamazoo, Michigan, 2009) or similar devices. Normal compartment pressures range from 0 to 15 mmHg. Tissue pressures greater than 35–45 mmHg suggest impaired capillary blood flow, produce clinically significant muscle ischemia, and may indicate the need for fasciotomy (American College of Surgeons Committee on Trauma, 2008). Standard laboratory indicators of muscle injury are CK, CPK, LDH, AST/ALT, and urine myoglobin. Patients with multiple trauma may have many sources of tissue injury, making elevations of these labs less reliable in pinpointing compartment syndrome.

Ongoing hemorrhage

Ongoing hemorrhage may not be apparent until the patient is resuscitated and peripheral vasoconstriction eases. Expanding hematomas

Table 10.7 Extremity nerve assessment.

Nerve assessments

Nerve	Function	Examination
Radial	Sensation	Pinprick and two-point discrimination (separate two ends of a paper clip by 5 mm) over the dorsal surface of the thumb web space)
	Motion	Extend the wrist and the MP joint
Ulnar	Sensation	Pinprick and two-point discrimination over the distal fat pad of the little finger
	Motion	Compare the strength of the fingers as the patient spreads them to the side. Flex the distal joint of the little and ring fingers against resistance. Adduct the thumb
Median	Sensation	Pinprick and two-point discrimination over the index, middle, and ring fingers. Coin discrimination
	Motion	Flex the wrist and PIP joints of the thumb and index finger against resistance
Axillary	Motion	Abduction of the upper arm at the shoulder
Femoral	Sensation	Pinprick discrimination over the median and anterior surface of the thigh and knee
	Motion	Extension of the leg at the knee
Tibial	Sensation	Pinprick discrimination over the medial and lateral surfaces of the sole of the foot
	Motion	Plantar flexion of the foot
Peroneal	Sensation	Pinprick discrimination over the lateral surface of the great toe and medial surface of the second toe
	Motion	Dorsiflexion of the foot

(or those with blush on contrast CT), diminished distal pulses, unanticipated edema, hemodynamic instability despite pelvic stabilization, and dropping hemoglobin/hematocrit values are all possible signs. Each long bone fracture generally results in the loss of several units of blood; bleeding in excess of that should be investigated (Smith & Scalea, 2006). Angiography is the diagnostic tool of choice. Level I/II recommendations are (i) major pelvis fracture with signs of ongoing bleeding after nonpelvic sources are ruled out; (ii) major pelvis fracture whose bleeding at the time of laparotomy cannot be controlled; (iii) evidence of arterial extravasation of intravenous contrast in the CT imaging of the pelvis; or (iv) patients > 60 years of age with significant pelvis fractures regardless of hemodynmaic stability (Cullinane et al., 2011, p. 1862). Definitive intervention may include transcatheter embolization, direct ligation, or bypass grafting.

Pelvic fractures

Pelvic fractures present a unique set of issues for trauma patients. Due to the forces involved and location of organs adjacent to the pelvis, major fractures are often accompanied by genitourinary organ damage or vascular injury and bleeding. Major pelvic injuries include traumatic fractures and involving innominate and sacral bones, joints, ligaments and major vascular support and due to the valveness nature of veins in the pelvis, considerable blood loss can occur even without arterial involvement (Rajab, Weaver, & Havens, 2013). Bleeding is one of the more serious complications seen in pelvic fractures. Retroperitoneal bleeding is mainly venous; 80% of the blood loss requiring transfusion in pelvic fracture is from the fracture site. Pelvic stabilization with sheet wraps or pelvic binders can help tamponade bleeding sites. Bladder and urethral injury is assumed until proven otherwise. Vaginal or bowel injury, fat emboli, other bone fractures and soft tissue injury, and sepsis from infection in open fractures put patients at risk after major pelvic fractures and require continuous monitoring and surveillance by the team.

Crush syndrome management

Crush syndrome is a complication seen in blunt trauma associated with orthopedic injuries. Compression of tissues either with extreme force or for prolonged periods of time often causes release of toxins that can cause systemic consequences. Release of pressure and reperfusion of the area may result in lactic acid, potassium, myoglobin, and uric acid uptake in the systemic circulation in quantities not normally found in the bloodstream. Muscle ischemia followed by reperfusion is the fundamental pathophysiologic mechanism of rhabdomyolysis (Malinoski, Slater, & Mullins, 2004). Myoglobin is released, and this large protein molecule is unable to be filtered by the kidney, and renal failure can result. Dark, tea-colored urine that is dipstick-positive for blood despite the absence of red blood cells (RBCs) on microscopy is suggestive of myoglobinuria and rhabdomyolysis (Malinoski, *et al.*, 2004). Management strategies are targeted at dilution and avoidance of cellular toxicity. Large volumes of crystalloid temper the intravascular deficits caused by fluid initially sequestered in the injured muscle and the hyperkalemia of cellular rupture. Sodium bicarbonate may be added to the intravenous fluids to increase myoglobin solubility, decrease renal cast formation, and force alkaline urine excretion. Mannitol may also be added for its volume expansion and oxygen-free radical scavenger properties. Studies are conflicting regarding the true efficacy of these additives and certainly both have risks. IV fluid delivery at a rate that yields urinary outputs of 200–300 ml/h for adults is suggested for the first 24 h to flush the kidneys of myoglobin (Vanholder, 2011). Ongoing monitoring for fluid overload and hyperkalemia and the cardiac effects is essential. Hypocalcemia is not corrected unless there is significant symptomatology as the majority of infused calcium will be deposited into the injured muscle tissues leading to severe rebound hypercalcemia as it is released approximately 24 h post injury (Malinoski, Slater, and Mullins, 2004; Vanholder, 2011).

Pain management in orthopedic injury

Pain control is also essential for patients with orthopedic injuries in order to promote mobility as part of an attempt to prevent complications from bedrest. Bone fractures are painful, and pain control can often best be achieved with nonsteroidal anti-inflammatory drugs (NSAIDs) such as ketorolac (Toradol). But due to anticoagulant properties of this drug class

and the risk for hindering bone healing, many patients cannot tolerate this agent for pain control. Narcotics are most frequently used for pain control in this group of injuries.

Burns

Significant burns are generally managed at burn centers; however, trauma priorities may require that some burn injuries will need management at a nonburn center and a brief summary of management and monitoring principles follows.

Burn classification

Burns can result from various mechanisms: thermal, electrical, chemical, radiation, and inhalation. Thermal burn mechanisms are well known. Electrical/lightning burns will have tissue damage along the path of current from entrance to exit. Current follows the path of least resistance, with blood vessels, muscles, and nerves sustaining more damage than the external appearance might suggest. Fractures secondary to the muscle contractions may be missed in the intial evaluation. Chemical burns require copious irrigation/decontamination. Alkali agents will cause ongoing damage even after removal of the actual substance. Inhalation injuries result from a combination of superheated and toxic gases. Among the foci of care for the burn population are: fluid replacement/management, ventilation, local and end organ cellular perfusion, tissue coverage, and preventing infection.

Depth of burn is an important assessment. Partial thickness burns include the epidermis and upper level of the dermis. Those elements of the dermis needed for reepithelialization and nerve endings remain intact. The partial thickness wound will appear wet, is painful, and blanches to pressure. Full thickness burns cause destruction of cell reproduction and will require a skin graft for coverage. The full thickness burn will appear dry, leathery, and is insensate.

Total body surface area (TBSA) is used as the measure of tissue involvement. The Rule of Nines or the Lund–Browder chart for infants gives a general measure of TBSA (see Figure 10.3). In the

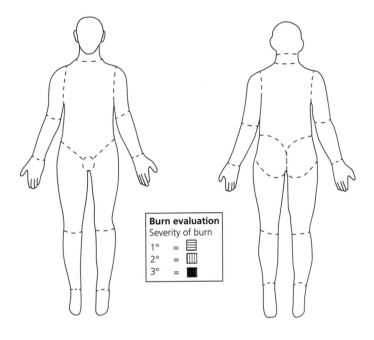

Lund and browder chart								
Area	Age—Years					% 2°	% 3°	% Total
	0–1	1–4	5–9	10–15	Adult			
Head	19	17	13	10	7			
Neck	2	2	2	2	2			
Ant. Trunk	13	17	13	13	13			
Post. Trunk	13	13	13	13	13			
R.Buttock	$2^{1/2}$	$2^{1/2}$	$2^{1/2}$	$2^{1/2}$	$2^{1/2}$			
L.Buttock	$2^{1/2}$	$2^{1/2}$	$2^{1/2}$	$2^{1/2}$	$2^{1/2}$			
Genitalia	1	1	1	1	1			
R.U.Arm	4	4	4	4	4			
L.U.Arm	4	4	4	4	4			
R.L.Arm	3	3	3	3	3			
L.L.Arm	3	3	3	3	3			
R.Hand	$2^{1/2}$	$2^{1/2}$	$2^{1/2}$	$2^{1/2}$	$2^{1/2}$			
L.Hand	$2^{1/2}$	$2^{1/2}$	$2^{1/2}$	$2^{1/2}$	$2^{1/2}$			
R.Thigh	$5^{1/2}$	$6^{1/2}$	$8^{1/2}$	$8^{1/2}$	$9^{1/2}$			
L.Thigh	$5^{1/2}$	$6^{1/2}$	$8^{1/2}$	$8^{1/2}$	$9^{1/2}$			
R.Leg	5	5	$5^{1/2}$	6	7			
L.Leg	5	5	$5^{1/2}$	6	7			
R.Foot	$3^{1/2}$	$3^{1/2}$	$3^{1/2}$	$3^{1/2}$	$3^{1/2}$			
L.Foot	$3^{1/2}$	$3^{1/2}$	$3^{1/2}$	$3^{1/2}$	$3^{1/2}$			
					Total			

Figure 10.3 Burn evaluation and Lund/Browder chart. From Wiegard (2011). © Elsevier.

absence of a chart, the patient's palm can be used to approximate 1% TBSA.

Fluid management in burn therapy

Fluid management is guided by several formulas and guidelines. Direct and indirect losses will cause a fluid shift from the vascular space. This begins shortly after the burn, peaks in 6–8 h and can last up to 48 h (Pham & Gibran, 2007). Once approximated, the TBSA is utilized in the following resuscitation formula:

- Parkland formula: 2–4 cc lactated Ringer's solution/kg/% TBSA partial or full thickness burns. One half of this volume is infused over the first 8 h post burn. The other half is infused over the next 16 h. This is an approximate volume and should be titrated to urinary output, which remains the best outcome measure for these patients (0.5 cc/kg/h for adults; 1 cc/kg/h for pediatrics).
- Pediatric patients will need supplemental isotonic fluids with dextrose due to their low glycogen stores (Pham and Gibran, 2007).

Ventilation support will often be required via mechanical ventilation or pressure support and hyperbaric oxygen is used in some settings (Pham and Gibran, 2007). Many centers adopt low-volume, low–airway pressure ventilation as their standard and then move to oscillator mode if ineffective (Pham & Gibran, 2007). Monitoring will include workup of breathing, arterial blood gases, SpO_2, carboxyhemoglobin levels, and outcome measures of resuscitation mentioned in the foregoing section.

Cellular perfusion is maximized by volume replacement and by limiting peripheral constriction. Serial monitoring should include distal nerve/motor function and pulse quality. Compartment syndrome, caused by circumferential eschar, may limit perfusion and require escharotomy to release the constriction and reestablish distal flow. Airway pressures should drop with chest escharotomy and distal circulation, motor and sensory function return with extremity procedures.

Injured muscle may lead to myoglobin and potassium release, causing obstruction of the renal tubules with resultant rhabdomyolysis or cardiac dysrhythmias, respectively.

Myoglobinuria is identified by direct measurement or port-wine urine that has no RBCs on analysis. Urinary output goals increase to 100 ml/h until the urine clears and an osmotic diuretic may be added to limit intrarenal failure (Miller, 2009; Pham and Gibran, 2007). Early surgical debridement of necrotic muscle may be needed if the myoglobinuria and acidosis does not resolve with aggressive resuscitation measures.

Pain management is essential. Dressing changes are painful. Patients who have daily dressing changes may tolerate pain with NSAIDs, acetaminophen, and limb elevation. Patients who require multiple daily dressing changes and therapy sessions will generally require narcotics and anxiolytics. Positioning to limit edema is especially important for both pain control and tissue perfusion (Miller, 2009).

Aseptic wound care is critical to avoiding infection and promoting tissue coverage. Employ personal barrier precautions and asepsis until all burns are cleansed and covered with dry sterile dressings and/or clean, dry sheets. Use a mild soap and water for cleaning. Avoid substances such as povidone-iodine solution or chlorhexidine gluconate solution as they may hamper the healing process. Leave blisters intact and only debride loose tissue. Practitioners may aspirate large blisters or those over a major joint, leaving the roof intact (Miller, 2009).

A variety of topical antibiotics exist that penetrate eschar and limit underlying tissue necrosis. Those most commonly used are silver- or sulfa-based. Bacitracin is recommended for the face. Do not apply cream directly to wound. Recommended procedure is to "butter" the dressing with the topical cream and apply the dressing to the wound. This provides the correct amount of cream (not too thick) and is far less painful to the patient. Dressing removal will also provide mechanical debridement instead of having to scrape the cream off of the skin. Primary excision and grafting are standard management for full thickness burns (Miller, 2009; Pham & Gibran, 2007). Removal of eschar within 2–4 days of the initial burn followed by graft placement results in less overall sepsis and improved adherence of grafts. Anemia is common secondary to dilution, surgical debridement, bone marrow suppression, and frequent lab draws. Red cell replacement is dependent on hemoglobin level, patient tolerance, and risk factors.

Summary

In this chapter, evidence-based guidelines supporting specific injury identification and management have been reviewed. Clinical pearls of wisdom gleaned from years of hands-on experience with trauma patients where "refereed evidence" does not exist were also offered. Monitoring the trauma patient can involve exponential amounts of technology and complexity. The data obtained can be extremely valuable but can also distract the APN and trauma practitioners from the essential elements of physiologic monitoring principles embedded in clinical practice. Basic monitoring including volume status, heart rate, clinical neurologic exam, fever, pain perception, elicited tenderness, and a high index of suspicion are the key elements to monitor progress or relapse of the trauma patient and should not be ignored in favor of complex technology, but rather augment it. Nothing can replace a direct, hands-on assessment of the patient.

References

A Joint Project of the Brain Trauma Foundation and American Association of Neurological Surgeons, Congress of Neurological Surgeons and AANS/CNS Joint Section on Neurotrauma and Critical Care (2007) *Guidelines for the Management of Severe Traumatic Brain Injury*, 3rd edn, Mary Ann Liebert, New York.

Adewale, A. (2009) Fluid management in adult and pediatric trauma patients. *Trauma Reports*, **10** (3), 1–12.

Ahmed, O. and Zangan, S. (2012) Emergent management of empyema. *Seminars in Interventional Radiology*, **29**, 226–230.

American College of Surgeons Committee on Trauma (2008) *Advanced Trauma Life Support for Doctors, ATLS, Student Course Manual*, 8th edn, American College of Surgeons, Chicago.

Balogh, Z.J. and Butcher, N.E. (2010) Compartment syndromes from head to toe. *Critical Care Medicine*, **38** (9), S445–S451.

Biffl, W.I., Harrington, M.D., and Cioffi, W.G. (2003) Implementation of a tertiary survey decreases missed injury. *Journal of Trauma*, **54** (1), 38–44.

Boldt, J. (2008) Fluid choices for resuscitation in trauma. *International Trauma Care (ITACCS)*, **18**, 57–65.

Bourdin, G.B. (2010) The feasibility of early physical activity in intensive care unit patients: a prospective observational one-center study. *Respiratory Care*, **55**, 400–407.

Brain Trauma Foundation (BTF) (2007) Guidelines for the management of severe traumatic brain injury. *Journal of Neurotrauma*, **24** (Suppl 1), S1–S106.

Bullock, M.R., Chesnut, R., Ghajar, J. *et al.* (2006) Guidelines for the surgical management of traumatic brain injury. *Neurosurgery*, **58** (3), S2–vi.

Center for Disease Control (2010) Deaths: leading causes for 2006. *Morbidity and Mortality Weekly Report*, **58** (14), 1–20, http://www.cdc.gov/nchs/data/nvsr/nvsr58/nvsr58_14.pdf (accessed July 24, 2014).

Coplin, W.M. (2001) Intracranial pressure and surgical decompression for traumatic brain injury: biological rationale and protocol for a randomized clinical trial. *Neurological Research*, **23**, 277–290.

Cullinane, D.C., Schiller, H.J., Zielinski, M.D., *et al.* (2011). Eastern Association for the Surgery of Trauma Practice Management Guidelines for hemorrhage in pelvic fracture—Update and systematic review. *The Journal of Trauman, Injury, Infection, and Critical Care*, **71**, 1850–1868.

Cushman, J.G., Agarwal, N., Fabian, T.C. *et al.* (2001) Management of mild traumatic brain injury. *Journal of Trauma*, **51** (5), 1016–1026.

Dudley, R.R., Aziz, I., Bonnici, A. *et al.* (2010). Early venous thromboembolic event prophylaxis in traumatic brain injury with low-mollecular-weight heparin: risks and benefits. *Journal of Neurotrauma*, **27**, 2165–2172.

Dunham, C.M., Bosse, M.J., Clancy, T.V. *et al.* (2001). *Practice Management Guidelines for the Optimal Timing of Long Bone Fracture Stabilization in Polytrauma Patients: The EAST Practice Management Guidelines Work Group*, http://www.east.org/tpg/longbone.pdf (accessed July 24, 2014).

Hoff, W.S., Bonadies, J.A., Cachecho, R., and Dorlac, W.C. (2011) East Practice Management Guidelines Work Group: update to practice management guidelines for prophylactic antibiotic use in open fractures. *The Journal of Trauma*, **70** (3), 751–754.

Hollingsworth-Fridlund, P. (2001) Reasons why trauma patients have missed injuries or delays in diagnosis. *Journal of Trauma Nursing*, **8** (4), 112–115.

Johnson, M.D. and Walsh, R.M. (2009 Current therapies to shorten postoperative ileus. *Cleveland Clinic Journal of Medicine*, **76**, 641–648.

Kress, J. (2009) Clinical trials of early mobilization of critically ill patients. *Critical Care Medicine*, **37** (Suppl 10), S442–S447.

Leeper, B. (2006) Monitoring and hemodynamics. *Critical Care Clinics of North America*, **18** (2), xiii–xiv.

Malinoski, D.J., Slater, M.S., and Mullins, R.J. (2004) Crush injury and rhabdomyolysis. *Critical Care Clinics*, **20**, 171–192, http://www.ncbi.nlm.nih.gov/pubmed/14979336 (accessed July 24, 2014).

McQuillan, K.A., Flynn-Makic, M.B., and Whelan, E. (2008). *Trauma Nursing: From Resuscitation to Rehabilitation*, 4th edn, Saunders, Philadelphia.

Miller, S. (2009) Optimizing outcomes in the adult and pediatric burn patient. *Trauma Reports*, **10** (2), 1–12.

Nassar Jr, A.P., Queiroz da Silva, F.M., and De Cleva, R. (2009) Constipation in intensive care unit: incidence and risk factors. *Journal of Critical Care*, **24**, 630.e9–630.e12.

Paffrath, T., Wafaisade, A., Lefering, R. *et al.* (2010) Venous thromboembolism after severe trauma: incidence, risk factors and outcome. *Injury, the International Journal of Care of the Injured*, **41**, 97–101.

Pham, T.N. and Gibran, N.S. (2007) Thermal and electrical injuries. *The Surgical Clinics of North America*, **87**, 185–206.

Rajab, T.K., Weaver, M.J., and Havens, J.M. (2013) Technique for temporary pelvic stabilization after trauma. *The New England Journal of Medicine*, **369** (17), e22.

Schirmer, C.M., Ackil, A.A., and Malek, A.M. (2008) Decompressive craniectomy. *Neurocritical Care*, **8**, 456–470.

Shaz, B.H., Dente, C.J., Nicholas, J. *et al.* (2010) Increased number of coagulation products in relationship to red blood cell products transfused improves mortality in trauma patients. *Transfusion*, **50**, 493–500.

Simon, B., Ebert, J., Capella, J. *et al.* (2012) Management of pulmonary contusion and flail chest: an Eastern Association for the Surgery of Trauma practice management guideline. *The Journal of Trauma and Acute Care Surgery*, **73**, S351–S361.

Smith, L.C. and Scalea, T.M. (2006) Pelvic Trauma. *Trauma Reports*, **7** (1), 1–11.

Stryker Corporation, Kalamazoo, MI. (2009) *Intra-Compartmental Pressure Monitor System*, Retrieved from http://www.stryker.com/en-us/GSDAMRetirement/index.htmstellent/groups/public/documents/web_content/127368.pdf (accessed August 8, 2014).

Tisherman, S.A., Barie, P., Bokari, F. *et al.* (2004). Clinical practice guideline: endpoints of resuscitation. *Journal of Trauma*, **57**, 899–912.

Vanholder, R.A. (2011). *Crush-Related Acute Kidney Injury*, http://www.uptodate.com/contents/crush-related-acute-kidney-injury-acute-renal-failure?source=seelink (accessed July 24, 2014).

Waibel, B.H. and Rotondo, M.F. (2010) Damage control in trauma and abdominal sepsis. *Critical Care Medicine*, **38** (9), S421–S430.

Webb, L.X. (2002) New techniques in wound management: vacuum-assisted wound closure. *Journal of the American Academy of Orthopedic Surgery*, **10**, 303–311.

Wiegard, D.L.M. (2011) *AACN Procedure Manual for Critical Care*, Elsevier, Philadelphia.

CHAPTER 11

Oncologic emergencies in critical care

Lisa M. Barbarotta

Smilow Cancer Hospital at Yale-New Haven, New Haven, CT., USA

Evolution of oncology critical management

Cancer is the second leading cause of death in the United States and a leading cause of death worldwide (Kochanek *et al.*, 2011). Enhanced critical care capabilities, sophisticated technology, new oncology treatment strategies, and earlier detection of complications have contributed to improved survival of cancer patients. Survival rates for critically ill cancer patients have improved dramatically with a 20% decrease in overall mortality between the years 1978 and 1998 (Thiery *et al.*, 2005).

Improvements in survival may also be attributed to better selection of oncology patients appropriate for intensive care settings. Investigators have tried to define objective criteria for critical care admission (Groeger and Aurora, 2001). These criteria include postoperative care, management of medical emergencies related to cancer or its treatment, and monitoring during intensive cancer treatments. Other considerations for intensive care unit (ICU) admission should include the likelihood of survival and the patient's goals (Shelton, 2010). Performance status and the presence and number of comorbidities may also impact survival (Soares and Salluh, 2010). While factors impacting survival have been identified, the decision to admit an oncology patient to the ICU setting must be individualized. The need for and appropriateness of critical care should be reevaluated regularly throughout the ICU stay. The optimal duration of ICU admission has not been identified. Additional areas for further research include the impact of critical care on quality of life (Darmon and Azoulay, 2009).

The most common reasons for ICU admission in patients with cancer include respiratory failure, postanesthesia recovery, infection and sepsis, bleeding, and oncologic emergencies (Shelton, 2010). This chapter will address critical care of oncology patients with hematologic, infectious, and structural complications of cancer or its treatment.

Sepsis in the immunocompromised host
Physiologic guidelines

A normal neutrophil count is approximately 65% of the total white blood cell count. A neutrophil count of less than 2500/mm³ is considered abnormal. The risk for infection increases as the neutrophil count decreases. Severe neutropenia is defined as an absolute neutrophil count (ANC) of less than 500/mm³. Patients with an ANC < 100/mm³ are at greatest risk for infection. See Box 11.1 for calculation of the ANC. A patient may have a normal or high total white blood cell (WBC) count and be neutropenic; therefore, the ANC should always be calculated in at-risk patients. In addition to the neutrophil count, the duration of neutropenia is also a risk factor for infection; the longer a patient is neutropenic, the greater the risk for infection. In the oncology population, common causes of neutropenia include hematologic malignancies such as leukemia, myelodysplastic syndrome, lymphoma, myeloma; and chemotherapy, and radiation therapy to the pelvis, sternum, or femur.

The incidence of febrile neutropenia in cancer patients receiving intensive chemotherapy is

Critical Care Nursing: Monitoring and Treatment for Advanced Nursing Practice, First Edition. Edited by Kathy J. Booker.

Box 11.1 Calculating the absolute neutrophil count (ANC).

$$ANC = WBC \times \frac{(segs + bands)}{100}$$

Example: WBC = 3.0 or 3000; segs = 5 and bands = 0
3000 × (5 + 0)/100 = 3.0 × 0.05 = 150

between 70 and 100% (Danai *et al.*, 2006; Moerer and Quintel, 2009). Due to the high risk for infection in this population, sepsis is a common complication and is a leading cause of nonrelapse mortality (Penack *et al.*, 2011). Different sources have published definitions for sepsis which include an elevated WBC count. In the neutropenic patient, this criterion cannot be used to define sepsis. Therefore, any neutropenic patient with signs of a systemic inflammatory response that cannot be attributed to another cause (such as drug fever or transfusion reaction) should be presumed to have sepsis (Penack *et al.*, 2011). Negative blood cultures should not reduce suspicion of sepsis as only 30% of patients with febrile neutropenia have culture-proven bloodstream infections (Feld, 2008; Penack *et al.*, 2007).

In addition to severity and duration of neutropenia, other risk factors for neutropenic sepsis include disruptions in mucosal barriers from mucositis, central venous catheters, and invasive procedures. The incidence of infection is higher in patients with poor nutritional status (Penack *et al.*, 2011). In the neutropenic patient, fever is defined as a single oral temperature of 100.9 °F (38.3 °C) or a temperature of 100.4 °F (38 °C) sustained for 1 h (Legrand *et al.*, 2011). The presence of shaking chills should also warrant an evaluation for fever and infection.

Infections are commonly caused by gram-negative or gram-positive organisms. *Escherichia coli*, *Pseudomonas aeruginosa*, and *Klebsiella pneumonia* are the most common gram-negative organisms to cause infection in the neutropenic host. Coagulase-negative staphylococci, *Staphylococcus aureus*, and streptococci are the most common gram-positive organisms (Klastersky *et al.*, 2011). With increasing use of central venous catheters, gram- positive organisms are assuming prominence.

Assessment and monitoring in neutropenic patients

In neutropenic patients, a fever or chills is often the only sign of infection. Neutropenic patients cannot exhibit pus, sputum, or pulmonary infiltrates, or WBCs on a urinalysis. Clinical signs of infection will be much more subtle and require a careful, astute assessment. The skin must be examined carefully for any breaks in integrity, for rashes that may signal fungal, viral, or bacterial infections, and for changes in the appearance of line insertion sites. Central line infections may manifest only as tenderness or mild erythema at the insertion site. The oral mucosa should be examined with good light for the presence of erythema, oral thrush or lesions, and thickened or scant saliva. The perirectal area should also be examined carefully for erythema, induration, tenderness, and breaks in skin integrity. However, a rectal exam should never be performed in a neutropenic host. Any disruption in the mucosal barrier in the rectum can result in severe, life-threatening infections.

The assessment of abdominal pain in a neutropenic patient can be challenging. Necrotizing entercolitis or typhlitis can be a life-threatening complication of neutropenia. No clinical criteria for diagnosis have been established; however, fever and abdominal pain in the presence of neutropenia should raise suspicion. Bowel wall thickening on radiographic imaging can confirm suspicion. In a cohort study of 60 patients, median time from last chemotherapy to development of abdominal pain was 10 days. Hypotension and diarrhea were also associated with necrotizing enterocolitis. The 30- and 90-day mortality rates were 30 and 52%, respectively. Duration of neutropenia, lack of surgical intervention, and presence of severe sepsis led to a poorer overall survival rate (Badgwell *et al.*, 2008).

Neutropenia management

When a neutropenic patient develops a fever, the infectious workup must begin promptly. Blood cultures should be obtained as soon as possible, including one set of peripheral blood cultures and one set of blood cultures obtained from a central line, if present (Schiffer *et al.*, 2013). A urine culture should also be obtained. Once blood cultures are obtained, empiric antibiotics should begin immediately. The process of blood drawing and antibiotic initiation should be completed within 1h of fever presentation. Stool cultures and cerebrospinal fluid samples should be obtained based on clinical suspicion (Halfdanarson, Hogan, and Moynihan, 2006). A chest radiograph is often part of the febrile workup. However, findings are often negative.

Use of empiric antibiotics with broad- spectrum coverage is recommended. Antibiotics should continue until the neutrophil count recovers to over 500/µl for 2 days and for 48h after fever resolution (Legrand et al., 2011). Administration of effective antimicrobial therapy within the first hour of observed hypotension is associated with increased survival. In a study of more than 2000 patients, each hour of delay in antibiotic administration resulted in a 7.6% average decrease in survival (Kumar et al., 2006).

Monotherapy with a broad-spectrum antibiotic is as effective as dual therapy for gram-negative organisms and has fewer side effects. Acceptable drug choices for monotherapy include cefipime, ceftazidime, or carbapenem (Halfdanarson, Hogan, and Moynihan, 2006; Klastersky et al., 2011). Use of agents with gram-positive coverage should be considered in patients with known colonization with gram-positive bacteria, patients with central venous access devices, patients with skin or mucosal damage, patients with hypotension, and in patients who received prophylactic antibiotics for gram-negative bacteria (Halfdanarson, Hogan, and Moynihan, 2006). Vancomycin is the common drug of choice for empiric gram-positive coverage. Indwelling catheters should be removed if the catheter is the suspected source of infection (Legrand et al., 2011). Combination therapy with beta-lactams and an aminoglycoside may be appropriate for infections caused by resistant organisms such as P. aeruginosa or in patients at high risk for complications (Klastersky et al., 2011). Antifungal coverage should be considered in a patient on empiric antibiotics with persistent fever for 5 days or more.

Persistent fever with signs of clinical deterioration warrant a complete reassessment and collection of new culture data to look for new sources of infection (Legrand et al., 2011) (see

Fig. 11.1). Causes of persistent fever include inappropriate antibiotic dosing, *Clostridium difficile* infection, antibiotic-resistant organisms, fungal infections, parasitic infections (e.g., *Toxoplasma gondii*), viral infections including herpesviruses, parainfluenza, respiratory syncytial virus, and influenza viruses; persistent focus of infection (such as an indwelling catheter); and noninfectious causes including blood transfusions, venous thrombosis, drug-induced fever, graft-versus-host disease (GVHD), underlying malignancy, pancreatitis, and hemophagocytic lymphohistiocytosis (Legrand et al., 2011). The expected or median time to fever resolution in hospitalized patients with cancer is 5–7 days (Legrand et al., 2011).

Evidence-based guidelines

In 2010, the German Society of Hematology and Oncology published guidelines on the management of sepsis in neutropenic patients (Penack et al., 2011). These guidelines recommend empiric antimicrobial therapy with meropenem, imipenem/cilastin, or piperacillin/tazobactam monotherapy. The addition of an aminoglycoside is not recommended due to increased toxicity without added efficacy. Once an organism is identified, antimicrobial selection should be targeted to that organism.

Early goal-directed therapy is recommended to restore cardiac function and improve survival. Studies have demonstrated increased survival of patients with sepsis when interventions are initiated within the first 6h (Dellinger et al., 2013; Penack et al., 2011). Interventions include volume resuscitation with crystalloids or colloids to a mean arterial pressure of at least 65mmHg, central venous pressure of 8–12mmHg, pulmonary wedge pressure of 12–15mmHg, urinary output of at least 0.5ml/kg/h, and central or mixed venous oxygen saturation of 70% or more. Use of albumin is not recommended as there have been no studies demonstrating efficacy. If fluid resuscitation does not achieve these parameters, treatment with vasopressors, specifically norepinephrine, is indicated. There is no role for sodium bicarbonate therapy in the presence of lactic acidosis and pH>7.15.

For the treatment of pulmonary failure, Penack et al. (2011) recommend the use of

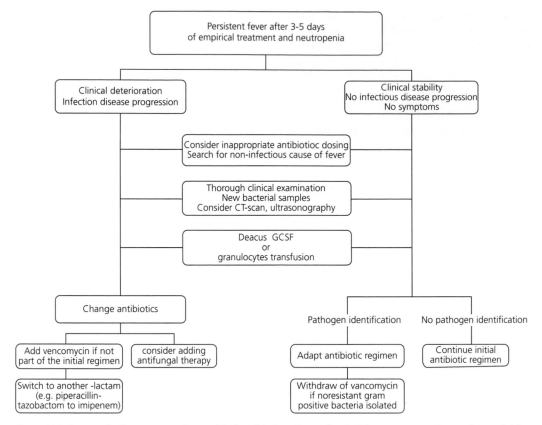

Figure 11.1 Suggested adjustments to the empirical antibiotic regimen after 3–5 days treatment. Source: Legrand, M., Max, A., Schlemmer, B., & Gachot, B. (2011). *Annals of Intensive Care, 1,* p. 6.

continuous positive airway pressure (CPAP) in a patient who is awake and cooperative with minor disturbances in gas exchange defined as a PaO_2/FiO_2 of more than 200. Noninvasive ventilation is preferred when feasible and initiated early as studies have demonstrated decreased need for intubation in the oncology population. Failure of noninvasive ventilation has been reported in 50% of critically ill hematology patients and is associated with increased mortality (Azoulay *et al.*, 2004).

Diagnostic bronchoscopy with bronchoalveolar lavage is not indicated as the diagnostic yield is, at best, 50% and often leads to mechanical ventilation, decreasing the chances for survival (Hummel *et al.*, 2008b; Rabbat *et al.*, 2008).

There are no specific recommendations related to management of renal dysfunction as there are no clear guidelines for the initiation of renal replacement therapy in the setting of neutropenic sepsis.

Nutritional recommendations include use of enteral over parenteral nutrition with an intake not exceeding 20–25 kcal/kg of ideal body weight until the recovery phase when intake can increase to 30 kcal/kg. Blood glucose levels should be maintained at less than or equal to 150 mg/dl. In non-neutropenic patients, glucocorticoids are a component of early goal-directed therapy. However, this intervention has not been studied prospectively in the neutropenic population and is not recommended by this group (Penack *et al.*, 2011). Similarly, activated protein C (APC) has been used effectively in non-neutropenic sepsis; however, the use of APC in the neutropenic population is often not feasible as thrombocytopenia usually accompanies neutropenia and APC is contraindicated with a platelet count of less than 30 000/μl. In patients with higher platelet counts, APC is recommended in patients with APACHE II scores of over 25 and at least two organs failing.

Routine use of growth factors such as granulocyte colony-stimulating factor (GCSF) is not recommended. In 2010, the European Organisation for Research and Treatment of Cancer (EORTC) updated guidelines for the use of GCSF to reduce the incidence of chemotherapy-induced febrile neutropenia in adult patients with cancer (Aapro et al., 2011). Regarding the use of GCSF in patients with existing febrile neutropenia, the EORTC recommends the following: "Treatment with G-CSF for patients with solid tumours and malignant lymphoma and ongoing FN is indicated only in special situations. These are limited to those patients who are not responding to appropriate antibiotic management and who are developing life-threatening infectious complications (such as severe sepsis or septic shock)" (Aapro et al., 2011, p. 21).

In 2009, the Infectious Diseases Society of America updated their clinical practice guidelines for the management of candidiasis. For neutropenic patients, empiric treatment for suspected invasive candidiasis should include caspofungin (loading dose of 70 mg, then 50 mg daily), lipid formulation Amphotericin B (3–5 mg/kg daily), or voriconazole (6 mg/kg intravenous [IV] twice daily for two doses then 3 mg/kg twice daily) (Pappas et al., 2009). For documented candidemia in neutropenic patients, an echinocandin such as caspofungin, micafungin, or anidulafungin or lipid formulation Amphotericin B is recommended (Pappas et al., 2009). For prevention of candidal infections in patients with chemotherapy-induced neutropenia or patients undergoing stem cell transplant, fluconazole 400 mg daily, posaconazole 200 mg three times daily, or caspofungin 50 mg daily is recommended (Pappas et al., 2009).

Research
Identification of biomarkers that may predict risk of severe infection in febrile neutropenic patients is being evaluated. Procalcitonin (PCT) and C-reactive protein (CRP) may be useful markers. In patients with hematologic malignancy, elevated PCT but not CRP was found to be predictive of severe infection (Massaro et al., 2007). Other cytokines such as interleukin 6 and interleukin 8 are also under investigation.

Stem cell transplant

Hematopoietic stem cell transplant (HSCT) is being used more frequently in the management of malignant illnesses. HSCT is a general term that includes bone marrow, peripheral blood, and cord blood as the possible sources of stem cells. Autologous transplant involves collecting and reinfusing the patient's own stem cells. Autologous transplant allows the delivery of high-dose chemotherapy and uses the patient's own stem cells to rescue the bone marrow and shorten the time to marrow recovery. Autologous stem cell transplant is most commonly used in the management of patients with lymphoma and multiple myeloma. Syngeneic transplant uses stem cells from an identical twin. Allogeneic transplant uses stem cells from a human leukocyte antigen (HLA) matched donor (Saria and Gosselin-Acomb, 2007). Allogeneic transplant involves administration of high doses of chemotherapy and/or total body radiation in order to treat the underlying malignancy and make space for the new donor cells to grow or engraft (Rimkus, 2009). The conditioning treatment can cause organ damage. Additionally, the immunosuppressive effects of treatment increase the risk for life-threatening infection. Allogeneic transplant is used to treat patients with leukemia, aplastic anemia, lymphoma, and, less frequently, multiple myeloma.

At least 15–40% of transplant patients will require critical care at some point during their transplant course (Afessa et al., 2003). Estimated mortality rates for HSCT patients admitted to the ICU range from 72 to 100% (Kasberg, Brister, and Barnard, 2011). Patients receiving autologous transplants have much lower mortality rates (5–10%) but higher relapse rates. Some studies suggest that early ICU admission may reduce mortality (Kasberg,

Brister, and Barnard, 2011). Risk factors for mortality have been identified and include the need for mechanical ventilation, vasopressor support for more than 4 h; higher number of comorbidities, and other organ damage (Kasberg, Brister, and Barnard, 2011). Prior to transplant, the potential risks of the procedure are explained to the patient in detail. The goal of allogeneic transplant is to cure the underlying disease and regain an acceptable quality of life (Saria and Gosselin-Acomb, 2007). Risk factors for post-transplant complications include renal or other organ disease, older age, obesity, donor type (match versus mismatch), and underlying disease (Rimkus, 2009). Complications requiring intensive care include infection, GVHD, hepatic veno-occlusive disease (VOD), and respiratory complications (Saria and Gosselin-Acomb, 2007). The risk for particular complications changes over time. These complications will be briefly discussed here.

Infection

Agents used for conditioning prior to infusion of stem cells result in profound myelosuppression. In addition, many of these agents result in inflammation and disruption of the gastrointestinal mucosa (Rimkus, 2009). Prophylactic antimicrobials including antiviral, antifungal, and antibacterial agents are commonly used to mitigate the risk of invasive infection. Despite advances in prophylactic strategies and supportive care, infection remains a leading cause of morbidity and mortality (Martin-Peña *et al.*, 2010). In a prospective study of infectious complications in allogeneic stem cell transplant recipients, the incidence of infection was 1.36 episodes per patient in the first year post transplant (Martin-Peña *et al.*, 2010). Risk for infection is highest during the pre-engraftment period and in the late phases post transplant (Martin-Peña *et al.*, 2010).

Fever during the period of neutropenia is managed as described earlier in the section "Neutropenic Fever." Catheter-related bloodstream infections, bacteremia, and pneumonia are the most common types of infection in the pre-engraftment period (Martin-Peña *et al.*, 2010). However, even after the neutrophil count recovers, allogeneic stem cell transplant recipients remain at high risk for infection due to the use of immunosuppressive medications to decrease the incidence of GVHD, as well as delayed lymphocyte and immunoglobulin level recovery (Kasberg, Brister, and Barnard, 2011). In the late phase post transplant, the presence of GVHD is a primary risk factor for development of infections (Martin-Peña *et al.*, 2010).

Graft-versus-host disease

GVHD results when the donor's immune system, specifically the T cells, recognizes the patient's body tissues as foreign and mounts an inflammatory reaction. GVHD may be acute or chronic, with acute GVHD occurring within the first 100 days post transplant and chronic GVHD occurring after 100 days. GVHD is suspected based on clinical findings and timing of presentation, and can be confirmed by tissue biopsy (Kasberg, Brister, and Barnard, 2011). Severity is described by a grading and staging system. Acute GVHD develops as a result of tissue damage from the conditioning regimen, which stimulates the release of cytokines, which in turn activate donor T cells, resulting in tissue destruction and necrosis (Kasberg, Brister, and Barnard, 2011). Development of moderate to severe GVHD is associated with a higher mortality rate, with acute GVHD accounting for 15–40% of deaths (Kasberg, Brister, and Barnard, 2011).

Acute GVHD involves the skin, gut, or liver. Acute GVHD of the skin is most common and manifests as a maculopapular rash, which may be pruritic (Kasberg, Brister, and Barnard, 2011). Hepatic GVHD is the second most common and manifests as abnormal liver function, specifically elevations in conjugated bilirubin and alkaline phosphatase. Acute GVHD of the gut is marked by diarrhea and abdominal discomfort (Kasberg, Brister, and Barnard, 2011; Newman, 2000).

Immunosuppressive agents including calcineurin inhibitors (cyclosporine, tacrolimus), methotrexate, and antithymocyte globulin are used prophylactically to decrease the risk of GVHD. Once GVHD develops, corticosteroids are the mainstay of treatment. Other agents used include rituximab, daclizumab, infliximab, sirolimus, and mycophenolate mofetil, and photopheresis may be used to treat acute

GVHD (Kasberg, Brister, and Barnard, 2011; Saria and Gosselin-Acomb, 2007).

Chronic GVHD can involve any organ or tissue type and is marked by dryness and fibrotic complications (Saria and Gosselin-Acomb, 2007). Chronic GVHD results from donor T cells inducing autoantibodies resulting in an "auto-immune-like state" (Kasberg, Brister, and Barnard, 2011, p. 357). The biggest risk factor for the development of chronic GVHD is the occurrence of acute GVHD. Chronic GVHD may occur as an extension of acute GVHD, occur after acute GVHD has resolved, or occur in the absence of acute GVHD. The most common organs involved with chronic GVHD include the skin, lungs, and liver (Kasberg, Brister, and Barnard, 2011). Chronic GVHD is classified differently than acute GVHD and is based on the number and extent of organs involved (Pallera & Schartzberg, 2004). (see Table 11.3). Management of chronic GVHD uses similar strategies and medications used to treat acute GVHD. High-dose steroids are typically used in first-line management (e.g., 2 mg/kg/day) with tapering of steroids once symptoms improve (Kasberg, Brister, and Barnard, 2011). Other agents as described earlier may be used in combination; however, the ideal combination has not yet been identified (Kasberg, Brister, and Barnard, 2011; Newman, 2000).

Hepatic veno-occlusive disease

Hepatic VOD, also known as sinusoidal obstructive syndrome (SOS), involves central venular occlusion and endothelial injury resulting in hepatocyte necrosis and inter-parenchymal fibrosis (Coppell, Brown, and Perry, 2003; Kasberg, Brister, and Barnard, 2011). Chemotherapy causes endothelial injury resulting in cytokine release (Coppell, Brown, and Perry, 2003). This complication occurs in 5–60% of transplant patients (Richardson et al., 2012). It is an early compli-cation and severity ranges from self-limiting to life-threatening. Mortality from severe VOD exceeds 50% (Richardson et al., 2012). The diagnosis of VOD is based on a classic triad of weight gain, tender hepatomegaly, and jaundice (Tuncer et al., 2012). Symptoms most commonly present within the first 3 weeks after transplant. Risk factors for the

development of VOD/SOS include pre-existing liver disease; history of VOD/SOS; hepatic radiation; recent use of gemtuzumab ozogamicin; condition regimens containing high-dose total body irradiation (>14 Gy), cyclophosphamide, busulfan, melphalan; or concomitant use of sirolimus during condi-tioning (Tuncer et al., 2012).

Clinical features include weight gain, increased abdominal girth, severe right upper quadrant pain, and hyperbilirubinemia. On exam, ascites and painful hepatomegaly may be present (Tuncer et al., 2012). Coagulation factor deficiencies and thrombocytopenia refractory to platelet transfusions may also be present (Saria and Gosselin-Acomb, 2007; Tuncer et al., 2012). Weight gain may be unresponsive to diuretics. Renal dysfunction may develop as a result of hepatorenal syn-drome, seen in 50% of patients with SOS (Tuncer et al., 2012). Transjugular liver biopsy is the gold standard diagnostic test; however, this may be contraindicated in patients with severe coagulopathy or thrombocytopenia (Saria and Gosselin-Acomb, 2007).

Prevention of VOD is critical as there are no effective treatments for VOD. Modification of risk factors including reducing chemo-therapy doses and fractionating total body irradiation may decrease the incidence of VOD. Supportive treatment includes ursodiol, analgesia, avoidance of nephrotoxins and hepatotoxins, aggressive fluid management, and blood product support (Johnson and Savani, 2012; Kasberg, Brister, and Barnard, 2011; Zhang, Wang, and Huang, 2012). Antithrombin III, prostaglandin E1, defib-rotide, and heparin have been examined in the prophylactic setting; however, none of these agents effectively decreased the risk of VOD/SOS development (Johnson and Savani, 2012; Richardson et al., 2012; Zhang, Wang, and Huang, 2012).

The goal of supportive care in patients who develop VOD/SOS is to maintain intravascular volume and optimize renal perfusion without causing fluid volume overload (Tuncer et al., 2012). Use of diuretics to manage fluid volume overload, paracentesis to manage large volume ascites, and hemodialysis may be used as clini-cally indicated (Richardson et al., 2012). There are no effective, evidence-based strategies for treating patients with severe VOD/SOS (Richardson *et al.*, 2012; Tuncer *et al.*, 2012). Defibrotide has demonstrated efficacy in treating VOD/SOS and improving survival in Phase II and III trials (Richardson *et al.*, 2012). However, there have been no prospective, randomized controlled trials examing the use of defibrotide in VOD management. Defibrotide is currently only available through a treatment investigational new drug (IND) study in the United States (Richardson *et al.*, 2012).

Pulmonary complications

Noninfectious pulmonary complications affect between 21 and 35% of allogeneic transplant patients (Kasberg, Brister, and Barnard, 2011). Complications include pulmonary edema, diffuse alveolar hemorrhage (DAH), idiopathic pneumonia syndrome, bronchiolotis obliterans organizing pneumonia, and pulmonary fibrosis (Kasberg, Brister, and Barnard, 2011; Saria and Gosselin-Acomb, 2007).

Respiratory complications are the most common cause of mortality in the transplant population (Sharma *et al.*, 2005). Development of respiratory failure requiring mechanical ventilation is associated with a poor prognosis (Kasberg, Brister, and Barnard, 2011).

DAH is characterized by cough, dyspnea, hypoxia, respiratory compromise, and fever without evidence for infection (Afessa, 2011a; Saria and Gosselin-Acomb, 2007). Hemoptysis is uncommon (Afessa, 2011a). DAH most commonly occurs within the first 30 days after transplant and carries a mortality rate of 76% (Afessa, 2011a). Bronchoscopy may establish the diagnosis. On chest radiograph, unilateral or bilateral alveolar infiltrates may be seen. Admission to the ICU and use of mechanical ventilation is usually warranted (Afessa, 2011a; Saria and Gosselin-Acomb, 2007). Management includes use of steroids to mediate inflammation (Saria and Gosselin-Acomb, 2007). The optimal steroid dose and schedule has not been identified (Afessa, 2011a). There are no prospective, randomized trials examining treatment of DAH in the transplant setting (Afessa, 2011a).

The idiopathic pneumonia syndrome (IPS) is usually a diagnosis of exclusion (Saria and Gosselin-Acomb, 2007). Afessa (2011b) states that "IPS is characterized by clinical features of pneumonia and diffuse lung injury in the absence of an identified infection" (p. 7). IPS is seen between days 21 and 87 post allogeneic stem cell transplant and carries a mortality rate up to 82% (Afessa, 2011b; Saria and Gosselin-Acomb, 2007). Risk factors include older age, total body irradiation, GVHD, +CMV (cytomegalovirus) serology of the donor, diagnosis other than leukemia, and pretransplant conditioning (Afessa, 2011b). Clinical symptoms may vary in intensity from asymptomatic to acute respiratory distress and may include dyspnea, dry cough, hypoxemia, and tachypnea (Saria and Gosselin-Acomb, 2007). Radiographic findings reveal diffuse, bilateral infiltrates (Afessa, 2011b; Saria and Gosselin-Acomb, 2007). Diagnosis may be confirmed by bronchoscopy with bronchoalveolar lavage. Other than supportive care, there are no definitive interventions (Saria and Gosselin-Acomb, 2007).

Bronchiolitis obliterans occurs in 10–15% of HSCT patients and is seen in patients who have developed chronic GVHD. Bronchiolitis obliterans syndrome (BOS) is defined as a fixed airflow obstruction that occurs within the first 2 years after allogeneic stem cell transplant (Bacigalupo *et al.*, 2012). The prognosis is poor, with a 5-year survival of 15% (Bacigalupo *et al.*, 2012). Clinical symptoms may include recurrent sinus and bronchial infections. Chronic cough unexplained by other causes is common (Saria and Gosselin-Acomb, 2007). Pulmonary function tests are the gold standard for diagnosis and reveal bronchodilator-resistant airway obstruction. The National Institutes of Health developed BOS diagnostic criteria, which include FEV1 < 75% and FEV1/VC ratio over 0.7 (Bacigalupo *et al.*, 2012). Treatment should be initiated once these criteria are met. Treatment involves immunosuppressive agents, such as steroids; however, many do not respond to therapy. Prednisone, 1 mg/kg of body weight, given once daily for 2 weeks with taper over 4 weeks is suggested (Bacigalupo *et al.*, 2012). BOS often develops in the setting of immunosuppression tapering. Reinitiation of immunosuppression, such as tacrolimus or sirolimus, may be recommended (Bacigalupo *et al.*, 2012).

Bronchodilators and inhaled steroids may be used as an adjunct to systemic therapy (Bacigalupo *et al.*, 2012).

Hematologic complications

Hemorrhagic complications

Patients with solid tumors and hematologic malignancies may experience bleeding complications that require critical care. Bleeding may result from thrombocytopenia, coagulation defects, or tumor invasion of blood vessels. Bleeding may manifest as localized bleeding or generalized bleeding. Appropriate management should target the underlying cause.

Thrombocytopenia

Thrombocytopenia is a common hematologic disorder in patients with cancer and is a common occurrence in the ICU, associated with a longer length of stay and increased mortality (Baughman *et al.*, 1993). Thrombocytopenia is caused by one of three possible mechanisms: (1) decreased platelet production, (2) increased platelet destruction, or (3) sequestration in the spleen. Decreased platelet production may result from nutritional deficiencies such as vitamin B12 or folate deficiency, or a disorder affecting bone marrow function including aplastic anemia, acute myeloid or lymphoid leukemias, myelodysplastic syndrome, lymphoma, or multiple myeloma. Decreased platelet production may also result from treatment with myelosuppressive agents, including chemotherapy and radiation therapy (see Box 11.2). Thrombocytopenia resulting from myelosuppressive therapy is usually predictable, occurring 6–14 days after treatment, and recovers 1–3 weeks following completion of therapy (Vadhan-Raj, 2009). Increased platelet destruction is seen in disorders such as disseminated intravascular coagulation (DIC), thrombotic thrombocytopenia purpura (TTP), immune thrombocytopenia purpura (ITP), medications, sepsis, and infection.

In drug-induced thrombocytopenia, there is an abrupt onset of severe thrombocytopenia (<20 000), usually with clinically relevant bleeding. Platelet recovery is seen within 1–2

Box 11.2 Chemotherapeutic treatments associated with thrombocytopenia (Fischer *et al.*, 2003; Jardim *et al.*, 2012).

Carboplatin
Dacarbazine
Fluorouracil
Doxorubicin and Ifosfamide
Fludarabine
Ifosfamide, Carboplatin, and Etoposide (ICE)
Mesna, Doxorubicin, Ifosfamide, Dacarbazine (MAID)
Melphalan
Mitomycin
Nitrosureas (Carmustine; lomustine)
Oxaliplatin
Streptozocin
Thiotepa

Box 11.3 Nonchemotherapy drugs associated with thrombocytopenia development (Sekhon and Roy, 2006).

Abciximab
Acetominophen
Carbamazepine
Chlorpropamide
Cimetidine
Danazol
Diclofenac
Digoxin
Efalizumab
Eptigibatide
Gold
Hydrochlorothiazide
Interferon-alpha
Methyldopa
Nalidixic acid
Quinidine
Quinine
Penicillins
Ranitidine/Rifampin
Tirofiban
Trimethprim/sulfamethoxazole
Vancomycin

days after drug discontinuation. See Box 11.3 for nonchemotherapy agents that may cause thrombocytopenia (George and Aster, 2009). Splenic sequestration may be seen in lymphoma, chronic lymphocytic leukemia, and myeloproliferative disorders. Patients may have more than one cause of thrombocytopenia at a given time (Carlson and DeSancho, 2010). The following will focus on thrombocytopenia resulting from cancer or anticancer therapies.

Monitoring elements

In order to identify the cause of thrombocytopenia, a thorough history must be obtained from the patient including the onset, duration, severity, and type of bleeding symptoms. A detailed review of the patient's medication list must also be obtained in order to identify agents that may be causing thrombocytopenia.

A complete blood count including the platelet count should be obtained. However, examination of the peripheral blood smear is a critical component in identifying causes of thrombocytopenia. In some instances, when using automated counting machines, platelet clumping may be mistaken for thrombocytopenia. When examined under a microscope, platelet clumping is easily identified. Examination of the peripheral smear may reveal schistocytes or microspherocytes, suggesting a destructive process (Carlson and DeSancho, 2010).

Spontaneous bleeding is not typically seen unless the platelet count is less than 10 000/mm^3. In patients with fever, sepsis, trauma, or untreated hematologic malignancy, bleeding may be seen at higher platelet counts. The most common site of bleeding is mucocutaneous including wet purpura, bleeding gums, petechiae, ecchymoses, epistaxis, gastrointestinal, or genitourinary bleeding (Carlson and DeSancho, 2010).

A thorough assessment including examination of the oral and nasal mucosa, skin, wounds, peripheral puncture sites, and central line entry sites for signs of bleeding should be conducted at least every 8 h. Examination of sputum, emesis, stool, urine, and any other drainage should be examined for occult and visible blood. A neurologic examination should be performed regularly. A patient with thrombocytopenia who complains of a new headache must undergo thorough evaluation for bleeding in the central nervous system as a headache may be the only warning sign. Changes in neurologic examination should also warrant a radiologic evaluation for bleeding.

Management

In cases of thrombocytopenia due to infection, sepsis, or DIC, the underlying cause must be identified and treated. In patients with thrombocytopenia due to a hematologic malignancy, bone marrow metastasis from a solid tumor, or a side effect of myelosuppressive therapy, bleeding must be prevented and managed supportively until the underlying disease is treated or until the bone marrow function recovers.

Platelet transfusion is the most effective treatment for patients with severe thrombocytopenia (Vadhan-Raj, 2009). However, there are no evidence-based guidelines outlining the best, safest parameter for platelet transfusion. Patients who are afebrile and asymptomatic may not require platelet transfusion unless the platelet count is less than 10 000/mm^3. Studies have indicated that a platelet threshold of 10 000/mm^3 is safe and well tolerated (Benjamin and Anderson, 2002). In febrile or septic patients, or in patients undergoing treatment for leukemia, transfusion may be required if the platelet count is less than 20 000/mm^3. For patients who are experiencing bleeding or require an invasive procedure such as placement of a central venous catheter, biopsy, lumbar puncture, thoracentesis, or paracentesis, platelet count should be maintained above 50 000/mm^3 (Carlson and DeSancho, 2010).

Platelet transfusions are available in different formulations including pooled donations, single-donor platelets, and HLA-matched platelets. Patients who have never received platelet transfusions before can be treated with pooled donations. If a platelet transfusion does not achieve the expected increase in platelet count (10 000 unit increase for every 1 unit transfused) or does not improve bleeding, one should suspect either continued platelet consumption, splenic sequestration, or alloimmunization (Carlson and DeSancho, 2010). Alloimmunization occurs when the patient's immune system recognizes the antigens on donated platelets as foreign and clears them from circulation. This concept can be tested by sending blood to the blood bank or the American Red Cross where they look for the presence of antiplatelet antibodies. Measuring the platelet count 1 h and 24 h after transfusion may also be helpful. If the 1 h platelet count is increased but not maintained at 24 h, a persistent consumptive or hemorrhagic process is likely. If neither the 1 h nor the

24 h count is increased, alloimmunization is the likely problem (Carlson and DeSancho, 2010). When alloimmunization has occurred, single-donor platelets or HLA-matched platelets will be necessary to appropriately increase the platelet count. In patients with hematologic malignancies or in patients who have undergone organ or stem cell transplants, irradiated platelets must be transfused in order to minimize the risk for transfusion-associated GVHD (Rühl, Bein, and Sachs, 2008; Treleaven *et al.*, 2012).

A number of cytokines have been studied in the setting of chemotherapy-induced thrombocytopenia in an effort to stimulate thrombopoesis. However, these agents have had only modest efficacy with unacceptable toxicity (Vadhan-Raj, 2009). Agents such as recombinant thrombopoeitin (TPO) and TPO-receptor agonists have been used effectively to treat ITP; however, use in chemotherapy-induced thrombocytopenia has not yet been established.

Thrombotic microangiopathy
Physiologic guidelines
Thrombotic microangiopathy (TMA) is a group of disorders characterized by microvascular thrombosis, thrombocytopenia, and end-organ damage (Blake-Haskins, Lechleider, and Kreitman, 2011). TMA includes TTP and hemolytic uremic syndrome (HUS). TTP and HUS are two distinct disorders, both involving microvascular damage and platelet destruction. TTP has classically been defined as a pentad of clinical symptoms including fever, anemia, thrombocytopenia, renal insufficiency, and neurologic changes. However, a minority of patients present with the entire pentad (Levandovsky *et al.*, 2008). George (2009) suggested that TTP be redefined as adults with "thrombocytopenia and microangiopathic hemolytic anemia without an alternative etiology" (p. 75) and that the term HUS be reserved for children with these symptoms as well as renal dysfunction. HUS is often preceded by a diarrheal illness and is characterized by microangiopathic hemolytic anemia, low platelets, and a clinical picture marked by renal insufficiency (Levandovsky *et al.*, 2008). The diagnosis of TTP is reserved for situations where neurologic symptoms predominate in comparison to HUS, in which renal dysfunction predominates (Blake-Haskins, Lechleider, and Kreitman, 2011). TTP and HUS associated with cancer or cancer therapies are characterized by both microvascular and macrovascular thrombus formation in comparison to idiopathic or human immunodeficiency virus (HIV)-associated disease, which is primarily microvascular with platelet-rich thrombosis.

Causes of TMA include medications, such as estrogen, quininine, cyclosporine, tacrolimus, ticlodipine, and clopidogrel; infections including *E. coli* 0157:H7, HIV, and pneumococcus; and idiopathic causes including pregnancy, autoimmune disorders, and stem cell transplant. Approximately, 3–15% of patients who develop TTP/HUS have an underlying malignancy (Benoit and Hoste, 2010). If a patient presents with TTP/HUS without a cancer diagnosis, a thorough evaluation for underlying malignancy should be employed, especially if the patient presents with an elevated lactate dehydrogenase (LDH) or is refractory to treatment. Cancer populations at risk for TMA include patients post stem cell transplant, patients with lung, breast, gastric, colon, pancreas, and prostate cancers and lymphomas (Benoit and Hoste, 2010; Carlson and DeSancho, 2010). Anticancer agents known to precipitate TTP/HUS include mitomycin-C, bleomycin, cisplatin, gemcitabine, and tamoxifen. Other medications include calcineurin inhibitors, which are frequently used as immunosuppressive therapy in the stem cell transplant population.

The pathophysiology of TTP begins with microvascular damage to endothelial cells with release of von Willebrand factor (vWF) molecules. In healthy conditions, vWF molecules are cleaved by ADAMTS13, regulating thrombus formation. In TTP, there is a severe deficiency of ADAMT13 (with ADAMTS13 activity <5% of normal) or an inhibitor of ADAMTS13 may be present (Blake-Haskins, Lechleider, and Kreitman, 2011). The development of antibodies that may act as an ADAMTS13 inhibitor may be induced by some drugs. If the ultralarge vWF molecules are not cleaved by ADAMTS13, the vWF molecules induce platelet aggregation in the microcirculation in areas of shear stress, resulting in increased platelet consumption and red blood cell (RBC) destruction. Platelet aggregation results in small-vessel microthrombi formation, which then results in impaired organ function, manifesting as renal impairment, respiratory compromise, and central nervous system impairment. In HUS, ADAMTS13 activity is usually preserved (Levandovsky et al., 2008) and there is selective endothelial damage in the kidneys (Carlson and DeSancho, 2010).

Recently, an entity called post-transplant TMA was described as distinctly different from classic HUS and TTP. Post-transplant TMA is defined as the presence of microangiopathic hemolysis with renal and/or neurologic dysfunction (Ho et al., 2005). There is an absence of severe ADAMTS13 deficiency and no evidence of systemic microthrombus formation (Ruutu et al., 2007). The incidence following allogeneic stem cell transplant varies from 0.5 to 76% (Fuge et al., 2001; Iacopino et al., 1999; Ruutu et al., 2002). The wide variation in incidence reflects the lack of a consistent definition of post-transplant TMA (Ho et al., 2005). Transplant patients often have anemia, thromobocytopenia, fever, renal dysfunction, and schistocytes for other reasons associated with transplant, which may complicate or confound the diagnosis of post-transplant TMA (Ho et al., 2005).

Two groups have developed criteria for defining post-transplant TMA. The Blood and Marrow Transplant Clinical Trials Network Toxicity Committee Consensus definition for post-transplant TMA includes the presence of RBC fragments (≥2 schistocytes per high power field on peripheral blood smear); concurrent elevated serum LDH; concurrent renal and/or neurologic dysfunction (renal dysfunction defined as doubling of serum creatinine or 50% decrease in creatinine clearance from baseline); and negative direct and indirect Coombs test (Ho et al., 2005). The International Working Group criteria include more than 4% schistocytes in blood; prolonged or progressive thrombocytopenia defined as a platelet count less than $50 \times 10^9/l$ or 50% or greater decrease in platelet count; sudden and persistent increase in LDH; decrease in hemoglobin concentration

or increased transfusion requirements; and decrease in serum haptoglobin (Ruutu et al., 2007). The sensitivity and specificity of the International Working Group criteria exceeds 80% (Ruutu et al., 2007). Distinguishing the definition of post-transplant TMA from TTP and HUS is critical as the treatment is different.

The onset of post-transplant TMA often occurs within the first 100 days after transplant. The median time to onset is 44 days with a range of 13–319 days (Ho et al., 2005). Risk factors include increased age, female sex, unrelated or mismatched donor, use of calcineurin inhibitors, use of sirolimus and tacrolimus in combination, GVHD, and viral or fungal infections (Ho et al., 2005).

Monitoring elements

TTP occurs more frequently in women (3:2 female to male ratio) and usually occurs in the fourth decade of life (Coppo and Veyradier, 2012). A characteristic constellation of clinical signs and symptoms is seen in TTP which may include fever, anemia, thrombocytopenia, renal dysfunction, and neurologic symptoms. Neurologic symptoms are most commonly seen in 50–80% of cases, and present first, including headache, vision changes, tinnitus, confusion, hemiparesis, seizures, and coma (Carlson and DeSancho, 2010; Coppo and Veyradier, 2012). A prodrome may precede the above symptoms, including fatigue, arthralgias, myalgias, and abdominal or back pain. Cardiac events may be seen including myocardial infarction, congestive heart failure, arrhythmias, cardiogenic shock, and sudden cardiac arrest (Coppo and Veyradier, 2012). Laboratory evaluation reveals schistocytes on the peripheral smear (mandatory for diagnosis), thrombocytopenia and anemia on the complete blood count, elevated LDH, increased reticulocyte count, elevated indirect bilirubin, decreased haptoglobin, and elevated creatinine. A direct antibody test will be negative. ADAMT13 activity level may be undetectable in TTP. Treatment should not be delayed while waiting for results of this test, as the test may take more than 24 h to process. Coagulation parameters are usually normal in TTP/HUS (Benoit and Hoste, 2010). In HUS, there is no fever or neurologic changes; the clinical picture is dominated by renal dysfunction including elevated creatinine and proteinuria. The patient may be oliguric. The differential diagnosis for TTP and HUS includes DIC, prosthetic valve hemolysis, malignant hypertension, vasculitis, infection, and Evan syndrome.

Management

Therapeutic plasma exchange (TPE) is the standard therapy for TTP. Prior to use of plasma exchange for TTP, mortality rates exceeded 90%. With the use of plasma exchange, mortality rates are reduced to less than 30%. Plasma exchange results in the removal of ADAMTS-13 inhibitor and replaces the patient's plasma with the active enzyme. The goal of plasma exchange is to correct the platelet count and reverse hemolysis. Complete response to TPE is defined as a platelet count of more than 100 000 on two consecutive evaluations, decreased LDH, and resolution of neurologic deficits (Levandovsky et al., 2008). It may take 1–2 weeks to accomplish these goals. Other authors identify remission as a normal platelet count for 30 days after discontinuation of TPE (Gcorgc, 2009). The number of plasma exchanges required to achieve remission is highly variable and may range from 3 to 89 (George, 2009). Complications of TPE are usually related to the central line required to perform the procedure and include infection and bleeding. Platelet transfusions should be avoided unless there is life-threatening bleeding.

Hemodialysis may be appropriate in patients with renal failure. Neurologic symptoms may improve before renal function. Other therapies with known activity include vincristine, Rituximab, Eculizumab, and IV immune globulin (Blake-Haskins, Lechleider, and Kreitman, 2011; Carlson and DeSancho, 2010). Patients with acquired autoimmune ADAMTS13 deficiency may also require immunosuppressive therapy to maintain remission (George, 2009). Despite known effective therapies, the prognosis of cancer patients who develop TTP/HUS is poor.

In a cohort study over 24 years with 178 patients, plasma exchange resulted in an 80% response rate and survival rates over 90%. The presence of renal insufficiency was associated with decreased risk for relapse. Longer time to initial response was associated with increased risk for relapse. The main predictor of mortality was the presence of an underlying disorder (Levandovsky et al., 2008).

Optimal treatment for drug-induced TMA remains unproven (Blake-Haskins, Lechleider, and Kreitman, 2011). Prompt discontinuation of the offending agent is the first step in the treatment. Case studies have demonstrated safe use of plasmapheresis and plasma exchange. In patients refractory or unresponsive to plasma exchange, eculizumab has demonstrated efficacy in a small number of cases (Blake-Haskins, Lechleider, and Kreitman, 2011; Gruppo and Rother, 2009; Nümberger et al., 2009; Scheiring, Rosales, and Zimmerhackl, 2010). Rituxan has also demonstrated responses in refractory cases (Blake-Haskins, Lechleider, and Kreitman, 2011; De La Rubia et al., 2010).

In post-transplant TMA, the primary intervention is discontinuation of calcineurin inhibitor therapy (Ho et al., 2005). Plasma exchange has not been proven to be effective in this population (George et al., 2011; Ho et al., 2005; Ruutu et al., 2007). For drugs such as tacrolimus and cyclosporine, which may be necessary in the transplant population, reintroduction at a lower dose may be safe and may not necessarily result in recurrent or worsening TMA (Blake-Haskins, Lechleider, and Kreitman, 2011).

Hyperviscosity syndromes
Physiologic guidelines

Hyperviscosity is defined as "an increased intrinsic resistance of fluid to flow" (Halfdanarson, Hogan, and Moynihan, 2006, p. 841). Increased blood viscosity can occur as a result of malignancies including Waldenstrom macroglobulinemia (WM), multiple myeloma, and acute leukemias. In a healthy blood sample, hematocrit is the most important factor contributing to serum viscosity and fibrinogen is the major protein component. In hyperviscosity syndrome (HVS), excessive amounts of immunoglobulins, which are large proteins, are produced. IgM is the largest immunoglobulin and is the most common cause of hyperviscosity. Waldenstrom macroglobulinemia is the disorder in which

IgM is produced in abnormally large quantities (Mullen and Wang, 2007). The proteins accumulate in the intravascular space, forming aggregates that increase osmotic pressure and increase resistance to blood flow. This leads to microvascular congestion, decreased tissue perfusion, and end-organ damage (Behl, Hendrickson, and Moynihan, 2010). IgA and IgG proteins can be overproduced in multiple myeloma; however, less than 7% of patients with newly diagnosed myeloma have hyperviscosity (Kyle *et al.*, 2003).

There is no relationship between the amount of serum viscosity and the severity of clinical symptoms (Behl, Hendrickson, and Moynihan, 2010). The normal range for serum viscosity is 1.2–2.8 centipoise (cP). It is unusual to see clinical symptoms with serum viscosities less than 3 cP. In patients with WM, one-third of patients with a serum viscosity of 4 cP or greater will be asymptomatic. Symptoms are seldom seen in patients with IgM levels less than 4 g/l; however, some patients will develop symptoms with IgM levels between 3 and 4 g/l (Halfdanarson, Hogan, and Moynihan, 2006; Mullen and Wang, 2007).

Monitoring elements
The classic triad of symptoms in HVS includes visual changes, neurologic changes, and bleeding (Mullen and Wang, 2007). The onset of symptoms is usually gradual (Halfdanarson, Hogan, and Moynihan, 2006). Neurologic changes may include headache, confusion, vertigo, ataxia, and paresthesias. Visual changes result from vascular changes in the retina. A fundoscopic exam should be performed in all patients with suspected HVS and will reveal dilated, engorged veins referred to as " 'sausage-like' hemorrhagic retinal veins which are pathognomic" for HVS (Higdon and Higdon, 2006, p. 1877). This is a condition known as fundus paraproteinaemicus. If untreated, this leads to retinal vein occlusion and "flame-shaped" hemorrhages (Behl, Hendrickson, and Moynihan, 2010, p. 197). Clinically, the patient may report blurred vision, decreased visual acuity, and blindness if left untreated. Mucosal bleeding of the gingiva, nasal mucosa, gastrointestinal tract, or uterus may result as the proteins coat the platelets and interfere with clot formation. Other life-threatening consequences of HVS

include congestive heart failure, acute tubular necrosis, pulmonary edema, and multiorgan system failure. A thorough assessment for signs and symptoms of bleeding, as well as changes in neurologic, cardiac, renal and visual function, should be performed every 8 h.

Lab parameters including electrolytes, serum viscosity, and quantitative immunoglobulin measures should be monitored at least once daily. Hyponatremia and hypercalcemia may be seen. Hyponatremia is a false value due to artifact from hyperproteinemia and does not require interventions to correct hyponatremia.

Management
Plasmapheresis is the fastest way to decrease plasma viscosity, especially in cases of elevated IgM because most of the IgM is intravascular (Halfdanarson, Hogan, and Moynihan, 2006). In WM, a single pheresis session can effectively decrease the serum viscosity and improve symptoms. Conversely, in cases of IgA- or IgG-associated HVS, multiple pheresis sessions may be required to achieve the same results. In centers where plasmapheresis is not available, phlebotomy of 100–200 ml of whole blood has demonstrated efficacy in improving symptoms acutely.

Hydration with normal saline until euvolemia or hypervolemia is achieved followed by loop diuretics may also reduce serum viscosity. Definitive treatment of hyperviscosity must involve treatment of the underlying disorder, usually with chemotherapy agents. Blood transfusions for anemia must be used judiciously and avoided if possible during periods of hyperviscosity as packed RBCs can increase serum viscosity and lead to life-threatening vascular alterations (Behl, Hendrickson, and Moynihan, 2010).

Hyperleukocytosis and leukostasis
Physiologic guidelines
Hyperleukocytosis is defined as a WBC count of 100 000/μl or more. Leukostasis is a result of high WBC counts, contributing to increased viscosity. Hyperleukocytosis with leukostasis is seen in acute leukemias, including ALL with 11q23 translocations and AML subtypes M3, M4, and M5. Up to 30% of adult AMLs can present with hyperleukocytosis. Symptomatic

leukocytosis is more common in AML versus ALL (Halfdanarson, Hogan, and Moynihan, 2006). A high WBC count is a negative prognostic indicator. In ALL, patients who present with a WBC greater than 30 000/µl have a poorer prognosis (Hoelzer *et al.*, 1988). Symptomatic leukostasis is rarely seen in chronic myelogenous leukemias and chronic lymphoid leukemias even in the presence of very high WBC counts (Halfdanarson, Hogan, and Moynihan, 2006).

Increases in circulating leukocytes can increase serum viscosity, resulting in sludging and decreased perfusion in the microvasculature. This is called leukostasis. Leukemic blasts also interact with the vascular endothelial cells with enhanced aggregation of blasts. There may also be increased expression of adhesion molecules on lymphoblasts and myeloblasts, increasing the incidence of leukostasis.

Monitoring elements

The presentation of leukemic patients with leukostasis is similar to patients with HVS. Most commonly, the presenting symptoms are respiratory and neurologic. Pulmonary symptoms include dyspnea on exertion or at rest, chest pain, decreased oxygen saturation, and tachypnea. Arterial blood gases may not be helpful as pseudohypoxia can be seen due to rapid consumption of plasma oxygen from large numbers of leukocytes. A chest X-ray should be performed to evaluate respiratory symptoms. Findings can vary from normal to diffuse infiltrates.

Neurologic manifestations can range from mild confusion to somnolence. Focal neurologic deficits can be seen and intracranial hemorrhage must be ruled out. Other symptoms can include visual changes due to retinal hemorrhage or thrombosis, myocardial infarction, limb ischemia, renal vein thrombosis, and DIC. Fevers are also common and may be high. The combination of pulmonary symptoms and fever presents a challenge as it may be difficult to distinguish from infection. Infection should always be ruled out and usually requires empiric management. There are no specific tests to diagnose leukostasis. The diagnosis is based on the WBC count correlated with clinical symptoms.

Management

Reduction of the WBC count can be achieved quickly with leukopheresis. There are no evidence-based guidelines for the initiation of leukopheresis. A blast count greater than 100 000/µl with clinical symptoms is an appropriate finding to initiate decision making. In AML, the goal is to reduce the WBC count to less than 50 000/µl. In ALL, leukopheresis is usually not necessary unless the blast count is over 200 000/µl (Behl, Hendrickson, and Moynihan, 2010).

Supportive measures include aggressive IV hydration and careful monitoring of fluid balance with strict input/output (I/O) documentation. Transfusions must be avoided unless critical as transfusions will further increase viscosity and worsen symptoms. The key to decreasing the WBC is initiation of effective therapy. For myeloid leukemias, hydroxyurea is initiated in a dosage of 50–100 mg/kg/day to provide cytoreduction until chemotherapy can be initiated. Patients with high WBC are at very high risk for tumor lysis and must be managed accordingly (see Section "Tumor lysis syndrome"). Cranial radiation is rarely considered in patients with acute mental status changes although there is no good evidence to support this practice (Halfdanarson, Hogan, and Moynihan, 2006).

Tumor lysis syndrome
Physiologic guidelines

Tumor lysis syndrome (TLS) is a life-threatening metabolic emergency that can occur spontaneously, in response to chemotherapy, or, less frequently, radiation (Cortes *et al.*, 2010). Tumor lysis results from the massive release of intracellular contents from tumor cells into the bloodstream as the cells die. Intracellular anions (phosphate), cations (potassium), and nucleic acids (uric acid) are released into circulation in high volumes resulting in hyperphosphatemia, hyperkalemia, and hyperuricemia (Benoit and Hoste, 2010). Phosphorous binds to calcium resulting in hypocalcemia. The rapid, massive release of electrolytes into the bloodstream overwhelms and exceeds the ability of the kidneys to filter and excrete (Varon and Acosta, 2010). Calcium–phosphate and uric acid crystals can deposit in the renal tubules, leading to acute kidney injury (AKI). TLS is a common cause of AKI in critically ill patients (Benoit and Hoste, 2010; Darmon *et al.*, 2007). Other sequelae of acute electrolyte imbalances include heart failure, cardiac arrhythmias, pulmonary edema, seizures, and death (Abu-Alfa and Younes, 2010).

Risk categories can be divided into low, intermediate, and high. High-risk factors include patients with aggressive forms of lymphoma including Burkitt's and lymphoblastic lymphomas; acute lymphoblastic leukemia (ALL), ALL with a WBC count greater than or equal to 100 000/μl, or acute myeloid leukemia with WBC ≥ 50 000/μl. The intermediate risk category includes diffuse large B cell lymphoma, ALL with WBC count 50 000–100 000/μl, chronic lymphocytic leukemia with WBC count 10 000–100 000/μl treated with fludarabine, or any other highly chemosensitive tumor. Low-risk factors include other non-Hodgkin's lymphoma types and other cancers with low growth rates (Coiffer *et al.*, 2008). Other risk factors for tumor lysis include high LDH (>2× upper limit of normal), preexisting renal disease, dehydration, sepsis, and use of other nephrotoxic agents (Abu-Alfa and Younes, 2010; Mughal *et al.*, 2010).

Monitoring

The first step in monitoring patients for TLS is to identify patients at risk. Early recognition can lead to improved outcomes (Kennedy and Ajiboye, 2010). As previously mentioned, patients with high tumor burden who receive effective treatment are those most at risk. TLS can develop within hours of initial treatment and up to 7 days thereafter (Cairo and Bishop, 2004). A baseline complete blood count will help identify the degree of risk based on WBC. A baseline LDH, potassium, uric acid, creatinine, phosphorous, and urinalysis will help determine the need for interventions. Laboratory monitoring should be performed at baseline, prior to initiation of treatment, and every 6–12 h depending on the patient's baseline uric acid and renal function. If the patient has an elevated creatinine at baseline in addition to other risk factors, such as elevated WBC or elevated uric

Table 11.1 Laboratory and clinical findings in tumor lysis syndrome.

Laboratory TLS: two or more of the following values within 3 days prior to or 7 days after the initiation of cancer treatment

- Uric acid ≥ 8 mg/dl or 25% increase from baseline
- Potassium ≥ 6.5 mEq/l or 25% increase from baseline
- Phosphorous ≥ 4.5 mg/dl or 25% increase from baseline
- Calcium ≤ 7 mg/dl or 25% decrease from baseline

Clinical TLS: laboratory TLS + one or more of the following items:

- Serum creatinine ≥ 1.5× upper limit of normal adjusted for age
- Cardiac arrhythmia or sudden death
- Seizure

Adapted from Cairo and Bishop (2004). Cairo and Bishop (2004).

acid, electrolytes should be checked as frequently as every 6 h for the first 48–72 h of chemotherapy or anticancer treatment. Lab results should be evaluated for results in relation to normal as well as trends (see Table 11.1 for laboratory definition of TLS). Lab results should be correlated with the patient's clinical findings.

Commonly, the patient with TLS presents without symptoms and the condition is detected based on lab results. Signs and symptoms develop as a result of electrolyte imbalance and AKI (see Table 11.2) and can develop within 24–48 h of starting therapy, with the exception of hyperkalemia, which can occur as early as 6 h from the start of anticancer treatment (Holmes Gobel, 2006). With hyperuricemia, symptoms do not develop until uric acid levels exceed 10 mg/dl, resulting in fatigue, nausea, vomiting, and flank pain. When uric acid levels exceed 20 mg/dl, the patient may exhibit signs of renal failure including oliguria, anuria, hypertension, and edema (Lydon, 2005). Symptoms related to elevated phosphate are usually a manifestation of impaired renal function (Holmes Gobel, 2006). The nurse should assess for signs of renal dysfunction such as oliguria but also must assess for signs and symptoms of hypocalcemia. Serum potassium levels exceeding 6.5 mEq/l may have cardiac sequelae including tachycardia, P and T wave changes, ventricular tachycardia, and ventricular fibrillation. Baseline and daily electrocardiograms (ECGs) should be

Table 11.2 Signs and symptoms of tumor lysis syndrome.

Electrolyte imbalance	Symptoms	Clinical signs
Hyperkalemia	Lethargy Weakness, irritability Syncope Paresthesias Muscle cramps Nausea/vomiting	Decreased deep tendon reflexes Paralysis Hyperactive bowel sounds Diarrhea Cardiac arrhythmias Cardiac arrest Early ECG changes: tachycardia, prolonged QT interval and ST segment, inversion of T wave Late ECG changes: bradycardia, peaked T waves, depressed R waves progressing to widened QRS, prolonged PR, loss of P wave; ventricular tachycardia, ventricular fibrillation, heart block
Hyperuricemia	Lethargy Fatigue Weakness Flank or back pain Malaise Nausea, vomiting Pruritis	Hematuria Gout (painful, red, inflamed joints) Nephrolithiasis Urate nephropathy Hypertension Fluid volume overload Pulmonary and peripheral edema
Hyperphosphatemia		Anuria Oliguria Azotemia Edema Hypertension Acute renal failure
Hypocalcemia	Irritability/restlessness Hallucinations, confusion Weakness Depression, anxiety Twitching Muscle cramps Paresthesias	Carpopedal spasm Tetany Ventricular arrhythmias ECG changes (prolonged QT interval, inverted T waves; heart block) Facial grimacing Laryngeal spasm Psychosis Intestinal cramps Chronic malabsorption Seizures Respiratory arrest

Sources: Abu-Alfa and Younes (2010); Holmes Gobel (2006); Kennedy and Ajiboye (2010).

performed and repeated in the setting of hyperkalemia. Patients with potassium levels higher than 6 should be monitored continuously for the development of arrhythmias.

The nurse should thoroughly assess for signs and symptoms of TLS including uremic symptoms in patients with elevated creatinine (mental status changes), fluid volume overload unresponsive to diuretics, and severe acidosis. Volume status must be evaluated regularly including meticulous I/O measurements, often requiring the use of indwelling urinary catheters and checking daily weight.

Daily urinalysis for the presence of blood and crystals should be performed. Patients with oliguria must have a renal ultrasound performed to rule out obstructive uropathy (Mughal et al., 2010).

Treatment

The mainstay of treatment is the recognition of at-risk patients, prevention, and early intervention. Prevention of TLS includes vigorous IV hydration with judicious use of diuretics if needed. Aggressive volume repletion should be implemented immediately at the time of presentation to minimize delays in initiation of effective anticancer treatment. Expanding plasma volume facilitates renal blood flow and therefore urine flow, promoting excretion of potassium, phosphate, and uric acid. Clearance of uric acid crystals is directly dependent on the glomerular filtration rate, so optimization of renal blood flow is critical. The goal is to maintain a urine output of $80–100\,ml/m^2/h$. This goal may not be realistic or safe in individuals with congestive heart failure and may necessitate the use of diuretics to achieve the goal (Abu-Alfa and Younes, 2010). Diuretics may only be used if the patient has been hyperhydrated; the use of diuretics in patients with hypovolemia or obstructive uropathy may exacerbate renal insufficiency (Kennedy and Ajiboye, 2010). Furthermore, use of diuretics has not demonstrated improved outcomes such as survival, or decreased the need for hemodialysis (Karajala, Mansour, and Kellum, 2009).

Management of electrolyte imbalances

Hyperkalemia
Review the patient's medication list for other medications that may increase serum potassium levels including supplemental potassium, angiotensin-converting enzyme (ACE) inhibitors, direct rennin inhibitors, aldosterone antagonists, potassium-sparing diuretics (spironolactone), and nonsteroidal anti-inflammatory drugs. A low potassium diet should be implemented. Care should be used to monitor for potassium amounts in dietary supplements and enteral and parenteral nutrition formulations (Holmes Gobel, 2006).

Medications to lower potassium levels should be employed when the patient is symptomatic or the potassium level is above normal. Sodium polystyrene sulfonate resin (Kayexalate®) can be employed (60 g orally or via retention enema); however, this agent takes several hours to take effect and should not be the sole or first measure used in an acute setting. This agent works by exchanging potassium for sodium in the colon, resulting in potassium losses through stool output.

There is no strong evidence to support the use of this agent in the acute setting (Abu-Alfa and Younes, 2010). Contraindications to Kayexalate use include serum potassium less than 5 mmol/l, history of hypersensitivity to polystyrene sulfonate resins, and obstructive bowel disease (Kayexalate prescribing information, 2010). Contraindications to enema use include low platelet count and neutropenia. Loop diuretics such as furosemide lower potassium quickly by enhancing urinary excretion. These agents will also help to prevent fluid volume overload due to hyperhydration. Regular human insulin (10 units) and glucose (50 ml of 50% solution) administered intravenously also work to lower potassium. The insulin load results in shifting of potassium from the extracellular space back into the cell. Glucose is administered concominantly to avoid hypoglycemia. This intervention works within 20 min and lasts as long as 6 h. Inhaled beta agonists (10–20 mg of nebulized albuterol) may also be given to lower serum potassium, acting in a similar fashion to insulin, driving potassium back into the cell. Calcium gluconate 10 ml of 10% solution (1 g) IV over 5–10 min is often administered intravenously in patients with symptomatic hyperkalemia. The calcium temporarily antagonizes the cardiac effects of hyperkalemia, stabilizing the cardiac membrane. The calcium has an onset of 1–3 min and lasts up to 1 h. Sodium bicarbonate (50 mEq IV over 5–10 min) causes a temporary shift of potassium into the cells in the setting of acidosis. The effects and duration of action are variable (Mughal *et al.*, 2010). Refractory and symptomatic hyperkalemia may require hemodialysis.

Hyperphosphatemia with secondary hypocalcemia
High levels of phosphate in the blood are primarily managed with the administration of oral phosphate binding agents, forced diuresis, and dietary restriction of phosphorous. If possible, avoid providing calcium replacement (unless the patient has symptomatic hypocalcemia) as any supplemental calcium will increase the opportunity for phosphorous–calcium precipitation (Abu-Alfa and Younes, 2010). Patients

with serum calcium levels less than 8 mg/dl should be placed on seizure precautions (Holmes Gobel, 2006).

Hyperuricemia

Aggressive IV hydration to promote urine output of 80–100 ml/m²/h is the goal to maintain urinary excretion of excess uric acid. Uric acid becomes more soluble in an alkaline environment. However, urinary alkalinization is controversial because calcium–phosphate crystals are more soluble in an acidic urine environment. Therefore, urinary alkalinization may lead to increased calcium–phosphate crystallization. In the past, the addition of sodium bicarbonate to IV fluids was a mainstay of practice in order to achieve an alkine urine pH. However, this practice is no longer recommended due to lack of strong data to support safety and efficacy (Kennedy and Ajiboye, 2010; Mughal *et al.*, 2010). Hydration using an isotonic solution such as normal saline is recommended.

Use of medications to prevent and manage hyperuricemia is critical. Allopurinol is a xanthine oxidase inhibitor that inhibits the conversion of hypoxanthine to xanthine and xanthine to uric acid, resulting in the accumulation of these precursors and preventing the accumulation of uric acid. Xanthine and hypoxanthine are substances that are 5–10 times more soluble in urine than uric acid. Allopurinol must be instituted early, before elevations in uric acid occur, in order to effectively mitigate the risk of hyperuricemia. As described earlier, allopurinol changes nucleic acid metabolism but cannot metabolize uric acid that has already accumulated.

Allopurinol is available in oral and IV formulations. Allopurinol should be started 24–48 h prior to the start of anticancer therapy. Recommended daily dosing of IV allopurinol is 200–400 mg/m² or 600–800 mg/day in divided doses for oral allopurinol. Allopurinol must be dose-adjusted for renal dysfunction. Side effects include rash, hypersensitivity reactions, and renal lithiasis secondary to xanthine accumulation (Abu-Alfa and Younes, 2010). If a rash develops in a patient receiving allopurinol, it must be discontinued as severe cutaneous reactions have been reported. Allopurinol interferes with the cytochrome p450 system

and will interact with other drugs with similar activity (Kennedy and Ajiboye, 2010).

Febuxostat is a newer xanthine oxidase inhibitor that is more effective than allopurinol in treating hyperuricemia (Becker *et al.*, 2005). The daily dose is 120 mg, taken orally. The drug does not require dose adjustments for renal insufficiency. Side effects include liver function abnormalities, nausea, arthralgia, and rash (Uloric® prescribing information, 2009).

Rasburicase is an enzyme that breaks uric acid down into allantoin, a substance 5–10 times more soluble than uric acid. Rasburicase is Food and Drug Administration (FDA)-approved for the prevention and management of hyperuricemia in adults and children with cancer at a dose of 0.20 mg/kg IV over 30 min as a single daily dose for up to 5 days (Elitek® package insert). Rasburicase provides control of uric acid levels more rapidly than allopurinol (Cortes *et al.*, 2010). Other benefits to rasburicase include lack of drug interactions and no requirements for dose adjustments in renal dysfunction (Kennedy and Ajiboye, 2010). Contraindications to rasburicase use include G6PD deficiency, pregnancy, and breastfeeding (Abu-Alfa and Younes, 2010). Studies have examined the efficacy and different dosing schedules for rasburicase (Campara, Shord, and Haaf, 2009; Hummel *et al.*, 2008a; Hutcherson *et al.*, 2006; Kennedy and Ajiboye, 2010; Lee *et al.*, 2003; Liu, Sims-Mccallum, and Schiffer, 2005; Malaguarnera *et al.*, 2009; McDonell *et al.*, 2006; Reeves and Bestul, 2008; Trifilio *et al.*, 2006). Hummel *et al.* (2008a) demonstrated that a lower dose (0.04 mg/kg) for 1–2 doses is effective. Other researchers have looked at fixed dosing schedules ranging from 3 to 9 mg/dose (Campara, Shord, and Haaf, 2009; Malaguarnera *et al.*, 2009; McDonell *et al.*, 2006; Reeves and Bestul, 2008). Giraldez and Puto (2010) performed a retrospective study examining a 6 mg fixed dose in 15 patients with TLS. This single dose effectively reduced uric acid levels. In practice, the lowest effective dose in the fewest doses necessary to lower uric acid to below normal should be employed. Many centers are now using 6 mg fixed-dosing schedules and repeating the dose after 24 h if needed. Side effects of rasburicase include hypersensitivity reactions, hemolysis, and methemoglobinemia if given to patients with G6PD deficiency, and rash (Kennedy and Ajiboye, 2010).

There are no large-scale randomized controlled trials comparing rasburicase dose and frequency or absolute threshold levels for rasburicase use. Additionally, there are no data on the impact of rasburicase on outcomes including AKI, renal failure, hemodialysis use, or mortality (Kennedy and Ajiboye, 2010).

Acute kidney injury

In the event of AKI in the patient with impending or actual TLS, a nephrology consult should be placed. The goals are to minimize delays in anticancer therapy and optimize renal function. The tenets of AKI management include managing volume status, correcting electrolyte abnormalities, avoiding nephrotoxins, and adjusting medications for renal function (Abu-Alfa and Younes, 2010). The development of AKI may exacerbate preexisting electrolyte abnormalities, particularly hyperkalemia and hyperuricemia (Benoit and Hoste, 2010). Hemodialysis or renal replacement therapy may be considered in patients with large tumor burden, elevated WBC count, chronic kidney disease, end-stage renal disease, or AKI at the time of presentation, or congestive heart failure. Other authors have suggested that renal replacement therapy be employed when hyperphosphatemia continues for more than 6 h after the initiation of vigorous hydration (Darmon, Roumier, and Azoulay, 2009). The use of hemodialysis in this setting is not well studied and cannot be routinely recommended.

Suggested criteria for hemodialysis include the following parameters unresponsive to other measures (Mughal et al., 2010; Varon and Acosta, 2010):

- Potassium ≥ 6 mEq/l
- Uric acid ≥ 10 mg/dl
- Phosphorous ≥ 10 mg/dl
- Fluid volume overload unresponsive to diuretics
- Symptomatic hypocalcemia
- Severe acidosis
- Uremic symptoms such as mental status changes

Evidence-based treatment guidelines

In 2008, evidence-based guidelines for the prevention and treatment of TLS in adults and children were published (Coiffer et al., 2008). The guidelines are the first to outline specific roles for both allopurinol and rasburicase (Mughal et al., 2010). An algorithm based on TLS risk was developed. For low-risk patients, no interventions for prevention are recommended. For intermediate-risk patients, hydration and allopurinol are recommended as initial therapy to prevent hyperuricemia. Allopurinol should start 12 h prior to anticancer therapy and continue until the patient is considered to be at low risk. If hyperuricemia develops with these interventions in place, rasburicase should be instituted. For high-risk patients, hydration and rasburicase use upfront is recommended (Coiffer et al., 2008).

Clinical Pearls

Blood samples for patients who have received rasburicase must be sent to the lab on ice. Failure to do so results in falsely low levels of uric acid as rasburicase will continue to break down uric acid in the blood sample if not chilled (Abu-Alfa and Younes, 2010; Elitek package insert).

Structural emergencies

Traditional oncologic emergencies such as superior vena cava syndrome and spinal cord compression rarely require transfer to intensive care settings. Improvements in preventive strategies and improved diagnostic techniques have transferred the management of these conditions to oncology or medical surgical units (Demshar, Vanek, and Mazanec, 2011). However, patients at risk for these conditions may require intensive care for other diseases or treatment-related complications. Therefore, the critical care advanced practice registered nurse should be aware of signs and symptoms of impending structural emergencies, including superior vena cava syndrome and spinal cord compression. Presenting signs and symptoms, diagnostic techniques, and management strategies for each are outlined in Table 11.3.

Table 11.3 Traditional oncologic emergencies.

Emergency	Signs and symptoms	Diagnosis	Management
Hypercalcemia	Vague and nonspecific Confusion, lethargy Nausea, vomiting, constipation, abdominal pain Polyuria, elevated creatinine Shortened QT interval on ECG, arrhythmias	Corrected serum calcium > 10.5 mg/dl	Hydration with normal saline at rates between 200 and 300 ml/h if not contraindicated by cardiovascular status Once volume replete, loop diuretics can be used to induce calcium excretion Bisposphonate therapy: pamidronate (60–90 mg IV, caution in renal dysfunction) or zoledronic acid (4 mg IV, adjust for renal dysfunction) Calcitonin for fast effect but has short duration and leads to tachyphylaxis Steroids may be useful in selected cases of Vitamin D3–induced hypercalcemia
Syndrome of inappropriate antidiuretic hormone	Fatigue Difficulty concentrating Poor memory Headache Muscle cramps Dysgeusia In cases of severe hyponatremia: Confusion Hallucinations Seizures Coma	Serum osmolality < 275 mOsm/kg in a euvolemic patient Urine osmolaltiy > 100 mOsm/kg FENa > 1%	Treat underlying cause Fluid restriction of 0.5–1 l of free water per day Increased salt intake If symptoms are severe, use 3% saline intravenously with caution Be careful not to correct sodium too quickly, can result in central pontine myelinosis Correct serum sodium no more quickly than 8–10 mmol/l in 24 h Furosemide use contraindicated with 3% saline
Superior vena cava syndrome	Upper body edema Dyspnea, stridor Dysphagia Superficial venous dilatation Headaches Confusion	CT scan Plain radiography Venography	Treat underlying malignancy Emergent situations (presence of CNS symptoms): Stent placement, radiation therapy, corticosteroids, diuretics Elevate head of bed Supplemental oxygen
Malignant spinal cord compression	Back pain Radicular pain Motor weakness Gait disturbance Bowel and bladder dysfunction	MRI	Glucocorticoids (Dexamethasone initial bolus of 10–16 mg followed by 4 mg every 4–6 h) Radiation therapy Surgery

Sources: Behl, Hendrickson, and Moynihan (2010); Demshar, Vanek, and Mazanec (2011); Halfdanarson, Hogan, and Moynihan (2006); Higdon and Higdon (2006); Kaplan (2006).

Cardiac tamponade
Physiologic guidelines
Cardiac tamponade is a life-threatening oncologic emergency that results from excessive fluid accumulation in the pericardium. The fluid accumulation is referred to as a pericardial effusion and precedes tamponade. Excess fluid exerts pressure on the cardiac chambers, restricting the filling capacity of the ventricles. The end result is decreased cardiac output and hemodynamic instability (Turner Story, 2006). Tamponade can occur with fluid volumes as little as 50–80 ml

and as much as 2 l (Behl, Hendrickson, and Moynihan, 2010; Turner Story, 2006).

Patients with cancer can develop pericardial effusions as a result of tumor cell invasion into the pericardial fluid, as a side effect of anticancer treatment, or as a result of tumor extension into the pericardial space (Behl, Hendrickson, and Moynihan, 2010). Mesothelioma is the most common primary tumor type that involves the pericardium and is a difficult disease to treat. Other primary tumors of the heart include malignant fibrous histiocytoma, rhambdomyosarcoma, and angiosarcoma (Turner Story, 2006). Most effusions develop from lung or breast cancer; other causes include melanoma, leukemia, or lymphoma (Higdon and Higdon, 2006). Tumor obstruction of mediastinal lymph nodes can interfere with lymph drainage from the pericardium, leading to fluid accumulation. This is the most common cause of pericardial effusion in malignancy. Malignant effusions progress to tamponade more often than nonmalignant effusions because the presence of tumor cells stimulates the pericardium to produce excessive fluid (Turner Story, 2006). Tumors may also cause bleeding in the pericardial space, allowing rapid accumulation of fluid and increasing the risk for tamponade (Flounders, 2003). Many patients have metastatic disease in other sites at the time of presentation with pericardial effusion; the mean interval from diagnosis to development of tamponade is 17.4 months (Cozzi et al., 2010). Radiation therapy with doses of 4000 cGy or more to the chest is associated with the development of pericardial effusions. The majority of cases occur in the first year after radiation therapy (Miaskowski, 1999).

Chemotherapy and biotherapy agents can also cause pericardial effusions. Other conditions that may increase risk include underlying heart disease, systemic lupus erythematosus, rheumatoid arthritis, scleroderma, myxedema, tuberculosis, bacterial endocarditis, and pericarditis (Turner Story, 2006).

Pericardial effusions are classified by fluid type. Transudative fluids are low in protein and are the result of abnormal capillary permeability caused by benign mechanical factors such as cirrhosis. Transudative fluid is defined as having LDH levels less than 200 IU/l and protein levels less than 35 g/dl. Exudative effusions are protein-rich and are caused by leaking blood vessels due to increased capillary permeability. Exudative fluid has LDH levels greater than 200 IU/l and protein levels greater than 35 g/dl. Most malignant pericardial effusions are exudates.

Monitoring

Identification of tamponade is critical as unrecognized, untreated tamponade has a mortality rate of 65% (Miaskowski, 1999). The presence and severity of symptoms depend on how quickly the fluid has accumulated. The classic Beck triad of symptoms includes distended neck veins, silent precordium, and hypotension. These symptoms are rarely seen in malignancy as fluid tends to accumulate slowly over time (Behl, Hendrickson, and Moynihan, 2010; Schairer et al., 2011). Patients may report dyspnea; dull, diffuse chest pain, or heaviness that does not change with position; palpitations; nonproductive cough; dizziness; and fatigue (Higdon and Higdon, 2006). Symptoms may be mistaken for right heart failure and treated with diuretics. Diuretics will further decrease cardiac output and worsen hemodynamic instability; therefore, diuretics should be avoided until the cause of the symptoms is confirmed. As tamponade progresses, dyspnea worsens and confusion may ensue. Relief of symptoms may be achieved by sitting up and leaning forward.

A thorough exam reveals distant or quiet heart sounds, a narrow pulse pressure, and pulsus paradoxus. Patients at risk for cardiac tamponade should be placed on continuous cardiac monitoring to assess for changes in cardiac rhythm. Additionally, a 12-lead ECG should be performed. ECG changes consistent with tamponade include low-voltage complexes with nonspecific ST-T changes. Electrical alternans may be seen in patients with large effusions or tamponade (Behl, Hendrickson, and Moynihan, 2010; Lau et al., 2002). ECGs assist in diagnosing tamponade and also guide the need for interventions (see Fig. 11.2).

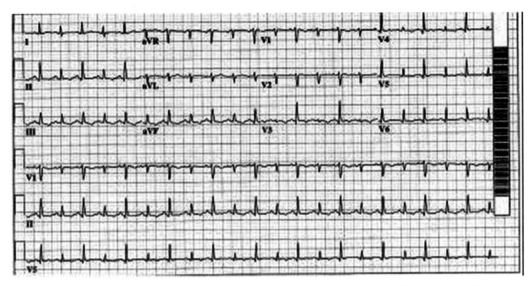

Figure 11.2 Electrical alternans in malignant cardiac tamponade. Twelve-lead electrocardiogram shows electrical alternans. Note the alternating amplitude and vector of the P waves, QRS complexes, and T waves. Reprinted with permission from Lau *et al.* (2002). Cardiac Tamponade and Electrical Alternans, *Texas Heart Institute Journal.,29.* 66–67. Copyright 2002 by the Texas Heart Institute".

Management

Successful treatment of pericardial effusion in patients with cancer may improve both quality and quantity of life (Cozzi *et al.*, 2010). There is no "gold standard" for the management of malignant pericardial effusion and treatment decisions must be individualized to the patient. Options for patients with malignant pericardial effusion include pericardial sclerosing, pericardial window, radiotherapy, and intrapericardial instillation of cystostatic agents (Maisch, Ristic, and Pankuweit, 2010). In patients with cancer, invasive strategies may be contraindicated by coagulopathies or coexisting cytopenias. Platelet transfusions can be used to increase the platelet count to an acceptable level (generally above 50 000). Cozzi *et al.* (2010) described a case series of seven patients with malignant effusions treated with pericardiocentesis. Patients tolerated the procedure well with no cardiovascular complications. Symptoms resolved rapidly and there were no cases of recurrence at 30 days. However, most cases of pericardial effusion will recur if further definitive therapy is not instituted (Cozzi *et al.*, 2010).

For chemosensitive tumors, management of the underlying disease is essential. Systemic chemotherapy may be helpful. Intrapericardial installation of chemotherapy has been used in an attempt to sclerose the pericardial space to prevent fluid reaccumulation. Agents including bleomycin, carboplatin, cisplatin, and mitomycin-C have been used for this purpose (Kaira *et al.*, 2005; Maisch, Ristic, and Pankuweit, 2010; Maruyama *et al.*, 2007; Moriya *et al.*, 2000). Sclerosis is safe and effective with minimal systemic side effects.

Randomized, case–control studies are needed to assess the best management strategies for malignant pericardial effusion. However, aggressive management of malignant pericardial effusion may result in improved quality of life and improved life expectancy, with minimal toxicity (Cozzi *et al.*, 2010).

Malignant airway obstruction
Physiologic guidelines

Obstructions in the airway can be caused by intrinsic tumors growing inside the tracheo-bronchial tree, or by compression or extension into the airway by extrinsic tumors (Chan, 2011). Primary bronchogenic carcinomas including small cell and non-small cell lung cancers that cause extrinsic compression are the most common cause of malignant airway obstruction (Behl, Hendrickson, and Moynihan, 2010; Chan, 2011). Primary intrinsic tumors of the trachea and bronchi are rare (Chan, 2011). Other primary cancers such as thyroid, esophageal, and lymphadenopathy from lymphoma can result in airway obstruction. The incidence of malignant central airway obstruction is 80 000/year (Chen, Varon, and Wenker, 1998). Approximately 35–40% of patients die from complications, and early intervention can improve quality of life and extend survival (Chan, 2011).

Central airway obstruction may be misdiagnosed as asmtha or chronic obstructive pulmonary disease (COPD). To distinguish between central airway obstruction and asthma, administration of inhaled bronchodilators or steroids can aid in the diagnosis. Patients with central airway obstruction will not improve with administration of these agents (Chen, Varon, and Wenker, 1998).

Monitoring

The severity of symptoms depends on the size and location of the tumor as well as the rate of tumor growth (Chan, 2011). Symptoms may have a gradual onset if the tumor is slow-growing or may present acutely in rapidly growing tumors. Dyspnea and hemoptysis are the most common presenting symptoms (Chen, Varon, and Wenker, 1998). Symptoms worsen in the supine position. In severe cases, the supine position can decrease right ventricular output, causing cardiac arrest (Chen, Varon, and Wenker, 1998). Early symptoms may include dyspnea and tachycardia. Later symptoms may include stridor, cough, hemoptysis, anxiety, impending doom, increased work of breathing, and diaphoresis (Chan, 2011). Physical exam may reveal decreased or absent breath sounds, stridor, wheezing, or use of accessory muscles. Chest excursion may be asymmetric; palpation of the chest wall may reveal decreased tactile fremitus over the involved area. Percussion of the involved area reveals dullness (Chen, Varon, and Wenker,

1998). Assess the skin for pallor, cyanosis, and diaphoresis. Assess the heart rate; bradycardia, perioral or acral cyanosis, and obtundation signal severe airway compromise (Chan, 2011; Chen, Varon, and Wenker, 1998). Pneumonia is a common sequela of central airway obstruction; therefore, patients may also exhibit signs and symptoms of respiratory infection. Patients at risk for impending airway obstruction should be monitored via continuous oxygen saturation to assess the severity of hypoxemia.

Chest radiographs may be done in acute situations to rule out other causes of hypoxia including pneumothorax (Chan, 2011). Computed tomography (CT) is preferred over chest radiograph to evaluate tumor size, depth of invasion, and extent of obstruction (Chan, 2011). Bronchoscopy is also helpful in direct visualization of the airway and is considered the gold standard for evaluating central airway obstruction (Chan, 2011). Bronchoscopy allows visualization of the tumor, facilitates distinction between intrinsic and extrinsic obstruction, and allows the opportunity for tissue biopsy (Chan, 2011). Bronchoscopy also provides an opportunity for therapeutic intervention.

Management

Before embarking on an intervention for airway obstruction, consider the patient's comorbidities, hemodynamic stability, cancer type, overall prognosis, and availability of technology (Chan, 2011). A patient with a poor overall prognosis may still benefit from intervention in order to improve quality of life; however, less invasive strategies may be considered.

The most important intervention is to establish and maintain a patent airway (Behl, Hendrickson, and Moynihan, 2010). Patients with impending airway obstruction must have suction supplies set up at the bedside as well as intubation supplies with endotracheal tubes of different sizes, and a tracheostomy kit with a variety of tube sizes in case of emergent tracheotomy. Use of supplemental oxygen, nebulized bronchodilators, and IV steroids may help stabilize the patient and improve symptoms while a plan is developed (Chen, Varon, and Wenker, 1998). Intubation may be difficult and technique is selected based on the level of airway obstruction. Lesions in the upper airway may require a tracheostomy while lesions in the lower airway will require endotracheal intubation that allows the end of the tube to lie beyond the obstruction (Chen, Varon, and Wenker, 1998). Some tumor types are highly vascular and bleeding is a potential complication.

Maintaining spontaneous ventilation is a priority in patients with central airway obstruction. Strategies to maintain spontaneous ventilation include avoidance of agents that cause respiratory depression including opioids and muscle relaxants, avoidance of general anesthesia, and positive pressure ventilation (Chen, Varon, and Wenker, 1998). If sedatives are required, use of medications that do not suppress respirations, such as haldol, should be used (Chen, Varon, and Wenker, 1998). Avoid the supine position as it may exacerbate symptoms and result in decreased right ventricular output (Chen, Varon, and Wenker, 1998). Acceptable position changes include sitting, decubitus, and prone (Chen, Varon, and Wenker, 1998).

Use of helium–oxygen combinations (80% helium, 20% oxygen) have been used successfully in the management of patients with central airway obstruction (Curtis et al., 1986; Mizrahi et al., 1986; Orr, 1988). Helium–oxygen concentrations have an increased density, resulting in decreased work of breathing and therefore decreased energy requirements (Boorstein et al., 1989). Improvements in work of breathing should be seen within minutes of initiation of helium–oxygen therapy (Boorstein et al., 1989).

Therapeutic interventions for malignant central airway obstruction include bronchoscopy, balloon bronchoplasty, laser resection, argon-plasma electrocoagulation, stent insertion, surgical resection, and radiation therapy. Bronchoscopy involves the use of a rigid bronchoscope with a wide diameter to visualize and treat tumors while allowing ventilation (Chan, 2011). The sharp tip of the bronchoscope may be used to debulk the tumor and apply pressure to facilitate hemostasis. Risks include damaging healthy tissue and perforating the mediastinum (Chan, 2011). Use of a rigid bronchoscope requires sedation and can only be used in patients with enough respiratory capacity to safely tolerate sedation (Chan, 2011). Balloon bronchoplasty uses a balloon to dilate the compromised airway. Advantages are that the results are immediate and can be used for intrinsic or extrinsic compromise. Disadvantages include temporary effects and the need for additional interventions. Complications include pneumothorax, mediastinitis, and bleeding (Chan, 2011).

Laser resection uses Neodynium:yttrium aluminum garnet (Nd:YAG) laser to transmit light energy to tissue. Laser therapy is delivered using either a flexible or rigid bronchoscope. The thermal energy is absorbed by the tumor tissue and the blood vessels supplying the tumor. This results in devascularization of the tumor as well as vaporization of the tumor. The primary risk is damage to healthy surrounding tissue (Chan, 2011). Other complications include bleeding, hypoxemia, tracheobronchial perforation, infection, pneumothorax, fistula, and endobronchial burns (Han, Prasetyo, and Wright, 2007; Stanopoulos et al., 1993). While this modality is successful in demonstrating 76% decrease in dyspnea and 94% rate of hemoptysis management, the relief is temporary (Han, Prasetyo, and Wright, 2007). Laser therapy is most successful in cases of acute obstruction, partial obstruction, intrinsic obstruction without cartilage involvement, growth less than 4 cm axially, tumor visible through bronchoscope, and healthy lung tissue distal to obstruction (McElvein and Zorn, 1984). Laser therapy may not be appropriate in cases of highly vascular tumors, widespread metastatic disease, or aggressive tumor types (Gillis et al., 1983).

Argon-plasma electrocoagulation uses a probe with a spark at the end, with argon gas released at the tip, causing an ionized plasma that causes "coagulative necrosis" at the tumor site (Chan, 2011, p. 8). Argon-plasma electrocoagulation can treat tumors that may not be accessible by laser therapy. The disadvantage is that argon-plasma electrocoagulation does not penetrate tissue as deeply as laser energy. This mode may be preferable for superficial tumors (Chan, 2011).

Stents made of silicone, metal, or a combination of both may be used to relieve obstruction in patients with extrinsic tumor compression or tracheoesophogeal fistula.

While stenting does not improve survival, it does significantly improve symptoms (Wood *et al.*, 2003). Benefits include restoration of airway patency, improved ventilation, and facilitation of secretion clearance (Chan, 2011). Complications include stent migration, stent obstruction, granulation tissue growth, and perforation.

External beam radiation therapy (EBRT) is the preferred treatment modality to decrease tumor size and provide palliation (Chan, 2011; Chen, Varon, and Wenker, 1998). Palliative doses of EBRT for the treatment of airway obstruction are 3000 cGy in 10 daily fractions. Side effects include skin changes to the involved field and fatigue. Patients must be monitored closely for worsening of symptoms as radiation-induced edema may results in worsening of obstructive symptoms within the first few days of therapy (Chen, Varon, and Wenker, 1998).

Brachytherapy, which involves placement of a radioactive source directly at the tumor site, has been shown to decrease symptoms and improve quality of life. This mode is contraindicated with tumors that invade major arteries (Chan, 2011). Side effects include bronchitis, hemoptysis, bronchial stenosis, and bronchial fistula (Chan, 2011).

Surgical resection is typically reserved for patients with localized (i.e., nonmetastatic) disease and is a potentially curative option (Chan, 2011). Surgical resection is contraindicated if complete resection jeopardizes healing of the anastomosis, if the tumor length exceeds 50% of the trachea, or if vital structures such as the aorta are involved (Chan, 2011).

Before any of these interventions are employed, a discussion with the oncology team, the patient, and family should take place to discuss overall prognosis and goals of care. In patients with a curative intent, more aggressive interventions such as surgery followed by adjuvant therapy may be most appropriate, while patients with metastatic disease would benefit from palliative interventions that will improve quality of life and minimize suffering.

Carotid blowout syndrome
Physiologic guidelines
The clinical signs and symptoms of carotid artery rupture are referred to as carotid blowout syndrome (CBS; see Fig. 11.3) (Chang *et al.*,

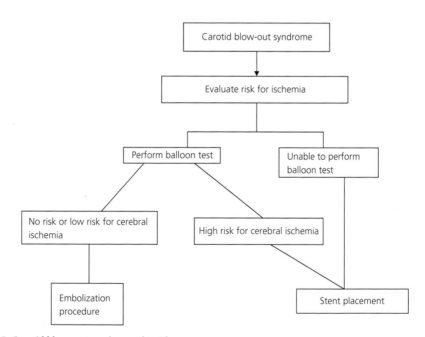

Figure 11.3 Carotid blow-out syndrome algorithm.

2007). Carotid artery rupture occurs in 3–4% of patients with head and neck cancer with a mortality rate of 40–50% (Chaloupka *et al.*, 1999; Citardi *et al.*, 1995; Garcia-Egido and Payares-Herrera, 2011; Macdonald *et al.*, 2000). The common carotid artery arises from the aorta on the left and the brachiocephalic artery on the right. The carotid arteries supply most of the blood to the head and neck. The carotids bifurcate at the level of the hyoid bone into internal and external branches. The bifurcation point is the thinnest and most vulnerable to rupture. The arteries have three layers: adventitia (connective tissue), media (smooth muscle), and intima (endothelial cells). The adventitia provides protection for the artery. The vasovasorium provides 80% of the nutrition to the arterial wall. If nutrition is interrupted by infection, ischemia, tumor invasion, radiation, or surgical damage, the arterial wall weakens, increasing the risk for pseudoaneurysm and rupture (Lesage, 1986). Radiation therapy creates free radicals, which cause fibrosis and weakening of the adventitia (Powitzky *et al.*, 2010).

Risk factors for CBS include radical neck resection, radiation therapy and postradiation necrosis, combined radio–surgery techniques, recurrent tumor with soft tissue invasion, infection, pharyngocutaneous fistula formation, poor wound healing, and flap necrosis with carotid exposure (Chaloupka *et al.*, 1996; Chang *et al.*, 2007; Garcia-Egido and Payares-Herrera, 2011; Macdonald *et al.*, 2000; Maran, Amin, and Wilson, 1989). History of radiation therapy is the most common risk factor and adds a 7.6-fold increase in the risk of carotid artery blowout in patients with head and neck cancer (Maran, Amin, and Wilson, 1989). Time from diagnosis to development of CBS ranges from as early as 6 months to 12 years, with an average time of 2.7 years (Chang *et al.*, 2007; Powitzky *et al.*, 2010).

There are three types of carotid artery rupture: type I (threatened), type II (impending), and type III (acute). In type I, there is exposure of the carotid artery because of a wound, fistula, or necrosis, or from neoplastic invasion of the carotid system with nonhemorrhagic pseudoaneurysm (Chang *et al.*, 2007; Powitzky *et al.*, 2010). Carotid artery rupture is inevitable

if tissue is not covered with healthy, vascularized tissue. Type II carotid artery rupture is classified by short episodes of acute hemorrhage that resolve spontaneously or with simple surgical packing or pressure (Chang *et al.*, 2007; Powitzky *et al.*, 2010). Impending rupture is almost certain to result in complete rupture if there is no intervention. Type III carotid artery rupture includes acute, profuse hemorrhage that is not self-limiting or controlled with surgical packing alone; there is complete rupture of the vessel (Chang *et al.*, 2007). Carotid artery rupture may occur in the internal carotid artery, the common carotid artery, the external carotid artery, or at the bifurcation.

Monitoring
CBS may occur without warning. At-risk patients should be closely monitored for signs and symptoms of impending rupture. Minor bleeding from the wound, flap site, tracheostomy, or mouth may signal slow tumor erosion of the vessel; visible pulsation of the artery, tracheostomy, or flap site; ballooning of an artery; irritability or restlessness. CBS may be instigated by increased pressure from coughing, retching, vomiting, or straining.

CT scan or magnetic resonance imaging (MRI) may be used to classify rupture type and identify patients who may benefit from early intervention. Angiography is the gold standard for diagnosis but is associated with an 8.5% complication rate (Powitzky *et al.*, 2010). A diagnostic grading system has been established to help identify patients who may benefit from early intervention. Grade 0 is no evidence of carotid disruption; Grade 1 is focal weakening or disruption of the vessel wall; Grade 2 is development of pseudoaneurysm; Grade 3 is extravasation from ruptured artery (Chang *et al.*, 2008). Ideally, intervention is initiated prior to progression to Grade 3.

Following intervention for CBS, the patient should be observed closely for neurologic deficits, which are the most common complications of CBS treatments (Lesage, 1986). Neurologic examination should include level of responsiveness, posture and motor activity, quality and size of pupils and reaction to light, and speech quality (Lesage, 1986). Neurologic sequelae of CBS treatment result from cerebral insufficiency and occur within the first 48 h (Lesage, 1986).

Management

The goal of CBS management is to recognize at-risk patients, use diagnostic studies to further determine risk, and treat in earlier stages to prevent acute (type III) rupture (Powitzky et al., 2010). The patient's risk for cerebral ischemia must be evaluated prior to treating. Ischemia risk can be determined by a balloon test. If the balloon test does not reveal risk for ischemia, embolization is the treatment option of choice. Endovascular therapy provides the best option for prevention and acute management of CBS in patients with head and neck cancer (Powitzky et al., 2010). Embolization with a balloon or coil is associated with decreased mortality and 15–20% neurologic morbidity (Chaloupka et al., 1996; Lesley et al., 2004; Powitzky et al., 2010). Open surgery with resection and reconstruction or carotid artery ligation has a high risk of hemodynamic instability and decreased cerebral perfusion with neurologic morbidity rates as high as 60% (Charbel et al., 1999; Citardi et al., 1995). Surgical management may also be challenging in the setting of previously irradiated tissue due to fibrosis and risk for poor wound healing (Chang et al., 2007). In the case of an exposed artery, flap placement may be necessary (Powitzky et al., 2010). If the balloon test identifies high risk for ischemia (decreased cerebral flow <20%) or if the patient is unable to tolerate the balloon test, stent placement is a more appropriate choice. Performing a balloon occlusion test may not be feasible in emergency cases or in cases of hemodynamic instability. Use of stents requires favorable anatomic conditions including patent femoral and iliac artery anatomy to allow placement of a large-bore sheath; nontortuous aortic arch and branches; no carotid stenosis; noncontaminated wound; and no contraindication to antiplatelet therapy (Chang et al., 2007; Powitzky et al., 2010). Self-expandable stents provide immediate hemostasis with minimal neurologic morbidity. Use of stents in the emergency setting may allow for stabilization of the patient and additional time to plan

further, definitive management (Chang et al., 2007). Immediate complications include stroke, asymptomatic thrombosis of the carotid artery; and long-term complications include rebleeding, brain abscess formation, and carotid thrombosis. Long-term safety of stents has been questioned based on rebleeding and thrombosis rates (Chang et al., 2007). Based on this information, stents should be reserved for emergency management. Further study on appropriate antimicrobial prophylaxis to minimize wound infection and optimize use of antiplatelet therapy is needed to improve long-term safety (Chang et al., 2007; Kim et al., 2006).

In the case of acute CBS, the provider should use a gloved finger to apply pressure to the site of bleeding until definitive treatment can be executed. The patient should be placed in Trendelenberg position (Lesage, 1986). Aggressive fluid resuscitation should be employed to maintain blood pressure and blood pressure should be monitored frequently. Mortality rates during ligation procedures are increased in the setting of hypotension and hypotension is the greatest predictor of poor outcomes (Powitzky et al., 2010). Any at-risk patient should have a proactive plan for managing CBS including prn orders for sedation and pain management. Additionally, supplies to manage CBS should be kept at or near the patient's bedside and include gloves, gown, face shield, and goggles; large sterile dressings; suction equipment; cuffed tracheotomy tube and 10 ml syringe; equipment to place and maintain a large-bore IV; oxygen equipment; and dark-colored towels. Emergency management may necessitate placement of a cuffed tracheostomy to protect the patient's airway and provide internal pressure on the source of bleeding. There is no evidence that bedrest prevents or delays rupture (Lesage, 1986). However, activities such as heavy lifting and straining should be avoided. Preventative management should include strategies to minimize straining (e.g., Bowel regimens), coughing (antitussives), and nausea/vomiting (antiemetics). The experience of a CBS is often stressful and traumatic for patients, family, and staff. Appropriate supportive resources should be employed including pastoral care and social work.

There are no prospective or comparison studies examining the most appropriate management of CBS. The available data are based on small studies, many of them retrospective. Larger, prospective studies are needed to help define best practices.

Monitoring and treatment of oncology-related critical care is complex. Interdisciplinary planning and treatment require continual surveillance of patient symptoms and attention to subtle changes. This chapter has reviewed the literature and recommended best practices for a wide range of conditions affecting oncology patients. Research continues and changes in practice evolve daily.

References

Aapro, M.S., Bohlius, J., Cameron, D.A. *et al.* (2011) 2010 update of EORTC guidelines for the use of granulocyte-colony stimulating factor to reduce the incidence of chemotherapy-induced febrile neutropenia in adult patients with lymphoproliferative disorders and solid tumors. *European Journal of Cancer*, **47**, 8–32.

Abu-Alfa, A.K. and Younes, A. (2010) Tumor lysis syndrome and acute kidney injury: evaluation, prevention, and management. *American Journal of Kidney Diseases*, **55** (Suppl 3), S1–S13.

Afessa, B. (2011a) Diffuse alveolar hemorrhage in hematopoietic stem cell transplant recipients and patients with hematologic malignancy, in *Pulmonary Involvement in Patients with Hematologic Malignancies* (ed. E. Azoulay), Springer-Verlag, Heidelberg/New York, pp. 437–444.

Afessa, B. (2011b) Noninfectious pulmonary involvement in hematopoietic stem cell or bone marrow transplant recipients, in *Pulmonary Involvement in Patients with Hematologic Malignancies* (ed. E. Azoulay), Springer-Verlag, Heidelberg/New York, pp. 63–76.

Afessa, B., Tefferi, A., Dunn, W.F. *et al.* (2003) Intensive care unit support and Acute Physiology and Chronic Health Evaluation III performance in hematopoietic stem cell transplant recipients. *Critical Care Medicine*, **31** (6), 1715–1721.

Azoulay, E., Thiery, G., Chevret, S. *et al.* (2004) The prognosis of acute respiratory failure in critically ill cancer patients. *Medicine (Baltimore)*, **83**, 360–370.

Bacigalupo, A., Chien, J., Barisione, G., and Pavletic, S. (2012) Late pulmonary complications after allogeneic hematopoietic stem cell transplantation: diagnosis, monitoring, prevention, and treatment. *Seminars in Hematology*, **49**, 15–24.

Badgwell, B.D., Cormier, J.N., Wray, C.J. *et al.* (2008) Challenges in surgical management of abdominal pain in the neutropenic cancer patient. *Annals of Surgery*, **248**, 104–109.

Baughman, R.P., Lower, E.E., Flessa, H.C., and Tollerud, D.J. (1993) Thrombocytopenia in the intensive care unit. *Chest*, **104**, 1243–1247.

Becker, M.A., Schumacher Jr, H.R., Wortmann, R.L. *et al.* (2005) Febuxostat compared with allopurinol in patients with hyperuricemia and gout. *New England Journal of Medicine*, **353**, 2450–2461.

Behl, D., Hendrickson, A.W., and Moynihan, T.J. (2010) Oncologic emergencies. *Critical Care Clinics*, **26**, 181–205.

Benjamin, R.J. and Anderson, K.C. (2002) What is the proper threshold for platelet transfusion in patients with chemotherapy-induced thrombocytopenia? *Critical Reviews in Hematology-Oncology*, **42**, 163–171.

Benoit, D.D. and Hoste, E.A. (2010) Acute kidney injury in critically ill patients with cancer. *Critical Care Clinics*, **26**, 141–179.

Blake-Haskins, J.A., Lechleider, R.J., and Kreitman, R.J. (2011) Thrombotic microangiopathy with targeted cancer agents. *Clinical Cancer Research*, **17**, 5858–5866.

Boorstein, J.M., Boorstein, S.M., Humphries, G.N., and Johnston, C.C. (1989) Using helium-oxygen mixtures in the emergency management of acute upper airway obstruction. *Annals of Emergency Medicine*, **18**, 688–690.

Cairo, M.S. and Bishop, M. (2004) Tumour lysis syndrome: new therapeutic strategies and classification. *British Journal of Haematology*, **127**, 3–11.

Campara, M., Shord, S.S., and Haaf, C.M. (2009) Single-dose rasburicase for tumor lysis syndrome in adults: weight-based approach. *Journal of Clinical Pharmacy Therapeutics*, **34**, 207–213.

Carlson, K.S. and DeSancho, M.T. (2010) Hematologic issues in critically ill patients with cancer. *Critical Care Clinics*, **26**, 107–132.

Chaloupka, J.C., Putman, C.M., Citardi, M.J. *et al.* (1996) Endovascular therapy for the carotid blowout syndrome in head and neck surgical patients: diagnosis and managerial considerations. *AJNR American Journal of Neuroradiology*, **17**, 843–852.

Chaloupka, J.C., Roth, T.C., Putman, C.M. *et al.* (1999) Recurrent carotid blowout syndrome: diagnostic and therapeutic challenges in a newly recognized subgroup of patients. *AJNR American Journal of Neuroradiology*, **20**, 1069–1077.

Chan, E. (2011) Malignant airway obstruction: treating central airway obstruction in the oncologic setting. *UWOMJ*, **80**, 7–9.

Chang, F.C., Lirng, J.F., Luo, C.B. *et al.* (2007) Carotid blowout syndrome in patients with head-and-neck cancers: reconstructive management by self-expandable stent-grafts. *AJNR American Journal of Neuroradiology*, **28**, 181–188.

Chang, F.C., Lirng, J.F., Luo, C.B. *et al.* (2008) Patients with head and neck cancers and associated postirradiated carotid blowout syndrome: endovascular therapeutic methods and outcomes. *Journal of Vascular Surgery*, **47**, 936–945.

Charbel, F.T., Gonzales-Portillo, G., Hoffman, W., and Cochran, E. (1999) Distal internal carotid artery pseudoaneurysms: technique and pitfalls of surgical management: tow technical case reports. *Neurosurgery*, **45**, 643–648.

Chen, K., Varon, J., and Wenker, O.C. (1998) Malignant airway obstruction: recognition and management. *The Journal of Emergency Medicine*, **16**, 83–92.

Citardi, M.J., Chaloupka, J.C., Son, Y.H. *et al.* (1995) Management of carotid artery rupture by monitored endovascular therapeutic occlusion (1988–1994). *Laryngoscope*, **106**, 1086–1092.

Coiffer, B., Altman, A., Ching-Hon, P. *et al.* (2008) Guidelines for the management of pediatric and adult tumor lysis syndrome: an evidence-based review. *Journal of Clinical Oncology*, **26** (16), 2767–2778.

Coppell, J.A., Brown, S.A., and Perry, D.J. (2003) Veno-occlusive disease: cytokines, genetics, and hemostasis. *Blood Reviews*, **17**, 63–70.

Coppo, P. and Veyradier, A. (2012) Current management and therapeutical perspectives in thrombotic thrombocytopenic purpura. *Press Medicale (Paris, France: 1983)*, **41** (3), e163–e176.

Cortes, J., Moore, J.O., Maziarz, R.T. *et al.* (2010) Control of plasma uric acid in adults at risk for tumor lysis syndrome: efficacy and safety of rasburicase alone and rasburicase followed by allopurinol compared with allopurinol alone—results of a multicenter phase III study. *Journal of Clinical Oncology*, **28**, 4207–4213.

Cozzi, S., Montanara, S., Luraschi, A. *et al.* (2010) Management of neoplastic pericardial effusions. *Tumori*, **96** (6), 926–929.

Curtis, J.L., Mahlmeister, M., Fink, J.B. *et al.* (1986) Helium-oxygen gas therapy: use and availability for the emergency treatment of inoperable airway obstruction. *Chest*, **90**, 455–457.

Danai, P.A., Moss, M., Mannino, D.M., and Martin, G.S. (2006) The epidemiology of sepsis in patients with malignancy. *Chest*, **129** (6), 1432–1440.

Darmon, M. and Azoulay, E. (2009) Critical care management of cancer patients: cause for optimism and need for objectivity. *Current Opinion in Oncology*, **21**, 318–326.

Darmon, M., Thiery, G., Ciroldi, M. *et al.* (2007) Should dialysis be offered to cancer patients with acute kidney injury? *Intensive Care Medicine*, **33**, 765–772.

Darmon, M., Roumier, M., and Azoulay, E. (2009) Acute tumor lysis syndrome: diagnosis and management, in *Yearbook of Intensive Care and Emergency Medicine* (ed. L. Vincent), Springer-Verlag, Berlin/New York, pp. 819–827.

De la Rubia, J., Moscardo, F., Gomez, M.J. *et al.* (2010) Efficacy and safety of rituximab in adult patients with idiopathic relapsing or refractory thrombotic thrombocytopenia purpura: results of a Spanish multicenter study. *Transfusion Apheresis Science*, **42**, 299–303.

Dellinger, R. P., Levy, M. M., Rhodes, A. et al. (2013) Surviving sepsis campaign: International guidelines for management of severe sepsis and septic shock: 2012. *Critical Care Medicine*, **41**, 580–637.

Demshar, R., Vanek, R., and Mazanec, P. (2011) Oncologic emergencies: new decade, new perspectives. *AACN Advanced Critical Care*, **22** (4), 337–348.

Elitek® (package insert) Manufactured by Sanofi-Aventis U.S. LLC. U.S. License No. 1752, © 2011 Sanofi-Aventis U.S. LLC, www.elitek.us (accessed September 12, 2014)..

Feld, R. (2008) Bloodstream infections in cancer patients with febrile neutropenia. *International Journal of Antimicrobial Agents*, **32**, S30–S33.

Fischer, D.S., Knobf, M.T., Durivage, H.J., and Beaulieu, N.J. (2003) *The Cancer Chemotherapy Handbook*, Mosby, Philadephia.

Flounders, J.A. (2003) Cardiovascular emergencies: pericardial effusion and cardiac tamponade. *Oncology Nursing Forum*, **30**, E48–E55.

Fuge, R., Bird, J.M., Fraser, A. *et al.* (2001) The clinical features, risk factors, and outcome of thrombotic thrombocytopenic purpura occurring after bone marrow transplantation. *British Journal of Haematology*, **113**, 58–64.

Garcia-Egido, A.A. and Payares-Herrera, M. (2011) Managing hemorrhages in patients with head and neck carcinomas: a descriptive study of six years of admissions to an internal medicine/palliative care unit. *Journal of Palliative Medicine*, **14**, 124–125.

George, J.N. (2009) The thrombotic thrombocytopenic purpura and hemolytic uremic syndromes: evaluation, management, and long-term outcomes experience of the Oklahoma TTP-HUS Registry, 1989–2007. *Kidney International*, **75** (Suppl 112), S52–S54.

George, J.N. and Aster, R.H. (2009) Drug-induced thrombocytopenia: pathogenesis, evaluation, and management. *Hematology/the Education Program of the American Society of Hematology*, **153–158**. doi: 10.1182/asheducation-2009.1.153

George, J.N., Terrell, D.R., Vesely, S.K. *et al.* (2011) Thrombotic microangiopathic syndromes associated with drugs, HIV infection, hematopoietic stem cell transplantation, and cancer. *La Presse Medicale*, **41**, e177–e188.

Gillis, T.M., Shapsay, S.M., Vaughan, C.W. *et al.* (1983) Laser bronchoscopic surgery. *Journal of Otolaryngology*, **12**, 217–222.

Giraldez, M. and Puto, K. (2010) Letter to the editor: a single, fixed dose of rasburicase (6 mg maximum) for treatment of tumor lysis syndrome in adults. *European Journal of Haematology*, **85**, 177–179.

Groeger, J.S. and Aurora, R.N. (2001) Intensive care, mechanical ventilation, dialysis, and cardiopulmonary resuscitation. Implications for the patient with cancer. *Critical Care Clinics*, **17**, 991–997.

Gruppo, R.A. and Rother, R.P. (2009) Eculizumab for congenital atypical hemolytic-uremic syndrome. *New England Journal of Medicine*, **360**, 544–546.

Halfdanarson, T.R., Hogan, W.J., and Moynihan, T.J. (2006) Oncologic emergencies: diagnosis and treatment. *Mayo Clinic Proceedings*, **81**, 835–848.

Han, C.C., Prasetyo, D., and Wright, G.M. (2007) Endobronchial palliation using Nd:YAG laser is associated with improved survival when combined with multimodal adjuvant treatments. *Journal of Thoracic Oncology*, **2**, 59–64.

Higdon, T.L. and Higdon, J.A. (2006) Treatment of oncologic emergencies. *American Family Physician*, **74**, 1873–1880.

Ho, V.T., Cutler, C., Carter, S. *et al.* (2005) Blood and marrow transplant clinical trials network toxicity committee consensus summary: thrombotic microangiopathy after hematopoietic stem cell transplantation. *Biology of Blood and Marrow Transplantation*, **11**, 571–575.

Hoelzer, D., Thiel, E., Loffler, H. *et al.* (1988) Prognostic factors in a multicenter study for treatment of acute lymphoblastic leukemia in adults. *Blood*, **71**, 123–131.

Holmes Gobel, B. (2006) Tumor lysis syndrome, in *Understanding and Managing Oncologic Emergencies: A Resource for Nurses* (ed. M. Kaplan), Oncology Nursing Society, Pittsburgh, pp. 285–304.

Hummel, M., Reiter, S., Adam, K. *et al.* (2008a) Effective treatment and prophylaxis of hyperuricemia and impaired renal function in tumor lysis syndrome with low doses of rasburicase. *European Journal of Hematology*, **80**, 331–336.

Hummel, M., Rudert, S., Hof, H. *et al.* (2008b) Diagnostic yield of bronchoscopy with bronchoalveolar lavage in febrile patients with hematologic malignancies and pulmonary infiltrates. *Annals of Hematology*, **87**, 291–297.

Hutcherson, D.A., Gammon, D.C., Bhatt, M.S., and Faneuf, M. (2006) Reduced-dose rasburicase in the treatment of adults with hyperuricemia associates with malignancy. *Pharmacotherapy*, **26**, 242–247.

Iacopino, P., Pucci, G., Arcese, W. *et al.* (1999) Severe thrombotic microangiopathy: an infrequent complication of bone marrow transplantation. Gruppo Italiano Trapianto Midollo Osseo (GITMO). *Bone Marrow Transplant*, **24**, 47–51.

Jardim, J.L., Rodrigues, C.A., Novis, Y.A.S. *et al.* (2012) Oxaliplatin related thrombocytopenia. *Annals of Oncology*, **23**, 1937–1942.

Johnson, D.B. and Savani, B.N. (2012) How can we reduce hepatic veno-occlusive disease-related deaths after allogeneic stem cell transplantation? *Experimental Hematology*, **40**, 513–517.

Kaira, K., Takise, A., Kobayashi, G. *et al.* (2005) Management of malignant pericardial effusion with instillation of Mitomycin-C in non-small cell lung cancer. *Japan Journal of Clinical Oncology*, **35**, 57–60.

Kaplan (2006) Hypercalcemia of malignancy. In Kaplan, M., (Ed.) Understanding and Managing oncologic Emergencies. A Resource for Nurses. Pittsburgh, PA: Oncology Nursing Society.

Karajala, V., Mansour, W., and Kellum, J.A. (2009) Diuretics in acute kidney injury. *Minerva Anesthesiology*, **75**, 251–257.

Kasberg, H., Brister, L., and Barnard, B. (2011) Aggressive disease, aggressive treatment: the adult hematopoietic stem cell transplant patient in the intensive care unit. *AACN: Advanced Critical Care*, **22**, 329–364.

Kayexalate® (Sodium Polystyrene Sulfonate, package insert and label information) prescribing information (2010). Manufactured by Sanofi-Aventis U.S. LLC, http://www.accessdata.fda.gov/drugsatfda_docs/label/2009/011287s022lbl.pdf. Last revised June 22, 2012 (accessed September 12, 2014)., Inc.

Kennedy, L.D. and Ajiboye, V.O. (2010) Rasburicase for the prevention and treatment of hyperuricemia in tumor lysis syndrome. *Journal of Oncology Pharmacy Practice*, **16**, 205–213.

Kim, H.S., Lee, D.H., Kim, H.J. *et al.* (2006) Life-threatening common carotid artery blowout: rescue treatment with a newly designed self-expanding covered nitinol stent. *The British Journal of Radiology*, **79**, 226–231.

Klastersky, J., Awada, A., Paesmans, M., and Aoun, M. (2011) Febrile neutropenia: a critical review of the initial management. *Critical Reviews in Oncology/Hematology*, **78**, 185–194.

Kochanek, K.D., Xu, J., Murphy, S.L. *et al.* (2011) Deaths: preliminary data for 2009. *National Vital Statistics Reports*, **59** (4), 1–51.

Kumar, A., Roberts, D., Wood, K.E. *et al.* (2006) Duration of hypotension beforeinitiation of effective antimicrobial therapy is the critical determinant of survival in human septic shock. *Critical Care Medicine*, **34**, 1589–1596.

Kyle, R.A., Gertz, M.A., Witzig, T.E. *et al.* (2003) Review of 1027 patients with newly diagnosed multiple myeloma. *Mayo Clinic Proceedings. Mayo Clinic*, **78**, 21–33.

Lau, T.K., Civitello, A.B., Hernandez, A., and Coulter, S.A. (2002) Cardiac tamponade and electrical alternans. *Texas Heart Institute Journal*, **29**, 66–67.

Lee, A.C., Li, C.H., So, K.T., and Chan, R. (2003) Treatment of impending tumor lysis with single-dose rasburicase. *Annals of Pharmacotherapy*, **37**, 1614–1617.

Legrand, M., Max, A., Schlemmer, B. *et al.* (2011) The strategy of antibiotic use in critically ill neutropenic patients. *Annals of Intensive Care*, **1**, 1–9.

Lesage, C. (1986) Carotid artery rupture: prediction, prevention, and preparation. *Cancer Nursing*, **9**, 1–7.

Lesley, W.S., Chaloupka, J.C., Weigele, J.B. *et al.* (2004) Preliminary experience with endovascular reconstruction for the management of carotid blowout syndrome. *AJNR American Journal of Neuroradiology*, **24**, 975–981.

Levandovsky, M., Harvey, D., Lara, P., and Wun, T. (2008) Thrombotic thrombocytopenic purpura-hemolytic uremic syndrome (TTP-HUS): a 24 year clinical expericne with 178 patients. *Journal of Hematology & Oncology*, **1**, 23.

Liu, C.Y., Sims-Mccallum, R.P., and Schiffer, C.A. (2005) A single dose of rasburicase is sufficient for the treatment of hyperuricemia in patients receiving chemotherapy. *Leukemia Research*, **29**, 463–465.

Lydon, J. (2005) Tumor lysis syndrome, in *Cancer Nursing: Principles and Practice*, 6th edn (eds C.H. Yarbro, M.H. Frogge, and M. Goodman), Jones and Bartlett, Sudbury, pp. 220–230.

Macdonald, S., Gan, J., Mckay, A.J., and Edwards, R.D.(2000) Endovascular treatment of acute carotid blowout syndrome. *Journal of Vascular Interventional Radiology*, **11**, 1184–1188.

Maisch, B., Ristic, A., and Pankuweit, S. (2010) Evaluation and management of pericardial effusion in patients with neoplastic disease. *Progress in Cardiovascular Diseases*, **53**, 157–163.

Malaguarnera, M., Vacante, M., Russo, C. *et al.* (2009) A single dose of rasburicase in elderly patients with hyperuricemia reduces serum uric acid levels and improves renal function. *Expert Opinion Pharmacotherapy*, **10**, 737–742.

Maran, A.G., Amin, M., and Wilson, J.A. (1989) Radical neck dissection: a 19-year experience. *Journal of Laryngology and Otolaryngology*, **103**, 76—76.

Martin-Peña, A., Aguilar-Guisado, M., Espigado, I. *et al.* (2010) Prospective study of infectious complications in allogeneic hematopoietic stem cell transplant recipients. *Clinical Transplantation*, **25**, 468–474.

Maruyama, R., Yokoyama, H., Seto, T. *et al.* (2007) Catheter drainage followed by the instillation of bleomycin to manage malignant pericardial effusion in non-small cell lung cancer: a multi-institutional phase II trial. *Journal of Thoracic Oncology*, **2**, 65–68.

Massaro, K.S.R, Costa, S.F., Leone, C., and Chamone, D.A. (2007) Procalcitonin (PCT) and C-reactive protein (CRP) as severe systemic infection markers in febrile neutropenic adults. *BMC Infectious Disease*, **7**, 137.

McDonell, A.M., Lenz, K.L., Frei-Lahr, D.A. *et al.* (2006) Single-dose rasburicase 6 mg in the management of tumor lysis syndrome in adults. *Pharmacotherapy*, **26**, 806–812.

McElvein, R.B. and Zorn Jr, G.L. (1984) Indications, results, and complications of bronchoscopic carbon dioxide laser therapy. *Annals of Surgery*, **199**, 522–525.

Miaskowski, C. (1999) Oncologic emergencies, in *Oncology Nursing Assessment and Clinical Care* (eds C. Miaskowski and P. Buschel), Mosby, St. Louis, pp. 221–243.

Mizrahi, S., Yaari, Y., Lugassy, G., and Cotev, S. (1986) Major airway obstruction relieved by helium/oxygen breathing. *Critical Care Medicine*, **14**, 986–987.

Moerer, O. and Quintel, M. (2009) Definition, epidemiologie and ukonomische aspekte der sepsis bei erwchsenen. *Der Internist*, **50**, 788, 790–794, 796–798.

Moriya, T., Takiguchi, Y., Tabeta, H. *et al.* (2000) Controlling malignant pericardial effusion by intrapericardial carboplatin administration in patients with primary non-small cell lung cancer. *British Journal of Cancer*, **83**, 858–862.

Mughal, T.I., Ejaz, A.A., Foringer, J.R., and Coiffier, B. (2010) An integrated clinical approach for the identification, prevention, and treatment of tumor lysis syndrome. *Cancer Treatment Reviews*, **36**, 164–176.

Mullen, E.C. and Wang, M. (2007) Recognizing hyperviscosity syndrome in patients with Waldenstrom macroglobulinemia. *Clinical Journal of Oncology Nursing*, **11**, 87–95.

Neuman, J. (2000) Graft-versus-host disease (chapter 22, pp. 22.3–22.13). In P. Buchsel & P. M. Kapustay (Eds). *Stem Cell Transplant: A Clinical Textbook*.

Nümberger, J., Philipp, T., Witzke, O. *et al.* (2009) Eculizumab for atypical hemolytic uremic syndrome. *New England Journal of Medicine*, **360**, 542–544.

Orr, J.B. (1988) Helium-oxygen gas mixtures in the management of patients with airway obstruction. *Ear, Nose, Throat Journal*, **67**, 868–869.

Pallera, A. and Schwartzberg, L. (2004) Managing the toxicity of hematopoietic stem cell transplant. *Journal of Supportive Oncology*, **2**, 228–229.

Pappas, P.G., Kauffman, C.A., Andes, D. *et al.* (2009) Clinical practice guidelines for the management of candidiasis: 2009 update by the Infectious Disease Society of America. *Clinical Infectious Diseases*, **48**, 503–535.

Penack, O., Rempf, P., Eisenblatter, M. *et al.* (2007) Bloodstream infections in neutropenic patients: early detection of pathogens and directed antimicrobial therapy due to surveillance blood cultures. *Annals of Oncology*, **18**, 1870–1874.

Penack, O., Buccheidt, D., Christopeit, M. *et al.* (2011) Management of sepsis in neutropenic patients: guidelines from the infectious disease working party of the German Society of Hematology and Oncology. *Annals of Oncology*, **22**, 1019–1029.

Powitzky, R., Vasan, N., Krempl, G., and Medina, J. (2010) Carotid blowout in patients with head and neck cancer. *Annals of Otology, Rhinology, & Laryngology*, **119**, 476–484.

Rabbat, A., Chaoui, D., Lefebvre, A. *et al.* (2008) Is BAL useful in patients with acute myeloid leukemia admitted in ICU for severe respiratory complications? *Leukemia*, **22**, 1361–1367.

Reeves, D.J. and Bestul, D.J. (2008) Evaluation of a single fixed dose of rasburicase 7.5 mg for the treatment of hyperuricemia in adults with cancer. *Pharmacotherapy*, **28**, 685–690.

Richardson, P.G., Ho, V.T., Giralt, S. *et al.* (2012) Safety and efficacy of defibrotide for the treatment of severe hepatic veno-occlusive disease. *Therapeutic Advances in Hematology*, **3**, 253–265.

Rimkus, C. (2009) Acute complications of stem cell transplant. *Seminars in Oncology Nursing*, **25**, 129–138.

Rühl, H., Bein, G., and Sachs, U.G.H. (2008) Transfusion associated graft versus host disease. *Transfusion Medicine Reviews*, **23**, 62–71.

Ruutu, T., Hermans, J., Niederwieser, D. *et al.* (2002) Thrombotic thrombocytopenic purpura after allogeneic stem cell transplantation: a survey of the European Group for Blood and Marrow Transplantation (EBMT). *British Journal of Haematology*, **118**, 1112–1119.

Ruutu, T., Barosi, G., Benjamin, R.J. *et al.* (2007) Diagnostic criteria for hematopoietic stem cell transplantation-associated microangiopathy (TMA): results of a consensus process by an International Working Group. *Haematologica*, **92**, 95–100.

Saria, M.G. and Gosselin-Acomb, T.K. (2007) Hematopoietic stem cell transplantation: implications for critical care nurses. *Clinical Journal of Oncology Nursing*, **11**, 53–63.

Schairer, J.R., Biswas, S., Keteyian, S.J., and Ananthasubramaniam, K. (2011) A systematic approach to evaluation of pericardial effusion and cardiac tamponade. *Cardiology in Review*, **18**, 233–238.

Scheiring, J., Rosales, A., and Zimmerhackl, L.B. (2010) Clinical practice: today's understanding of the haemolytic uraemic syndrome. *European Journal of Pediatrics*, **169**, 7–13.

Schiffer, C.A., Mangu, P.B., Wade, J.C. *et al.* (2013) Central venous catheter care for the patient with cancer: American Society of Clinical Oncology clinical practice guideline. *Journal of Clinical Oncology: Official Journal of the American Society of Clinical Oncology*, **31** (10), 1357–1370.

Sekhon, S.S. and Roy, V. (2006) Thrombocytopenia in adults: a practical approach to evaluation and management. *Southern Medical Journal*, **99**, 491–498.

Sharma, S., Nadrous, H.F., Peters, S.G. *et al.* (2005) Pulmonary complications in adult blood and marrow transplant recipients: autopsy findings. *Chest*, **128** (3), 1385–1392.

Shelton, B. (2010) Admission criteria and prognostication in patients with cancer admitted to the intensive care unit. *Critical Care Clinics*, **26**, 1–20.

Soares, M. and Salluh, J.I.F. (2010) Response to: organ dysfunction in patients with cancer admitted to the intensive care unit. *Critical Care Medicine*, **38**, 1233.

Stanopoulos, I.T., Beamis, J.F., Martinez, F.J. *et al.* (1993) Laser bronchoscopy in respiratory failure from malignant airway obstruction. *Critical Care Medicine*, **21**, 386–391.

Thiery, G., Azoulay, E., Darmon, M. *et al.* (2005) Outcome of cancer patients considered for intensive care unit admission: a hospital-wide prospective study. *Journal of Clinical Oncology*, **23**, 4406–4413.

Treleaven, J., Gennery, A., Marsh, J. *et al.* (2012) Guidelines on the use of irradiated blood components prepared by the British Committee for Standards in Haematology blood transfusion task force. *British Journal of Haematology*, **152**, 35–51.

Trifilio, S., Gordon, L., Shingal, S. *et al.* (2006) Reduced-dose rasburicase (recombinant xanthine oxidase) in adult cancer patients with hyepruricemia. *Bone Marrow Transplant*, **37**, 997–1001.

Tuncer, H.H., Rana, N., Milani, C. *et al.* (2012) Gastrointestinal and hepatic complications of hematopoietic stem cell transplantation. *World Journal of Gastroenterology*, **18**, 1851–1860.

Turner Story, K. (2006) Cardiac tamponade, in *Understanding and Managing Oncologic Emergencies: A Resource for Nurses* (ed. M. Kaplan), Oncology Nursing Society, Pittsburgh, pp. 1–29.

Uloric® (Febuxostat) prescribing information (2009). Manufactured by Takeda Pharmaceuticals America, Inc., http://general.takedapharm.com/content/file. aspx?applicationcode=66b0b942-e82b-46ad-886a-f4aa59f5f33c&filetypecode=ULORICPI&cacheRand

omizer=077f6b6e-7191-4c76-9a2d-c30ce9c27118. Revised 2013 (accessed September 12, 2014).

Vadhan-Raj, S. (2009) Management of chemotherapy-induced thrombocytopenia: current status of thrombopoietic agents. *Seminars in Hematology*, **46** (Suppl 2), S26–S32.

Varon, J. and Acosta, P. (eds) (2010) Critical care oncology, in *Handbook of Critical and Intensive Care Medicine*, Springer Science+Business Media, LLC, New York, pp. 229–248.

Wood, D.E., Liu, Y.H., Vallieres, E. *et al.* (2003) Airway stenting for malignant and benign tracheobronchial stenosis. *Annals of Thoracic Surgery*, **76**, 167–172.

Zhang, L., Wang, Y., and Huang, H. (2012) Defibrotide for the prevention of hepatic veno-occlusive disease after hematopoietic stem cell transplantation: a systematic review. *Clinical Transplantation*, **26** (4), 511–519.

CHAPTER 12

End-of-life concerns

Kathy J. Booker

Millikin University, Decatur, IL., USA

Introduction

End-of-life (EOL) issues arise frequently in the care of critically ill patients. However, those who care for patients regularly in these units may feel ill-prepared for early discussions or management of differing opinions by patients and family members, especially when transition points develop regarding patient response to treatment. Despite published guidelines on EOL care (Truog *et al.*, 2008), many clinicians find communication surrounding limitations or withdrawal of care difficult. Even oncology practitioners have reported inadequate formal preparation in how to deliver and discuss bad health news (Baile *et al.*, 2000).

Assessment and communication issues

In a busy intensive care unit (ICU), assessments are often predominately focused on the physiological management of a patient's conditions. Understanding the totality of patient needs including psychosocial and spiritual issues is extremely important in critically ill adults. Guidelines on pain assessment for those unable to communicate, including adult patients who are intubated or those with dementia, have been published (Herr *et al.*, 2006). Ongoing assessment of behaviors or verbal indicators of pain is critical. Anticipation of pain when implementing known painful procedures in those with dementia or intubated/unconscious patients is important. Herr *et al.* (2006) noted that the poor correlation of vital sign changes with degree of pain makes assessment more

difficult. For patients who are intubated or unconscious, behavioral indicators may include facial grimacing, frowning, wincing, and physical movement or tearing and diaphoresis. Undertreatment of pain remains an issue in care and must be vigilantly assessed in patients both able and unable to express pain aloud. Guidelines advanced by Herr *et al.* (2006) include strategies for pain assessment incorporating potential causes, observations of behaviors, use of analgesic trials, and an overview of published behavioral assessment tools. For patients with dementia, examination of causes and behaviors associated with pain and the collaboration with families who know the patient well are recommended strategies to ensure pain is managed as an ethical imperative for all patients (Herr *et al.*, 2006).

Other symptoms, such as dyspnea, have also been reported to be undertreated by health-care providers. The American Thoracic Society (ATS) published clinical guidelines for palliative care in patients with respiratory diseases and critical illnesses (Lanken *et al.*, 2008). These are helpful in outlining the parameters of movement from curative–restorative forms of care to palliative care and the core competencies expected in pulmonary and critical care clinicians. Mularski *et al.* (2010) examined palliative care for dyspnea and reviewed over 40 instruments used for rating dyspnea, determining that none of these scales was ideal for use in palliative care. This review, commissioned by the Agency for Healthcare Research and Quality (AHRQ) and supported by the National Cancer Institute, was a project for the development of a framework for assessing EOL quality indicators in cancer care (Mularski *et al.*, 2010). These authors

Critical Care Nursing: Monitoring and Treatment for Advanced Nursing Practice, First Edition. Edited by Kathy J. Booker.

identified the Numerical Rating Scale, a ranking numerical scale from 0 to 10, similar to pain-rating scales commonly employed in many care areas, as it is easy for most patients to use and applicable across a number of settings, from critical care to hospice. Its major limitation is the use of a one-dimensionality assessment of dyspnea, which is often complex and involves additional symptoms concurrently.

Mularski *et al.* (2010) also identified the Respiratory Distress Observation Scale (RDOS) for potential use in cognitively impaired patients. Campbell, Templin, and Walch (2010) evaluated the RDOS in patients with respiratory conditions referred for inpatient palliative care. While a few of the patients had severe distress, the RDOS was found to accurately reflect changes in treatment reflective of respiratory symptoms and had acceptable reliability (Chronbach's alpha = 0.64). Since this tool does not require patient self-report and includes quick analysis of multiple observable symptoms, including heart rate, respiratory rate, respiratory effort and patterns, and nasal flaring, further testing in critically ill patients at the EOL is promising (Campbell, Templin, and Walch, 2010). It should not be used when patients are receiving paralytic agents or when self-report is possible.

Family presence

The American Association of Critical Care Nurses (AACN, 2013) provides resources online for evidence-based practice guidelines. Practice alerts compile literature support for issues important to quality care in critical care units. These guide critical care practitioners to examine policies and consider inclusion of family members for visitation, involvement in care, and allowing presence during resuscitation and invasive procedures (AACN, 2013). Permissive family presence during resuscitation is also endorsed in a review by Doolin *et al.* (2010). See also Chapter 1.

Advanced directives

Since the passage of the US Uniform Patient Self-Determination Act (PSDA) in 1990 (Omnibus Budget Reconciliation Act, 1990),

health-care organizations receiving funding through Medicare and Medicaid are required to inform patients upon admission about the right to refuse treatment and institutional policies regarding advanced directives. This action may be handled by admission personnel and is easily overlooked as patients are being admitted to critical care units due to intensive focus on patients' clinical condition and the need for rapid interventional care. In the midst of a critical event, identifying and supporting a patient's right to refuse treatment is difficult and often deferred in an effort to save a life. Johnson *et al.* (2012) studied reasons for noncompletion of advanced directives in 505 patients admitted to cardiac intensive care in North Carolina. They found that over 64% of the patients did not have an advanced directive upon admission but 45.5% of these patients had discussed their wishes with the person designated to serve as the power of attorney by North Carolina state guidelines. Patients with advanced directives on admission were more likely to be over 65, Caucasian, have higher numbers of comorbid conditions, and less likely to have a family member present upon admission. Johnson *et al.* (2012) noted the difficulty in having meaningful discussions of EOL issues during a stressful time such as admission to an ICU and recommended that recognition of cultural issues affecting individual decisions as well as supportive conversations guided better implementation of the PSDA requirement.

Surrogate decision making

In the absence of advanced directives and when patients are unable to make their own decisions, most states provide for surrogate decision making. Truog *et al.* (2008) reviewed the US court cases that have influenced this area of practice and observe that "when patients cannot make decisions for themselves, decisions are made on their behalf by surrogates, using either the 'substituted judgment standard' (if the patient's values and preferences are known) or the 'best interests standard' (if they are not). While these decisions are often reached by consensus with the patient and family, patients do have an opportunity to designate a specific individual as a healthcare proxy" (p. 954). Sadly, many adults do not plan ahead for such situations and the decision for care and treatment must occur at the bedside under less-than-ideal circumstances. Adequate time and resources must be made available to surrogates. Many hospitals have dedicated pastoral support, strong interdisciplinary care teams, and may also have ethics committees with representation across disciplines and from the lay community to assist in difficult decisions regarding critical care.

AACN offers a number of online resources to support clinicians in helping with patient and family EOL discussions (AACN, 2011). One resource offers discussion points on advance directives and talking points to assist patients and families in discussing and enacting documents (Westphal and Wavra, 2005). Another important reference is the published guidelines for quality palliative care (National Consensus Project for Quality Palliative Care, 2013).

As an essential element in effective treatment of patients and families in the critical care unit, communication skills are extremely important for critical care personnel. When EOL issues arise, prior communication patterns are often accentuated so that families who have unresolved issues prior to a loved one's critical illness will struggle with the decisions that must be made when decisional capacity is lost. Truog et al. (2008) discussed the ethical principles and strategies that may help clinicians improve communication in the ICU (see Table 12.1). Based on the primary ethical principles surrounding withholding versus withdrawing treatment, killing versus allowing to die, and intended versus unforeseen consequences of treatment, Truog et al. (2008) reviewed these issues from the perspective of life-sustaining treatments and decisions that must often be handled at the EOL in critical care units.

The use of strategies to improve communication and adherence to ethical standards assist all members of multidisciplinary teams to provide compassionate, sensitive care to those who need it in the critical care setting.

Table 12.1 Strategies for improving end-of-life communication in the intensive care units.

1 Communication skills training for clinicians.
2 ICU family conference early in ICU course (Lilly et al., 2000)
   Evidence-based recommendations for conducting family conference:
      Find a private location (Pochard et al., 2001).
      Increase proportion of time spent listening to family (McDonagh et al., 2004).
      Use "VALUE" mnemonic during family conferences (Lautrette et al., 2007).
        Value statements made by family members.
        Acknowledge emotions.
        Listen to family members.
        Understand who the patient is as a person.
        Elicit questions from family members.
      Identify commonly missed opportunities (Curtis et al., 2005; West et al., 2005).
        Listen and respond to family members.
        Acknowledge and address family emotions.
        Explore and focus on patient values and treatment preferences.
        Affirm nonabandonment of patient and family.
      Assure family that the patient will not suffer (Stapleton et al., 2006).
      Provide explicit support for decisions made by the family (Stapleton et al., 2006).
   Additional expert opinion recommendations for conducting family conference:
      Advance planning for the discussion among the clinical team.
        Identify family and clinician participants who should be involved.
        Focus on the goals and values of the patient.
        Use an open, flexible process.
        Anticipate possible issues and outcomes of the discussion.
        Give family support and time.
3 Interdisciplinary team rounds.
4 Availability of palliative care and/or ethics consultation (Campbell and Guzman, 2003; Schneiderman et al., 2003).
5 Development of a supportive ICU culture for ethical practice and communication (Hamric and Blackhall, 2007).

Strategies for improving end-of-life communication in the intensive care unit (ICU). From Truog et al. (2008). © LWW.

Delivering bad news

Giovanni (2012) reviewed policy issues affecting EOL care in the United States and identified the incongruence between many patients' wishes and the care often delivered in critical care units. Giovanni identified current US priorities for cost containment and the growth of hospice movements contrasted with wide geographical differences and disparity in acute care services. The participation of nurses in assisting families and the health-care team during difficult conversations and decision-making is crucial.

Baile *et al.* (2000) developed and tested a six-step model (SPIKES) for delivering bad news to cancer patients, noting the low degree of education and training among physicians for successful models to deliver bad news in a humane and caring way. The SPIKES model includes the following steps:

Step 1: S—SETTING UP the interview—arrange for some privacy; involve significant others; sit down; make connection with the patient; manage time constraints and interruptions.

Step 2: P—Assessing the patient's PERCEPTION— before discussing the medical findings, the clinician uses open-ended questions to create a reasonably accurate picture of how the patient perceives the medical situation.

Step 3: I—Obtaining the Patient's INVITATION— while a majority of patients express a desire for full information about their diagnosis, prognosis, and details of their illness, some patients do not.

Step 4: K—Giving KNOWLEDGE and information to the patient—warning the patient that bad news is coming may lessen the shock that can follow the disclosure of the bad news.

Step 5: E—Addressing the patient's EMOTIONS with empathic responses—when patients get bad news, their emotional reaction is often an expression of shock, isolation, and grief (Baile *et al.*, 2000, pp. 305–306).

This model may be applied to critical care situations and when working with families of critically ill adults who may have lost decisional capacity. It may be taught as a strategy for practitioners to systematically consider the impact of bad news so that a humane and caring approach is used in difficult situations.

Other resources for communicating with families are available via the web site of the Center to Advance Palliative Care (Weissman and Meier, 2011). One strong reference on the CAPC web site offers a program for communication of difficult information in the ICU. It incorporates the SPIKE framework as one element in discussing bad news in critically ill patients. The CAPC web site also offers many references including selected hospital protocols, pocket cards, and methods for establishing family conferences.

Weissman and Meier (2011) published a consensus report from the CAPC, which identifies the need for more systematic assessments to advance palliative care for those facing life-limiting episodes during acute hospitalizations. This document advances the development of palliative assessment triggers for admission and during each hospital stay for patients who present with a potentially life-limiting or life-threatening condition. Within this consensus document, recommendations include targeted indicators such as recurrent admissions, complex care, functional declines, failure to thrive, home oxygen therapy, out-of-hospital cardiac arrest, and limited social support. The use of such tools to address pending needs is strongly encouraged for daily rounding and interdisciplinary support.

Palliative care in the ICU

Palliative care is a philosophy of care that does not equate to "comfort" measures or any particular intervention of care. The ATS published a clinical policy statement on palliative care for patients with respiratory and critical illness aimed to relieve suffering and provide support to patients and families to enhance quality of life (Lanken *et al.*, 2008). Palliative care is not limited to terminal care and is not incompatible with critical care delivery.

A national project endorsed by a number of specialty medical and nursing organizations, the National Consensus Project for Quality Palliative Care (2013) has published the second edition of clinical guidelines. These guidelines offer a review of models of care that have been successfully implemented across the nation and clearly define variables and guidance for clinicians interested in expanding their acumen in this area. The guidelines outline the basic assumptions, eight domains of quality care, and a series of guidelines for each domain with a focus on strong interdisciplinary support for patients and families targeting professional behavior and delivery of excellence in each area. Domains and examples of each standard are incorporated into Table 12.2 (National Consensus Project for Quality Palliative Care, 2013). Within this document, each domain is supported with a strong recommended reading bibliography as well as exemplars from programs that have attained best practices in the recommended guidelines. This resource is important to programs seeking excellence in the development of comprehensive palliative care programming.

Palliative care is a philosophy of care and treatment rather than a process linked to clinical staging. Because of the long tradition of interventional care in the critical care unit, care providers may struggle with limitations to aggressive management of care that may be associated with palliative measures. However, deliberate consideration of caregivers' personal perspectives and a thorough understanding of published guidelines should be required as part of orientation programs prior to working in an ICU practice. The ATS clinical policy (Lanken *et al.*, 2008) distinctly addresses how to ethically and compassionately shift from a care modality of aggressive curative/restorative

Table 12.2 Domains of quality palliative care and overview of clinical practice guidelines.

Domains of quality palliative care	Examples of clinical practice guidelines	Multidisciplinary impact
1 Structure and processes of care	Nine guidelines are recommended, including plan of care suggestions, assessment of patient and family, needs-based physical environment	Goals, plan of care, and assessment all based on interdisciplinarity
2 Physical aspects of care	One guideline focused on symptom management and outcomes. Extensive bibliography of pain and associated symptom management and treatment references	Clear incorporation of patient, family, and interdisciplinary team to skillfully treat and evaluate symptoms
3 Psychological and psychiatric aspects of care	Two guidelines focused on education and skillful management of psychiatric comorbidities, including stress , anticipatory grieving, and coexisting psychiatric issues	Referrals to health-care professionals with mental health expertise, incorporation of family and interdisciplinary involvement, including grief and bereavement services
4 Social aspects of care	One guideline advising comprehensive social assessment to incorporate family and social service support	Includes routine family meetings, comprehensive social and cultural assessments, and interdisciplinary cohesion
5 Spiritual, religious, and existential aspects of care	One guideline advising regular, guided assessment of patient and family concerns in this area, including "life review, assessment of hopes and fears, meaning, purpose, beliefs about afterlife, guilt, forgiveness, and life completion tasks" (p. 58)	Advises referrals to professions in spiritual and existential issues, including those with specialized knowledge of rituals or spiritual traditions
6 Cultural aspects of care	One guideline focused on cultural understanding and incorporation of patient/family's cultural needs, particularly with respect to "cultural preferences regarding disclosure, truth telling, and decision making" (p. 65)	Strong emphasis on communication; incorporation of interpreters, family members, and recommendation that hiring practices reflect community cultural diversity
7 Care of the imminently dying patient	Three guidelines covering impending death: recognition, communication of end-of-life concerns honestly and respectfully; postdeath care is respectful and culturally appropriate; bereavement plan is activated	Interdisciplinary involvement is paramount; hospice referrals, education, referrals for funeral arrangements, and family support are all interdisciplinary
8 Ethical and legal aspects of care	Three guidelines covering general guidance for legal issues regarding surrogates, decisional capacity issues, and ethical issues surrounding debilitating illness and palliative care	Inclusion of professional advise on legal and regulatory issues, guardianship, and other legal concerns; palliative care team seeks to prevent ethical dilemmas whenever possible through interdisciplinary involvement and patient/family support efforts

Adapted from NCPQPC (2009).

Table 12.3 Core competencies in palliative care for pulmonary and critical care clinicians recommended by the *Ad Hoc* ATS End-of-Life Care Task Force.

Communication and relationship competencies
   Ability to communicate with empathy and compassion
   Ability to guide the family during the patient's final hours
   Ability to help the family during their period of grief and bereavement
   Ability to identify the patient's values, life goals, and preferences regarding dying
   Ability to identify psychosocial and spiritual needs of patients and families and resources to meet those needs
   Advance care planning with patient and family
   Coordination of care and ability to work effectively in an interdisciplinary team
   Cross-cultural sensitivity and cultural competence
   Information sharing, including ability to break bad news skillfully
Clinical and decision-making competencies
   Ability to apply sound ethical and legal decision making to situations arising from symptom management and withholding
     and withdrawing life-sustaining therapy
   Ability to resolve conflicts over futility, requests for physician-assisted suicide, or active euthanasia
   Establishing an overall medical plan including palliative care elements
   Ability to prognosticate survival and expected quality of life
   Managing withholding and withdrawing life-sustaining therapy and the patient's impending death
   Pain and nonpain symptom management, including dyspnea
   Using the shared decision-making model with families and other surrogates for patients lacking full decision-making capacity
     (President's Council)

Reprinted with permission of the American Thoracic Society from Lanken *et al.* (2008, p. 914, table 2). © American Thoracic Society.

care to a palliative care perspective. Table 12.3 highlights core competencies for clinicians recommended within this document.

Symptom management

Patients in the ICU often experience rapid deterioration due to the complexity of critical conditions, many of which may lead to multiorgan system failure. Early identification of patient and family position and thoughts regarding aggressive resuscitation efforts is important from the time of admission. When decisions are made to limit aggressive care, symptom control is often essential, including management of pain, dyspnea, temperature changes, heart rate, and blood pressure extremes. In many cases, anxiolytics and opioids are helpful in controlling symptoms. Clinical guidelines generally support the use of small intravenous doses with titration for control of symptoms.

Within the recommendations advanced by Truog *et al.* (2008), guidelines for opioids and sedatives are advanced to manage pain, dyspnea, and agitation. In addition, use of nonpharmacologic interventions is enlisted, including sleep promotion, reductions in noise and lighting, and encouraging family presence during periods of agitation or delirium.

The AACN has also been active in promoting nursing skills in palliative care including an e-learning course available online for a nominal fee for individuals to learn more about palliative and EOL care (AACN, 2011). This course uses interactive patient scenarios to bring to life modules on symptom management, communication, conflict resolution, and withdrawing and withholding life support.

The End-of-Life Nursing Education Consortium (ELNEC) (AACN, 2011) has facilitated the education of thousands of nurse educators, nursing students, and practicing nurses, focusing on improving communication among health professionals and highlighting nursing's key role in working to facilitate EOL decisions (Wittenberg-Lyles, Goldsmith, and Ragan, 2011). Over 12 000 nurses and other healthcare professionals have used the ELNEC materials, which consist of eight modules on nursing care at the EOL (AACN, 2011).

Brain death

Despite the aggressive life-saving efforts within the critical care unit, patients may progress to brain death. With the ability to maintain respiration on mechanical ventilators, the development of brain death is difficult for family members to understand and the critical care team is challenged to provide clear direction and support in these situations. Wijdicks *et al.* (2010) published guidelines on determining brain death in adults. In these guidelines, the lack of an evidence base for determining brain death is acknowledged, and important review of studies that have employed alternative diagnostic methods such as magnetic resonance imaging and computed tomography evidence of brain death and multiple differential diagnoses are presented to ensure that patients truly have irreversible causes of coma. With the lack of evidence for accepted medical standards, the authors propose a clinically based set of guidelines for determination of brain death, including methods for clinical evaluation and steps to ensure that appropriate methods are implemented. Documentation and determination of timing of brain death are also offered (see Table 12.4). These guidelines may promote a more consistent method of brain death determination.

In the United States, broadly changing health-care delivery is anticipated over the coming decade. With rising health-care costs

Table 12.4 Checklist for declaring brain death, consistent with these guidelines.

Checklist for determination of brain death

Prerequisites (all must be checked)
Coma, irreversible and cause unknown
Neuroimaging explains coma
CNS depressant drug effect absent (if indicated on toxicology screen; if barbituates given, serum level $<10\,\mu g/ml$)
No evidence of residual paralytics (electrical stimulation if paralytics used)
Absence of severe acid–base, electrolyte, endocrine abnormality
Normothermia or mild hypothermia (core temperature $>36\,°C$)
Systolic blood pressure $\geq100\,mmHg$
No spontaneous respirations

Examination (all must be checked)
Pupils nonreactive to bright light
Corneal reflex absent
Oculocephalic reflex absent (tested only if cervical spine integrity ensured)
Oculovestibular reflex absent
No facial movement to noxious stimuli at supraorbital nerve, temporomandibular joint
Gag reflex absent
Cough reflex absent to tracheal suctioning
Absence of motor response to noxious stimuli in all four limbs (spinally mediated reflexes are permissible)

Apnea testing (all must be checked)
Patient is hemodynamically stable
Ventilaor adjusted to provide normocarbia (PaCO$_2$, 34–45 mmHg)
Patient preoxygenated with 100% FiO$_2$ for $>10\,min$ to PaO$_2$ $>200\,mmHg$
Patient well oxygenated with a PEEP of 5 cm H$_2$O
Provide oxygen via a suction catheter to the level of the carina at 6 l/min or attach T-piece with CPAP at 10 mm H$_2$O
Disconnect ventilator
Spontaneous respirations absent
Arterial blood gas drawn at 8–10 min, patient reconnected to ventilator
PCO$_2$ $\geq60\,mmHg$, or 20 mmHg rise from normal baseline value
OR:
Apnea test aborted

Ancillary testing (only one needs to be performed) to be ordered only if clinical examination cannot be fully performed due to patient factors, or if apnea testing is inconclusive or aborted)
Cerebral angiogram
HMPAO SPECT
EEG
TCD
Time of death (DD/MM/YY) _____
Name of physician and signature _____

and increased percentage of the gross domestic product spent on health care, EOL care is under considerable scrutiny. Wunsch *et al.* (2009) compared the use of ICU services during terminal hospitalizations between England and the United States. While a greater percentage of deaths occurred during hospitalization in England, only 10% were experienced in ICUs compared with 47% in the United States, with the largest differences among elderly persons. Wunsch *et al.* (2009) identified the many factors that influence differing patterns, including legal decision making for those unable to make health-care decisions, cultural norms, and physician philosophies affecting aggressiveness of treatment. Clearly, shifts in ICU utilization can be anticipated in the near future in the United States, and these will be difficult decisions to make without considerable efforts to improve collaboration of all health-care providers, patients, and families to meet the palliative care needs and promote safe and high-quality care at the EOL.

In summary, EOL issues abound in the critical care unit and many resources exist to prepare clinicians to develop skills for promoting compassionate patient and family decision making. Working with difficult decisional issues is a continual challenge in the critical care environment but it also brings rewards when patients and families express satisfaction with respectful, competent care. While many models and guidelines have been developed, the commitment of the critical care team is central to improving EOL care. Further research is needed to evaluate interventional and communication patterns that support high-quality, ethically supportive, and effective EOL care.

References

American Association of Colleges of Nursing (AACN) (2011) *End of Life Nursing Education Consortium (ELNEC)*, http://www.aacn.nche.edu/ELNEC/ (accessed July 27, 2014).

American Association of Critical Care Nurses (AACN) (2013) *Promoting Excellence in Palliative and End-of-Life Care*, http://www.aacn.org/wd/elearning/content/palliative/palliative.pcms?menu=elearning&lastmenu=divheader_courses_for_individuals (accessed July 27, 2014).

Baile, W.F., Buckman, R., Lenzi, R. *et al.* (2000) SPIKES—a six-step protocol for delivering bad news: application to the patient with cancer. *The Oncologist*, **5**, 302–311.

Campbell, M.L. and Guzman, J.A. (2003) Impact of a proactive approach to improve end-of-life care in a medical ICU. *Chest*, **123**, 266–271.

Campbell, M.L., Templin, T., and Walch, J. (2010) A respiratory distress observation scale for patients unable to self-report dyspnea. *Journal of Palliative Medicine*, **13** (3), 285–290.

Curtis, J.R., Engelberg, R.A., Wenrich, M.D. *et al.* (2005) Missed opportunities during family conferences about end-of-liffe care in the intensive care unit. *American Journal of Respiratory and Critical Care Medicine*, **171**, 844–849.

Doolin, C.T., Quinn, L.D., Bryant, L.G. *et al.* (2010) Family presence during cardiopulmonary resuscitation: using evidence-based knowledge to guide the advanced practice nurse in developing formal policy and practice guidelines. *Journal of the American Academy of Nurse Practitioners*, **23**, 8–14.

Giovanni, L.A. (2012) End-of-life care in the United States: current reality and future promise—a policy review. *Nursing Economics*, **30**, 125–136.

Hamric, A.B. and Blackhall, I.J. (2007) Nurse-physician perspectives on the care of dying patients in intensive care units: collaboration, moral distress, and ethical climate. *Critical Care Medicine*, **35**, 422–429.

Herr, K., Coyne, P.J., Key, T. *et al.* (2006) Pain assessment in the nonverbal patient: position statement with clinical practice recommendations. *Pain Management Nursing*, **7**, 44–52.

Johnson, R.W., Zhao, Y., Newby, K. *et al.* (2012) Reasons for noncompletion of advance directives in a cardiac intensive care unit. *American Journal of Critical Care*, **2**, 311–319.

Lanken, P.N., Terry, P.B., DeLisser, H.M. *et al.* (2008) An official American Thoracic Society clinical policy statement: palliative care for patients with respiratory diseases and critical illnesses. *American Journal of Respiratory and Critical Care Medicine*, **177**, 912–927.

Lautrette, A., Darrmon, M., Megarbane, B. *et al.* (2007) A communication strategy and brochure for relatives of patients dying in the ICU. *New England Journal of Medicine*, **356**, 469–478.

Lilly, C.M., De Meo, D.L., Sonna, L.A. *et al.* (2000) An intensive communication intervention for the critically ill. *American Journal of Medicine*, **109**, 469–475.

McDonagh, J.R., Elliott, T.B., Engelberg, R.A. *et al.* (2004) Family satisfaction with family conferences about end-of-life care in the intensive care unit:

increased proportion of family speech is associated with increased satisfaction. *Critical Care Medicine*, **32**, 1484–1488.

Mularski, R.A., Campbell, M.L., Asch, S.M. *et al.* (2010) A review of quality of care evaluation for the palliation of dyspnea. *American Journal of Respiratory and Critical Care Medicine*, **181**, 534–538.

National Consensus Project for Quality Palliative Care (2013) *Clinical Practice Guidelines for Quality Palliative Care*, 3rd edn, Author, Pittsburgh, http://www.nationalconsensusproject.org (accessed August 8, 2014).

Omnibus Budget Reconciliation Act of 1990 (1990) Title IV, Section 4206. *Congressional Record*, October 26, 236:H12456–H12457.

Pochard, F., Azoulay, E., Chevret, S. *et al.* (2001) Symptoms of anxiety and depression in family members of intensive care unit patients: ethical hypothesis regarding decision-making capacity. *Critical Care Medicine*, **29**, 1893–1897.

Schneiderman, I.J., Gilmer, T., Teetzel, M.D. *et al.* (2003) Effect of ethics consultations on nonbeneficial life-sustaining treatments in the intensive care setting: a randomized controlled trial. *Journal of the American Medical Association*, **290**, 1166–1172.

Stapleton, R.D., Engelberg, R.A., Wenrich, M.D. *et al.* (2006) Clinician statements and family satisfaction with family conferences in the intensive care unit. *Critical Care Medicine*, **34**, 1679–1685.

Truog, R.D., Campbell, M.I.., Curtis, J.R. *et al.* (2008) Recommendations for end-of-life care in the intensive care unit: a consensus statement by the American College of Critical Care Medicine. *Critical Care Medicine*, **36**, 953–963.

Weissman, D.E. and Meier, D.E. (2011) Identifying patients in need of a palliative care assessment in the hospital setting. A consensus report from the Center to Advance Palliative Care. *Journal of Palliative Medicine*, **14** (1), 1–7.

West, H.F., Engelberg, R.A., Wenrich, M.D., and Curtis, J.R. (2005) Expressions of nonabandonment during the intensive care unit family conference. *Journal of Palliative Medicine*, **8**, 797–807.

Westphal, C. and Wavra, T. (2005) *Acute and Critical Care Choices Guide to Advance Directives*, http://www.aacn.org/WD/Practice/Docs/Acute_and_Critical_Care_Choices_to_Advance_Directives.pdf American Association of Critical-Care Nurses. (accessed August 8, 2014).

Wijdicks, E.F.M., Varelas, P.N., Gronseth, G.S., and Greer, D.M. (2010) Evidence-based guideline update: determining brain death in adults: report of the Quality Standards Subcommittee of the American Academy of Neurology. *Neurology*, **74**, 1911–1918.

Wittenberg-Lyles, E., Goldsmith, J., and Ragan, S. (2011) The shift to early palliative care: a typology of illness journeys and the role of nursing. *Clinical Journal of Oncology Nursing*, **15** (3), 304–310.

Wunsch, H., Linde-Zwirble, W.T., Harrison, D.A. *et al.* (2009) Use of intensive care services during terminal hospitalizations in England and the United States. *American Journal of Respiratory and Critical Care Medicine*, **180**, 875–880.

CHAPTER 13

Monitoring for overdoses

Linda M. Dalessio

Western Connecticut State University, Danbury, CT., USA

Introduction

General management of drug overdoses

The general management for all drug overdoses is to support airway, breathing, and circulation. Intubation and ventilation may be required. Circulatory support is generally accomplished with intravenous (IV) crystalloid fluids. If hypotension is unresponsive to fluid resuscitation, use of vasopressor agents may be needed. Finger stick glucose testing should be done in all patients with altered mental status. If opioid or benzodiazepine overdose is suspected, the use of naloxone or flumazenil (Romazicon) may be needed. In the case of tricyclic antidepressant (TCA) or antiarrhythmic overdose use of sodium bicarbonate, hypertonic saline, and/or hyperventilation may be warranted. All treatment centers for overdose management should check with Poison Control Centers designated by the state. This chapter is not intended to guide all treatment and management of overdoses or toxic exposure. However, monitoring critically ill patients for overdose symptoms and understanding the management of overdoses are helpful to critical care practitioners.

A detailed history should be obtained from the patient (if able), family or significant other, law enforcement, and Emergency Medical Service (EMS) personnel. If pertinent, efforts should be made to obtain prescription bottles, or empty bottles of substances to quantify amounts of drugs taken. It may be necessary to obtain pharmacy information to have a complete list of drugs prescribed and amounts filled. Most drug overdoses affect the cardiovascular and central nervous system (CNS). If at all possible, toxidromes should be identified as these can help identify the drug toxin, especially in circumstances in which the toxin is unknown. These will be explored within this chapter.

Drug screening

In most hospitals, drug screens usually only involve five primary substances: opioids, marijuana, amphetamines, barbiturates, and cocaine. There are thousands of toxic substances in the world. Certain drug tests are available for some toxic substances but may only be available at state-level toxicology centers. Poison Control Centers guide practitioners in identifying substances, monitoring parameters, and safety issues in treatment and follow-up. The most common toxic substance overdoses seen in critical care settings include acetaminophen, benzodiazepines, opioids, alcohol, antidepressants, certain street drugs, and stimulants. Separate testing is ordered for salicylate and acetaminophen levels. Hospital laboratories may need to test separately for methadone.

Activated charcoal, gastric lavage, and cathartics (whole bowel irrigation) may be beneficial in some instances of drug ingestion. Gastric lavage has fallen out of favor by most toxicologists due to its lack of benefit and risk of aspiration. Activated charcoal may be considered if drug ingestion has occurred within 1 h. Studies have shown that when charcoal is given within 30–60 min following ingestion, 50% of a drug may be recovered. Once the drugs have passed through the pylorus into the small intestine, amounts recovered are much

Critical Care Nursing: Monitoring and Treatment for Advanced Nursing Practice, First Edition. Edited by Kathy J. Booker.
© 2015 John Wiley & Sons, Inc. Published 2015 by John Wiley & Sons, Inc.

smaller (Gussow, 2009). Others have warned of a higher risk of charcoal aspiration, which can lead to chemical pneumonitis.

Charcoal works by binding drugs to its large surface area. The general rule is to give a 10:1 ratio of activated charcoal or 1–2 g/kg of body weight. Charcoal does not effectively bind organic salts such as iron or lithium. Gastric lavage should be employed if the benefit outweighs the risk. It should be done within the first couple of hours post ingestion using a large-bore nasal gastric tube. Risks include aspiration, esophageal perforation, hypoxia, laryngospasm, misplacement of tube into respiratory tract, and discomfort. Cathartics should be used following charcoal administration to prevent constipation. Whole-bowel irrigation using Golytely (2 l/h) can be used in instances of ingestion of sustained-release medications, iron, or enteric-coated substances (Givens and O'Connell, 2007). Collaboration with state Poison Control Centers should be considered for all instances of poisoning/ingestion of known and unknown substances. Dialysis or use of molecular adsorbent recirculating system (MARS) has been effective in overdoses of barbiturates, lithium, metformin, salicylates, theophylline, toxic alcohols, isopropanol, valproic acid, carbamazepine, diltiazem, phenytoin, and mushroom poisoning (DePont, 2007).

Additional issues may involve law enforcement in cases of intentional poisoning by others and notification of state agencies may be needed for the protection of children or patients with psychiatric disabilities. Social services within the hospital setting should be consulted. Mandatory referral is needed to psychiatry in all instances of overdose so it may be determined whether the overdose was accidental or deliberate and interventions may be started.

It is impossible to cover every possible overdose within this chapter and newer therapies are under investigation. Drug overdoses or toxin exposure may be accidental or intentional. Primary organic substance overdoses are reviewed. All emergency and critical care personnel should become familiar with local and regional Poison Control Center contacts.

New and emerging therapies

New and exciting research into the use of intravenous lipid emulsion (ILE) therapy for certain drug overdoses is under way. The mechanism of action of ILE is thought to be a reduction in free drug levels and toxicity. ILE works by expanding the liquid phase availability, which acts as a large vascular liquid component and soaks up the lipid-soluble toxin like a sponge. Another action is inhibition of drug transport across membranes and facilitation of fatty acids into the mitochondria. This results in maintenance of cellular energy and increased inotropic support for the poisoned myocardium. Antidotal use of ILE is investigative and is not approved by the Food and Drug Administration (FDA), but it has recently become part of several professional guidelines for the treatment and management of local anesthetic systemic toxicity (LAST). Drug overdoses in which this therapy may be used are TCAs, some atypical psychiatric drugs, calcium channel blockers (CCBs), beta blockers, aminodarone, barbiturates, and certain anesthetic drugs. There have been several case reports in which this therapy has been used when standard supportive protocols, advanced cardiac life support (ACLS) protocols, and conventional toxicology for overdose have not been effective in the initial resuscitative efforts with patients who have taken an overdose of a lipophilic cardiotoxin (Cave, 2011).

The most convincing body of evidence for treating LAST is in overdoses of bupivacaine and lidocaine. Complications from this disorder can include cardiovascular and CNS collapse, which has been generally treated with a prolonged course of cardiopulmonary resuscitation efforts that are often unsuccessful. Major anesthesia organizations have incorporated the use of ILE in the treatment of LAST. Current guidelines for administration are 1.5 ml/kg bolus followed by an infusion of 0.25 ml/kg/ min of ideal body weight of a 20% lipid emulsion. If hemodynamic instability is still present, boluses can be repeated up to three times, 3–5 min apart (Ozcan and Weinberg, 2011). Avoidance of vasopressin and use of low-dose epinephrine may also be effective in the setting of LAST (Rothschild *et al.*, 2010).

Lipid emulsions with long chain fatty acids have been shown to have an advantage over medium chain fatty acids. Adverse effects of ILE are rare and reporting has included elevated liver function tests (LFTs), amylase, and symptoms associated with acute respiratory distress syndrome, allergic reactions, and gross hematuria. At initial infusion, intralipid can increase body temperature and cause chills, nausea, and vomiting. If this occurs, therapy should be discontinued. Relative contraindications to therapy include egg allergy, impaired lipid metabolism, uncompensated diabetic mellitus, pancreatitis, liver insufficiency, hypothyroidism if in relation to hypertriglyceridemia. Case reports of fat emboli have also been reported (Muzawazi and Manickam, 2012). Lipid emulsion administration can also interfere with certain laboratory tests and cause falsely elevated levels of total hemoglobin and methemoglobin (Ozcan and Weinberg, 2011). If ILE is administered during cardiac arrest (dosages have ranged in case reports from 50 ml of 20% lipid emulsion to 200 ml), clinicians must be aware that it will also bind lipid-soluble cardiac resuscitative drugs such as amiodorone and lidocaine (Ozcan and Weinberg, 2011).

High-dose insulin/glucose euglycemia (HIE) therapy is also being used in calcium channel and beta blocker overdose. This therapy has not been approved but has worked in animal and case studies and appears safe. The mechanism of action is thought to be increased inotropic effects within the cardiovascular system that involves calcium and the P13K pathway. HIE therapy causes increased inotropic effects, increased intracellular glucose transport, and vascular dilatation. The vasodilatation effect of insulin is thought to be due to the enhancement of endothelial nitric oxide synthase activity and its effects on P13K, which is a major insulin-signaling pathway. Insulin also enhances microvascular perfusion at the capillary bed and decreases vascular resistance, which results in improved cardiac output (Engebretsen et al., 2011).

Doses suggested in case studies are 1 µ/kg insulin bolus followed by 1–10 µ/kg/h. This is run concurrently with dextrose infusion, which may be needed for up to 24 h after insulin therapy is completed (Page, Hacket, and Isbister, 2009). Major adverse side effects

are hypoglycemia and hypokalemia. Frequent monitoring of blood glucose levels and potassium levels is needed with this therapy. This therapy is recommended initially in beta blocker and CCB poisoning but pitfalls exist (Smollin, 2010).

Another newer therapy that is being used is octreotide for sulfonylurea overdose. Sulfonylureas are one of the most commonly prescribed antidiabetic agents. Estimated overdose numbers approximate 4000 patients annually who are reported to Poison Control Centers (Spiller and Sawyer, 2006). Overdose of sulfonylurea affects B cells in the pancreatic islets causing hypoglycemia and inhibition of potassium channels, which causes opening of voltage-gated calcium channel and an influx of calcium ions. This triggers a cascade of events that produces exocytosis and increased insulin secretion, resulting in a hyperinsulinemic state and hypoglycemia. Peak plasma levels usually occur within 1–8 h and hypoglycemia usually occurs within 8 h. In the case of renal failure, symptoms can be delayed by several days. Signs and symptoms include hypoglycemia, tachycardia, diaphoresis, and CNS symptoms. Activated charcoal can be given if ingestion is within 1–2 h. Treatment should be started early, and patients should be allowed to eat and drink. IV dextrose should only be given for blood sugars less than 60 mg/dl with symptoms. For hypoglycemia that is refractory to dextrose administration, octreotide should be administered. Actions of octreotide help bind somatostatin subtype G receptors in the pancreatic B cells, which inhibits the opening of the calcium channels and decreases calcium flux, which reduces the release of insulin from B cells (Roberts, 2010). Optimal dosages have not been established but effective treatment with 50–100 µg subcutaneously every 8 h for 24–48 h have been given with success (Lheureux et al., 2005).

Indexing of drug and toxins seen in overdoses

Common drug ingestions will be covered using the following summary categories
1 Drug overview
2 Symptoms of overdose

3 Diagnostic testing and monitoring
4 Antidotes/evidence-based treatment/use of binding agents
5 Clinical pearls for patient management and treatment

Acetaminophen
Drug overview
Acetominophen is an over-the-counter (OTC) analgesic that also comes in extended-release forms and is often combined with opiates or other cold and fever medications. It is rapidly absorbed with peak levels in 30–120 min. Therapeutic dose is no more than 4 g/24 h. Absorption may be delayed in extended-release forms. Elimination half-life is 1–3 h after ingestion and up to 12 h in acute overdose. A Tylenol nomogram should be used for prediction of hepatotoxicity after acute overdose, within a 24 h window of ingestion; this is widely available on the Internet.

Symptoms of overdose
Acute overdose may be seen with ingestion of more than 140 mg/kg or 7.5 g in a 24 h period or as a single amount. Symptoms may be non-specific or absent early and then progress to include nausea, vomiting, malaise, and anorexia. On day 3, elevated transaminases, jaundice, right upper quadrant pain, and elevations in bilirubin can occur. With massive overdose, altered mental status and metabolic acidosis can occur. If liver injury progresses to fulminant hepatic failure, symptoms of encephalopathy, lactic acidosis, and coagulopathy will develop. The patient will either enter the recovery phase or progress to hepatic failure and will need to be evaluated for a liver transplant. Referral should be made early in diagnosis to the gastrointestinal (GI) or hepatologic service.

Diagnostic testing and monitoring
Acetaminophen levels should be obtained every 6–8 h, and complete metabolic panel, baseline acetylsalicylic acid (ASA) and drug toxicology screening should be completed. LFTs and coagulopathy should be completed daily until acetaminophen levels are undetectable and risk of toxicity is over. Testing should be based on individual presentation.

Antidotes/binding agents
Mucomyst (*N*-acetylcysteine IV infusion or orally) is the antidote of choice and is ideally administered within 8–10 h of ingestion and can be given up to 16 h post ingestion (Chun *et al.*, 2009). Patients should also receive lactulose, Golytely, or any laxative/cathartic to induce diarrhea for overdoses with extended-release forms of acetaminophen. Activated charcoal can be given within 4 h of ingestion or there are co-ingestions of other drugs. Charcoal can absorb up to 50% of acetaminophen. Charcoal dose is 1 g/kg for a total of a 50 g dose. Mucomyst oral loading dose is usually 140 mg/kg of the 10–20% solution. Maintenance oral dose is usually 70 mg/kg every 4 h for 17 doses, which is usually for 72 h. IV dosing may be the preferred method. The loading dose is 150 mg/kg over 15 min followed by 50 mg/kg over 4 h, then 100 mg/kg over 16 h. New therapies for infusion are commonly given

---

Clinical Pearls

Approximately 10–20% of patients can develop an analphylactoid reaction to Mucomyst that consists of hives and urticaria. The infusion is usually stopped; the patient is given Benadryl 1 mg/kg up to 50 mg, then the infusion is restarted. If patients develop hypotension or respiratory distress from IV Mucomyst, oral dosing is usually tolerated better. If a patient vomits within 1 h of a dose, the dose should be repeated.

Treatment can be stopped when acetaminophen levels are undetectable, international normalized ratio (INR) is less than 2, and the Alanine Aminotransferase (ALT) has returned to normal or has decreased more than 50% of peak value. Elevation of INR by itself can be misleading as elevated acetaminophen levels and therapeutic levels of Mucomyst can cause elevation of INR. There are newer treatments for fulminent liver failure from acetaminophen and other causes that are available to select patients at several hospitals across the United States called MARS. This system uses an extracorporeal technique with albumin exchange for the removal of toxins that is similar to hemodialysis. Consultation with hepatology and referral to these trial facilities may be life-saving when liver for transplant is not immediately available (DePont, 2007).

Clinical use of Mucomyst in patients who present beyond the 10 h period of ingestion or in patients who are already showing signs and symptoms of liver injury is becoming more controversial due to a concern that late presenters may have changed kinetics to Mucomyst, which may reduce its efficacy and lead to adverse hemodynamic changes. This is postulated to cause impairment of regeneration in the liver (Athuraliya and Jones, 2009; Yang *et al.*, 2009).

over 21 h, with the loading dose given over 60 min to decrease the risk of anaphylactic reactions (Hodgman and Garrard, 2012). If acetaminophen levels continue to rise, dosing may be continued past 16 h.

Mucomyst acts as a sulfhydryl group donor and substitutes the liver's usual sulfhydryl donor, glutathione. Mucomyst is able to bind and detoxify the intermediates of metabolism and may reduce the toxic intermediates. Mucomyst is most effective when given early in the setting of overdose. Some of the side effects are nausea and vomiting, especially with oral preparations.

Salicylates and nonsteroidal anti-inflammatory drugs

Drug overview

Salicylates are a class of drug that includes a variety of medications used for their analgesic and anti-inflammatory properties. Aspirin (ASA) overdose commonly causes an increased anion gap acidosis. Toxic effects of nonsteroidal anti-inflammatory drugs (NSAIDs) usually occur within 1 h and patients who have diseases with low protein levels are at increased risk of toxicity due to protein binding and drug distribution. Usually symptoms of NSAID poisoning are mild and nonspecific. Toxic levels usually produce mental status changes. The half-life is 1–50 h depending on the NSAID ingested. ASA (aspirin) is hydrolyzed to salicylic acid, which stimulates the respiratory center and produces hyperventilation. Salicylates also cause uncoupling of oxidative phosphorylation at the cellular level. Salicylates are metabolized in the liver to inactive metabolites. The remaining amounts are excreted unchanged in the urine.

Nonsalicylate NSAIDs are rapidly absorbed after ingestion and metabolites are not saturable; they are highly protein-bound, and elimination follows first-order kinetics. Massive ingestion is usually 6 g in an adult.

Symptoms of overdose

Symptoms with salicylate overdose can begin within 1–2 h after ingestion but can be delayed in sustained-release formulas. Nausea, vomiting, tinnitus, hearing loss, coma, seizures, respiratory alkalosis followed by metabolic acidosis, increased levels of lactic acid, tachycardia, tachypnea, fever, hypotension, and acute renal insufficiency can occur. Symptoms may also include nausea, vomiting, tinnitus, tachycardia, diaphoresis, and abdominal discomfort.

Cases of moderate poisoning result in acid–base balance being either normal or alkaline. Electrolyte disturbances may show combined respiratory alkalosis and metabolic acidosis with increased anion gap. Common symptoms include an increase in GI and neurological symptoms. Signs and symptoms of severe poisoning include seizures, coma, shock, respiratory depression, and noncardiogenic pulmonary edema. Severe renal dysfunction may develop.

Monitoring

Serum salicylate levels should be obtained every 2 h for the first 4–8 h, then every 6–8 h once levels are declining. Serum concentrations over 20 mg/dl saturate the liver and elimination changes from first-order to zero-order kinetics. This causes the half-life to increase from 2.5 h to an upper limit of 40 h. Renal elimination is then conducted. Levels of more than 30 mg/dl are associated with mild toxicity. Severe levels are 75 mg/dl and levels greater than 90–100 mg/dl or signs and symptoms of end-organ damage are usually indicative of lethal levels. With levels this high, hemodialysis should be initiated. Aspirin levels may start out low and become toxic within 24 h depending on half-life and elimination. Absorption can continue for up to 24 h because of delayed dissolving of tablets or formation of gastric concretions (movable intraluminal mass of pills).

Urine ph and specific gravity may be useful. Close monitoring of acid–base status is essential. Electrocardiogram (ECG) monitoring, serial arterial blood gases (ABGs), serum electrolytes, glucose, BUN, and creatinine levels should be monitored every 4–6 h. Liver function tests should be monitored as needed. Monitoring and diagnostic testing for NSAID overdose is the same as salicylates. Pregnancy testing should be completed in all women of childbearing age.

Antidotes/binding agents/treatment

For both ASA and NSAID overdose, GI decontamination may be performed with activated charcoal if time of ingestion is known. Repeated doses of charcoal with rising levels may be needed with sustained-release formulas along with whole-bowel decontamination because of delayed absorption and gastric concretion. Endoscopy with gastric lavage has also been utilized in cases of increasing levels. Hemodialysis may be necessary in cases where serum levels are more than 100 mg/dl or with severe and progressive clinical deterioration that is unresponsive to urine alkaline diuresis; referral to a renal consultant should be made early.

Initial fluid management should be D5NS or D5W with 1 ampule (50 mEq) of sodium bicarbonate, with 1–3 l given within the first 2 h if levels are over 30 mg/dl. The goal is to alkalinize the urine to a pH > 7.5 and urinary output of 2–4 ml/kg/h. Salicylate removal is increased by alkalization of the urine. CNS hypoglycemia can occur despite normal serum blood glucoses and blood glucose monitoring should be instituted. Treatment with D50 may be needed in patients with altered mental status and CNS symptoms.

Supportive measures for airway and circulation should be instituted for coma and seizures and if profound organ dysfunction occurs. Ventilator support with positive end-expiratory pressure should be utilized in cases of noncardiac pulmonary edema. Diuretics are ineffective.

> **Clinical Pearls**
>
> Anion gap acidosis is common. See chapter summary for analysis of metabolic analysis of acid–base disorders (see mnemonic for "MUDPILES"). Tinnitus and hearing loss are the most common symptoms of ASA overdose.

Methemoglobin
Drug overview

Methemoglobin is an abnormal hemoglobin state in which a part of the iron of unoxygenated hemoglobin is in the ferric state instead of the ferrous state; thus, it is unable to carry oxygen or carbon dioxide. The presence of methemoglobin shifts the oxygen dissociation curve to the left, which increases the affinity of the remaining hemoglobin to oxygen, making hemoglobin less capable of releasing oxygen to the tissues. Methemoglobin may be acquired or congenital. The acquired form is caused by exposure to toxins or drugs that oxidize ferrous iron. Congenital forms are usually caused by hemoglobin M or NADH methemoglobin reductase enzyme system. Normal methemoglobin levels are 1% of total hemoglobin.

The most common drugs that cause methemoglobin elevations are local anesthetics such as benzocaine, which may be present in many OTC topical medications. Other drugs, such as nitrates, sulfonamide antibiotics, benzene derivatives, dinitrophenol (which is an industrial chemical used by body builders for rapid weight loss), methanol, methylene blue, mothballs, pyridium, phenytonin, silver nitrate, nitrophenol, toluidine, and chlorates may not be as common. Use of Dapson (an anti-infective agent used in the treatment of leprosy and pneumocystis) has been associated with 42% of cases noted (Skold and Klein, 2013).

Most causes of this clinical condition are due to adverse medication reactions or illegal recreational abuse of amyl nitrate (called poppers). Common street names are rush, snappers, or liquid gold. The drug is usually inhaled and gives the user a burst of energy along with a muscle relaxant and vasodilating effect. Amyl nitrate is also the antidote for cyanide poisoning. Death can occur in untreated cases when methemoglobin levels exceed 70%. Normal methemoglobin levels are less than 2% but can also be elevated in cigarette smokers. Levels at 15–20% can cause symptoms of cyanosis but the patient is generally asymptomatic.

Symptoms of overdose

Symptoms are related to decreased oxygen delivery to cellular tissue. Cyanosis, tachycardia, and tachypnea are common. Cyanosis occurs when levels exceed 1.5 g/dl, generally represented by a chocolate hue instead of the common blue of cyanosis, seen in the blood and tissue. Cardiac dysrhythmias can occur in severe poisoning. Hypotension can occur in the case of methemoglobin with the use of nitrates. Lethargy, confusion, seizures, and syncope may also occur. There have been reports of cardiac arrest and myocardial infarction with high methemoglobin levels.

Diagnostic testing and monitoring

ABGs and Methemoglobin levels should be measured with the use of a cooximeter as calculated oxygen saturation levels and pulse oximetry values are usually not accurate. Serum glucose-6-phosphate dehydrogenase (G6PD) determination can be done to ascertain the etiology of methemoglobinemia poisoning. Serum G6PD deficiency can worsen with administration of methemoglobinemia-causing drugs. Metabolic panel and assessment of anion gap acidosis are needed. A complete blood count (CBC) with peripheral smear and haptoglobin levels should be completed to assess for hemolysis.

Antidotes/binding agents/treatment

Treatment is supportive. Oxygen supplementation is usually needed by 100% non-rebreather face mask. Intubation may be needed. Activated charcoal (1–2 g/kg) can be used if a substantial dose or long-acting drug that causes Methemoglobin has been given such as Dapsone (Berlin *et al.*, 1985). The use of methylene blue may be needed depending on Methemoglobin levels. Treatment is usually started if Methemoglobin levels are 30% in an asymptomatic patient or lower in symptomatic patients or patients with anemia or cardiac disease. The dose is 1–2 mg/kg IV and may be repeated in 1 h. Methylene blue converts the Methemoglobin in red cells to hemoglobin (Plotkin *et al.*, 1997). In patients with G6PD deficiency, the use of methylene blue may aggravate Methemoglobinemia and precipitate hemolytic anemia (Mansouri and Lurie, 1993).

Clinical Pearls

Gyromitra mushrooms are found in the northern hemisphere and can cause hemolysis, seizures, and elevated Methemoglobin levels. This mushroom is usually poisonous when raw. Treatment is with methylene blue. It is common for patients to present with normal arterial PO_2 accompanied by cyanosis (Levine *et al.*, 2011).

Cautious use of methylene blue is advised in patients who are receiving selective serotonin reuptake inhibitors (SSRIs) such as Prozac and Cymbalta due to the increased risk of serotonin syndrome in these patients. Methylene blue inhibits the action of monoamine oxidase A (MAO), which breaks down serotonin. In patients receiving SSRIs, this causes serotonin to rise, leading to serotonin syndrome. Symptoms include mental status changes, twitching, hypertonia, myoclonus, hypertension, high fever, and hyperactivity (Lowes, 2011) (see Table 13.1).

Table 13.1 Methemoglobin levels and associated symptoms.

Concentration of methemoglobin (g/dl)	Percentage of total hemoglobin*	Symptoms
<1.5	<10	None
1.5–3.0	10–20	Cyanosis
3.0–4.5	20–30	Anxiety, lightheadedness, headache, tachycardia
4.5–7.5	30–50	Fatigue, confusion dizziness, tachypnea, increased tachycardia
7.5–10.5	50–70	Coma, seizures, arrhythmias, Acidosis
>10.5	>0	Death

Adapted from Harris (2006). © Elsevier.
Patients with lower HG levels may experience more severe symptoms.
*Assumes HG = 15 g/dl.

Iron
Drug overview
Iron is generally used in the treatment of anemia and is an ingredient in prenatal vitamins. It is a common leading fatal cause of poisoning in children. Iron has a direct corrosive effect on tissue and may cause acute hemorrhage. Ingestion of 60 mg/kg is generally considered lethal. Ingestions of less than 40 mg/kg of elemental iron do not typically produce toxic symptoms. Iron is absorbed in the small bowel and converted into a ferric state. It combines with ferritin to form complexes in the intestinal mucosa. Normal levels are 50–150 µg/dl. In cases of overdose, transferrin becomes saturated and excess iron exists as free ferric ions. These ions disrupt oxidative phosphorylation and catalyze the formation of oxygen free radicals, which leads to lipid degradation and cell death. Other effects are increased capillary permeability and venodilation, which causes a shift to anerobic metabolism through mitochondrial dysfunction and production of hydrogen ions. Peak iron levels are seen within 4–6 h but may be delayed in sustained-release formulas.

Symptoms of overdose
Damage to GI mucosa causes massive volume depletion and fluid losses. Metabolic acidosis, massive vasodilation, increased capillary permeability, and myocardial dysfunction may develop. Hepatic failure and necrosis may result from the formation of free radicals. Coagulopathy develops from inhibition of coagulation factors by iron, and later from hepatic failure.

Iron poisoning usually involves initial corrosive effects in the GI system followed by resolution of most GI symptoms. Progressive metabolic acidosis may be present in lab values. Patients may then enter into the third stage (6–48 h), which is progressive shock. This is caused from direct cytotoxic effects of the iron. In this stage, there may be an abrupt worsening of symptoms that lead to cardiovascular collapse, coma, coagulopathy, liver failure, and death. The need for aggressive interventions including hemodialysis and hemodynamic support is greatest in this stage.

Diagnostic testing and monitoring
Diagnosis is based on history of exposure, vomiting, diarrhea, bleeding, and hypotension. It is possible to see radiopaque pills on X-ray. Elevated serum white blood cell (WBC) and glucose is also common. Total serum iron levels should be trended. Toxic dose is frequently seen with levels higher than 450–500 µg/dl; levels higher than 800 µg/dl are associated with severe poisoning. Repeat serum levels should be obtained within 6–8 h of ingestion to check for sustained-release forms of medication. CBC, extended metabolic panel, ABGs, LFTs, prothrombin time/partial thromboplastin time (PT/PTT), and INR should be trended. Conservative management is usually done for levels less than 500 µg/dl. Levels greater than 1000 µg/dl are associated with significant morbidity.

Antidotes/binding agents/treatment
Chelation therapy is used to treat iron overdose. Gastric lavage, activated charcoal, and ipecac syrup are not effective. Whole-bowel irrigation has been shown to be effective in instances of visable opacities found on abdominal X-rays. Iron is radiopaque, but X-rays can also be negative despite significant toxicity (Hunter and Taljanovic, 2003). Deferoxamine (DFO) is used for iron overdose. It binds free iron and converts it to ferrioxamine. It readily crosses the cell membrane and removes iron from cells. Initial infusion begins at 15 mg/kg/h to a maximum dose of 6 g regardless of weight. Use of higher doses over a shorter duration is the preferred method. Acute renal failure and hypotension can occur with the use of DFO and chemistries should be monitored. There have also been instances of adult respiratory distress syndrome (ARDS) occurring with

> **Clinical Pearls**
>
> A normal iron level does not exclude toxicity. Significant signs and symptoms of toxicity have been seen in patients with levels less than 350 µg/dl. Measuring levels of total iron-binding capacity (TIBC) is not useful in the management of these patients. TIBC levels are usually falsely elevated in the presence of high serum iron levels and are neither sensitive nor specific (Siff, Meldon, and Tomassoni, 1999).

infusions lasting for more than 24h. Rusty-red urine during treatment of DFO is common but may not occur. Discontinuation of therapy is based on resolution of clinical symptoms and acidosis.

Drugs of abuse
Overview
The use of illicit drugs, including OTC and prescription drugs, remains a large problem both in urban and suburban health centers. Frequent drug abusers tend to mix medications with alcohol and frequently obtain prescription drug opiates from multiple physicians, friends, or purchase them illegally (Lessenger and Feinberg, 2008). Complications that can arise from these drugs are cardiovascular compromise, thoracic complications, neurological insult, infections, and kidney failure.

At times, the unavailability of an illicit drug of choice results in the substitution of prescription or OTC drugs. Common drugs of abuse are crack cocaine, Ritalin, methamphetamine derivatives, heroin, and other opiate derivatives. Complications may include acute aortic dissection or spinal infarct from the sympathomimetic effect of cocaine to acute lung injury from inhalation of crack or other substances (Gotway *et al.*, 2002).

Symptoms of overdose
If the route used is injection, infection of any organ or tissue is possible with subsequent abscess formation. Rapid absorption occurs with both inhalation (smoking) and IV injection and lasts for around 30 min. Because of these effects, cocaine is most addictive by these routes. Rapid peak concentrations occur in the brain, and behavioral and psychological effects have a shorter duration of action. Snorting cocaine produces a longer duration of action over several hours. Specific thoracic complications that can occur from illicit drug use are pneumonia, pulmonary hemorrhage, emphysema, cardiogenic and noncardiogenic pulmonary edema, acute lung injury, aspiration pneumonia, septic embolization, and talc-induced lung disease. Rhabdomyolysis, hypothermia or hyperthermia, and seizures are common (Gotway *et al.*, 2002).

Diagnostic testing
General testing should include ASA, acetaminophen, and standard urine drug panels that include methadone testing. Alcohol levels should also be obtained. Monitoring of airway and continuous and 12-lead ECG monitoring is warranted. CBC, extended lytes, troponin or creatine phosphokinase (CPK) levels, and ABGs should be monitored. False positives for opioids can occur from dextromethorphan (DMX), quinine, quinolones, rifamptin, poppy seeds and oil, and verapamil. False negatives can occur from low doses of semisynthetic and synthetic opioids and patients with rapid metabolism (McBane and Weigle, 2010).

> **Clinical Pearls**
>
> Sending blood or urine samples to toxicology centers is not feasible in many cases, especially if no criminal activity has been committed. There are also many designer and street-level drugs for which testing is not available. The most important information is history and physical assessment.

Benzodiazepines
Drug overview
These agents include lorazepam, Xanax, Valium, flurazapam, oxazepam, and clonazepam. These drugs are highly protein-bound and may take longer to disperse in obese individuals. They are usually prescribed for their antianxiety, sedative, or antispasmodic effects. Rohypnol (flunitrazepam) is commonly known as the "date rape drug." It is rapid-acting and causes significant CNS depression within 30 min. Rohypnol has a very slow elimination and prolonged coma is common. It is not detectable on routine drug screens but can be tested for specifically at designated labs. Benzodiazepines enhance the action of the inhibitory transmitter gamma-aminobutyric acid (GABA). This causes decreased spinal reflexes and depression of the reticular-activating system. This in turn can cause coma and respiratory arrest in overdose situations.

Symptoms of overdose
CNS depression and respiratory arrest are the most common symptoms of overdose. Ataxia can be present. Hypotension is uncommon.

Death is usually uncommon with older forms of benzodiazepines but more common with the shorter-acting more potent forms. Toxic effects are magnified when drugs are combined with other CNS depressants such as barbiturates or alcohol.

Diagnostic testing and monitoring
Urine drug toxicity screen will be positive for benzodiazepines. They can be detected in the urine for 2–7 days.

Antidotes/binding agents/treatments
Charcoal can be given in acute ingestions within the hour and care must be taken to avoid aspiration risk. Treatment of benzodiazepine overdose is supportive. IV infusion of crystalloids for hypotension is used. Flumazenil can be given at 0.2 mg IV for one dose. Additional doses can be given at 1 min intervals if needed for a total dose of 1 mg. In cases of chronic use of benzodiazepines and acute overdose, use of flumazenil is not recommended due to the risk of precipitating seizures. In the case of coingestions of certain drugs such as cocaine and amphetamines, benzodiazepine can be protective and their effects should not be reversed. If respiratory depression is present, the airway should be supported.

Clinical Pearls

Certain drugs such as Ativan (IV formula) and Valium contain a dilutent that contains propylene glycol (PG) and can cause metabolic acidosis with anion and osmolar gap if given in significant quantities. Since the dose is patient-specific, some patients develop complications at lower doses than others (Arbour, 2003). Drugs such as Rohypnol will not show up in a standard toxicology screen for benzodiazepines. Testing for Rohypnol is commonly done in toxicology kits for sexual assault. Patients can develop acute withdrawal after cessation of chronic benzodiazepine use. Symptoms are similar to acute alcohol withdrawal and include hypertension, tachycardia, acute confusion, seizures, and hyperactivity.

Opiods
Drug overview
Opioids are a general group of drugs classified as narcotics. They are the second leading cause of accidental death. Emergency room visits for opioid abuse have doubled from 2004 to 2008

and treatment program admissions increased 400% between 1998 and 2008 (Okie, 2010). Narcotics are available by both prescriptions such as methadone, morphine, Percocet, oxycodone, and dilaudid and illicit drugs such as heroin. DMX, an opioid derivative, has potent antitussive effects but no analgesic or addictive properties. At high doses, it is classified as a hallucinogen and may produce dissociative general anesthetic similar to ketamine and phencyclidine (PCP). If consumed in low recreational doses between 100 and 200 mg, it has a euphoric effect. With moderate doses around 400 mg it has an increased euphoric effect with hallucinations and at very high doses of 700–800 mg, it produces profound alterations in consciousness and temporary psychosis. Tramadol is a centrally acting synthetic analog of codeine used as an analgesic agent. It also inhibits the reuptake of norepinephrine and serotonin and has weak opioid receptor antagonism. It is generally a prescriptive drug that is used for moderate to severe pain and is thought to have less addiction potential than other opioid pain relievers. It can cause physical and psychological depression.

Symptoms of overdose
The major symptoms seen in overdose are respiratory depression and hypoxia, which can lead to the development of noncardiogenic pulmonary edema. This is frequently observed at autopsy for patients who do not receive treatment and are found deceased. The lungs may be three times the normal size. Frequently, these patients are found with a "foam cone" present on their faces as evidence of their acute pulmonary edema. The mechanism is thought to be from hypoxic-induced stress pulmonary capillary fluid leak. Diuresis does not help in these situations. Frequently seen are miosis, CNS depression, hypotension, bradycardia, hypothermia, and slow gastric transit times. Seizures can also be induced by certain opioids such as fentanyl, meperidine, and propoxyphene. Tramadol overdose in large amounts can cause convulsions and seizures with respiratory depression, nausea, vomiting, and tachycardia observed due to the sympathomimetic effect.

Diagnostic testing and monitoring

Urine testing is used for opiates/opioids. False positives in urine for opioids can occur with prior ingestion of DMX, papaverine, poppy seeds, quinine, quinolones, rifampin, and verapamil. Opioids/opiates are usually detected in the urine for 2–3 days. Prolonged monitoring of opioid levels in sustained-release derivatives may be necessary. CBC, chemistries, ABGs, and chest X-rays should be monitored. Aspiration is a frequent complication. Anoxic brain injury can occur in the setting of profound hypoxic states. Compartment syndrome and subsequent rhabdomyolysis can develop from prolonged immobility (Boyer, 2012).

Antidotes/binding agents/treatment

Treatment is to support the airway, ventilation, and oxygenation. Charcoal may be useful. If sustained-release formulations are suspected, cathartics should be administered. Naloxone 0.4 mg IV is initially used and this can be repeated every 2–3 min. Patients who respond to naloxone may require a continuous drip. Drips are usually mixed as 4 mg in 250 ml and started at a rate of 0.4 mg/h. Drips can be titrated up to maximum dose of 10 μg/kg/min. Oxygen administration, IV access, ECG monitoring, and administration of IV crystalloid infusion with use of vasopressors may be required. Tramadol treatment should begin with benzodiazapines. Propoxyphene can cause dose-dependent

---

Clinical Pearls

Poppy seeds in food can contain enough codeine and morphine to produce a positive drug result. False positives and false negatives depend on what assays are conducted within facilities. Body packers can carry large quantities of illicit drugs such as heroin and can suffer from leakage of packages and rapid absorption of large quantities of opioids. Body cavity searches, immediate X-rays, computed tomography (CT) scans, and surgical evaluation may be needed in patients who have been found to have drugs hidden in body cavities. Contrast-enhanced CT scans may be helpful. X-rays have a sensitivity of 85–90% and false positive studies may be due to bladder stones, inspissated stool, or intraabdominal calcifications (Traub, Hoffman, and Nelson, 2003). Critical care admission, decontamination with charcoal, and high-dose continuous infusion of naloxone may be needed. Surgery may be needed in the case of retained opioid/herion packages. There have also been cases of acute liver failure with tramadol overdose (Pothiawala and Ponampalam, 2011).

---

widening of the QRS complex, which is similar to TCA overdose. This QRS widening affects the fast sodium channels in the cardiac conduction system. Treatment can be managed with sodium bicarbonate 1–2 mEq/kg intravenous push (IVP) and repeated as needed to maintain a serum pH of 7.45–7.55. Tramadol overdose may cause tachycardia and hypertension and naloxone can be less effective and can cause seizures. Recent data on tramadol overdose with seizures recommend treatment of seizures with benzodiazapines and avoidance of prophylactic treatment with anticonvulsants (Shadnia *et al.*, 2012).

Cocaine

Drug overview

Cocaine is a sympathomimetic and local anesthetic. Cocaine promotes the release of the neurotransmitters dopamine and norepinephrine while also blocking the reuptake in the central and sympathetic nervous system. This effect produces a powerful euphoric state. Psychologic and physiologic tolerance develops after the first dose.

Forms of cocaine include crack and freebase cocaine. Cocaine is water-soluble and can be absorbed through any mucous membrane. Freebase cocaine is preferred for smoking and is made by dissolving cocaine salts in an aqueous alkaline solution and extracting the freebase solution with a solvent like ether. Crack is a freebase form of cocaine that is made by combining sodium bicarbonate (baking soda) to create an aqueous alkaline solution and is then dried out or cooked and formed into "rocks" that are smoked. Cocaine is metabolized by liver esterases, plasma cholinesterase, and nonenzymatic hydrolysis. Patients with impaired pseudocholinesterase may be at greater risk for toxicity. Toxic dose is highly variable. A typical "line" of cocaine contains 20–30 mg or more with assorted additives. A pellet or rock of crack cocaine usually contains 100–150 mg of cocaine with additives. Ingestion of more than 1 g is usually fatal. Clinical effects are related to the profound vasoconstriction and hypertension that occur. These are caused from the inhibition of catecholamine reuptake and decreased production of the vasodilator nitric oxide. Inhalation or IV use results in euphoric response within 3–5 min. Peak cardiovascular effects occur within the first 8–12 min and last for around 30 min. Cocaine snorting effects occur within the first 15–20 min, peak within 20–40 min, and can last for several hours. Initial euphoria is usually followed by anxiety, delirium, psychosis, muscle rigidity, and seizures. Seizures are usually brief in duration. If status epilepticus occurs, continued drug absorption should be suspected as in ruptured cocaine bags in the GI tract. Packet ingestion effects can be markedly prolonged and lead to death (DeMaria and Weinkauf, 2011).

Symptoms of overdose

Patients with severe toxicity may develop clonus, seizures, and malignant hyperthermia. Tachydysrhythmias and cardiovascular collapse with acute myocardial infarction due to coronary vasoconstriction can occur. Pupils may be dilated. Symptoms of tea-colored urine should prompt examination of CPK levels for the presence of rhabdomyolysis. Flaccid paralysis and spinal cord infarction may also occur due to the extreme vasoconstriction that can occur with cocaine use. Bronchospasm, pulmonary hemorrhage, and pulmonary infarction are also possible (DeMaria and Weinkauf, 2011).

A syndrome called crack cocaine lung can occur which presents as acute lung injury due to the decreased blood flow and oxygen caused from the smoke inhalation of this drug. This presents as cardiogenic and noncardiogenic pulmonary edema. Signs and symptoms of dyspnea, chest pain, cough, and fever typically occur within 48 h of heavy crack smoking.

Chest X-ray results may show abnormal signs such as hyperinflation, increased vascular markings, and tree in bud sign on CT scan. Laboratory abnormalities can include hypokalemia, leukocytosis, and hyperglycemia (Devlin and Henry, 2008). Agranulocytosis may occur due to the adulterants that are combined with cocaine. Levamisole is an anthelminthic and immunomodulator that belongs to a class of synthetic imidazothiazole derivatives. It is currently used in veterinary medicine as a dewormer in livestock. Levamisole has been found by the US drug enforcement to be present in the majority of cocaine samples seized. It has been implicated as a suspected etiological agent in rare cases of agranulocytosis following cocaine ingestion. Certain morphologic findings on bone marrow biopsy in the cases of unexplained agranulocytosis and cocaine use have been found including circulating plasmacytoid lymphocytes, increased bone marrow plasma cells, and mild megakaryocytic hyperplasia (Czuchlewski *et al.*, 2010). Other complications seen with levamisole use are vasculopathy syndrome, autoimmune mediated neutropenia, cutanous vascular complications, and leukoencephalopathy. There are case reports of treatment with granulocyte colony-stimulating factor (GCSF) in severe cases (Buchanan and Lavonas, 2012).

Diagnostic testing and monitoring

Patients usually have hemodynamic instability with toxic doses of cocaine and commonly develop acute lung injury, which requires intubation. Urine usually stays positive for 3 days but a negative result does not rule out toxicity as urine levels can be very low within the first few hours. Patients should have IV access, receive cardiac monitoring, and be watched for signs and symptoms of seizures. If seizures occur, treatment should consist of protection of the airway and intubation if needed along with benzodiazepine treatment of Ativan 1–4 mg IVP or Versed 2–5 mg IVP. Treatment with phenytoin is not effective for seizures and should be avoided. Propofol infusion and dexmedetomidine (Precedex) infusions are also safe to use for sedation and anxiety. Ketamine should be avoided due to its sympathomimetic properties and the potential to precipitate myocardial depression in the setting of limited catecholamine reserves. Status epileticus should be managed with short-acting barbitutes and general anesthesia can be employed in refractory cases. Succinylcholine should not be used because it may increase muscle contraction, and exacerbate hypokalemia and hyperthermia. Rocuronium (0.6 mg/kg) and Vecuronium (0.08–0.1 mg/kg) are the drugs of choice that can be used for paralytic agents (DeMaria and Weinkauf, 2011).

In the case of malignant hyperthermia, paralysis and cooling is the treatment of choice. CBC and complete electrolyte profile, blood, urea, nitrogen, and creatinine should be tested. CPK levels along with chest X-ray should also be monitored. Cardiac parameters and 12-lead ECG should be done in patients with critical illness and toxicity as the profound vasoconstriction of cocaine/crack use can frequently cause myocardial infarction from severe coronary vasospasm. Thiamine, folate, and multivitamins should also be administered as alcohol abuse is commonly seen with cocaine/crack use.

Tachyarrhymias and hypertension can be treated with CCBs (5–20 mg diltizem) IVP followed by an infusion at 5–15 mg/h, alpha adrenergic blockers such as phentolamine (treatment of adrenergic sympathetic excess) in doses of 1–2 mg/dose. IV vasodilators such as nitroglycerin drip or hydralazine 10–20 mg every 4 h can also be used to alleviate signs and symptoms of coronary vasospam and hypertension. Hypotension should be aggressively treated with fluid hydration. Beta-adrenergic blockers such as labetalol, metroprolol, esmolol, and propanolol should not be used because they may worsen coronary spasm. Unopposed alpha-mediated peripheral vasoconstriction with nonselective beta blockers is potentially catastrophic. Labetalol, which has both alpha and beta-blockage properties, has been shown to lower blood pressure but does not improve coronary blood flow. Dexmedetomidine has been postulated to alleviate coronary vasospasm via a central sympatholysis (Schwartz, Rezkalla, and Kloner, 2010). If signs and symptoms of intestinal obstruction are present, immediate surgical intervention is needed. If packets of cocaine are swallowed for diversion of drug, life-threatening injury can occur if the package leaks. Positive urine tests for cocaine can occur with the use of the coco leaf tea.

Antidotes/binding agents/treatment

There is no specific antidote for cocaine overdose. Charcoal is usually ineffective. Dialysis is ineffective and acidification of the urine may aggravate myoglobinuric renal failure.

Clinical Pearls

It is possible to see symptoms of "crack dancing" or "twisted mouth," which is acute dyskinesia that presents as repetitive eye blinking, lip smacking, and involuntary movements and contractions of the arms and legs in some patients. This usually resolves within a few hours to a few days. Body temperature above 104–105°F can be life-threatening and patients should be cooled immediately with external or internal cooling devices. Substances that are added to cocaine before it is sold on the street can include talc, lactose, mannitol, sucrose, caffeine, heroin, phencyclidine, lidocaine, procaine, and strychnine. Some of these substances can also cause toxicity. The combined use of cocaine and ethanol forms cocaethylene in the liver, a substance that intensifies and lengthens cocaine's euphoric effects while possibly increasing the risk of sudden death (Farre *et al.*, 1997).

Amphetamines
Drug overview

Amphetamines and other similar drugs activate the sympathetic nervous system. The four mechanisms involved are catecholamine release from neurons, inhibition of monoamine neurotransmitter uptake of catecholamines, binding to extracellular catecholamine receptors, and inhibition of monoamine oxidase. Amphetamines are capable of altering neurotransmitter release. Each can affect different chemicals in the brain and have multiple effects. Some stimulant actions such as methylenedioxymethamphetamine (MDMA) (ecstasy) and bupropion (Wellbutrin) have not been fully explained. Amphetamines can be used to treat certain disorders such as narcolepsy and attention deficit disorders. Amphetamines can be ingested as an illicit drug such as methamphetamine, Ecstasy, and lysergic acid diethylamide (LSD). People can develop "meth mouth," which is erosion of the teeth from chronic methamphetamine use.

Amphetamines are generally well absorbed orally and have a large volume of distribution. Half-life varies depending on the drug ingested.

Symptoms of overdose

Generally, symptoms have to do with CNS overstimulation. Symptoms of euphoria, agitation, aggression, anxiety, hallucinations, seizures, coma, hyperthermia, all forms of cardiac dysrhythmias, myocardial infarction from vasospasm, extreme muscular rigidity and hyperactivity, mydrosis, and hypertension can lead to acute hemorrhagic intracranial bleeding. Rhabdomyolysis with acute renal failure is possible.

Diagnostic testing and monitoring

Diagnosis is usually based on history. Amphetamines are usually detected in the urine for 2–3 days. Suspicion should be high for any patient that comes in with seizures, muscular rigidity, fever, and rhabdomyolysis. Drug urine toxicology screen should be sent for amphetamines. There can be some cross reactivity to other substances such as pseudoephedrine and its derivatives, including OTC antihistamines. Most drug screens for amphetamines may not pick up toxicology for Ecstasy, which may need to be a specific separate test. Check with the hospital lab department or Poison Control Center.

Antidotes/binding agents/treatments

Treatment is supportive. Charcoal can be given if treatment is sought within 2h of ingestion. Patients may need aggressive cooling, fluids, support of airway, cardiac monitoring, and treatment of seizures and muscle rigidity with benzodiazepines. Antipyretics have no use in therapy for this type of hyperthermia, as the action is a lowering of the hypothalamic set point, which is not relevant in amphetamine overdose (Eyer and Ziker, 2007). If treatment is needed for hypertension, nitroprusside or nitroglycerin can be used. Esmolol or short-acting beta blockers can be used for tachyarrhythmias. Generally, the effects of amphetamines are not longlasting and few act for longer than 24h. Dialysis and hemoperfusion are ineffective in the elimination of amphetamines. Continuous cardiac monitoring, 12-lead ECG, CBC, complete metabolic panel, CPK, and cardiac isotopes with troponin-I levels are recommended.

Clinical Pearls

Methamphetamine use is endemic to some rural areas. It can be smoked, snorted, injected, or taken orally. It is relatively cheaper than other drugs of abuse. It is usually used in a binge and crash pattern and has a longer duration of effect than cocaine. Smoking produces a longlasting high, and 50% of the drug is removed from the body within 12h as opposed to cocaine, which is gone within 1h. Long-term use can lead to addiction with both psychological and long-term molecular changes in the brain. Psychotic changes in behavior along with hallucinations are common. Designer amphetamines such as Ecstasy have serotonergic activity and in the setting of other SSRIs or TCAs can produce serotonin syndrome (Meehan, Bryant, and Aks, 2010). False positive urine tests can occur with the use of poppy seeds and ephedrine (Neerman and Uzoegwu, 2010).

Phencyclidine

Drug overview

PCP is a dissociative anesthetic with hallucinogenic properties. Phencyclidine can cause extreme agitation and aggressive behavior. Patients may need to be chemically sedated and ventilated to handle behavioral issues and injuries.

This agent primarily acts by N-methyl-D-aspartate (NMDA) receptor antagonism and modulating serotonin antagonism. It is structurally related to ketamine (Meehan, Bryant, and Aks, 2010). PCP is readily absorbed by all routes, highly protein-bound, and metabolized in the liver. It has a rapid onset of action, effects last 6–24h, and alterations in perception can occur for up to 3 days. It is usually detected in the urine for up to 2 weeks and in some instances up to 1 month.

Symptoms of overdose

PCP causes a dissociative state with loss of reality. Perceptions are altered and visual and auditory hallucinations are frequent. Patients can appear intoxicated, agitated, calm, or comatose. Multidirectional nystagmus may be present. Hypertension, tachycardia, and hyperthermia may be present. Behavior may be violent and unpredictable. Muscle twitching, rigidity, and neuromuscular hyperactivity can occur. Rhabdomyolysis can occur from neuromuscular hyperactivity. Patients rarely present to medical providers and usually present due to coingestion of other substances or from trauma experienced from the effects of the drugs.

Diagnostic testing and monitoring

Vital signs, ECG monitoring, and tests to rule out other neurological conditions should be done. Drug screening for PCP, blood glucose testing, CBC, CPK, and complete metabolic panel should be done. Physical and chemical restraints may be needed for violent and aggressive behavior. Complications can occur including aspiration pneumonia, multisystem organ failure from hyperthermia, trauma, and extreme hyponatremia from water intoxication.

Antidotes/binding agents/treatments

Activated charcoal can be given within the first 1–2h. Care is supportive. Advanced life support measures should be instituted if needed such as intubation, chemical paralysis, cooling measures for hyperthermia, and aggressive fluid resuscitation. Benzodiazepines can be given for acute psychosis. Monitoring of airway, oxygen saturation, and end tidal CO_2 monitoring must be done.

Clinical Pearls

Use of large doses of DMX can cause a false PCP result in urine. Typically, PCP is added to other drugs for smoking or ingestion to enhance effects (Neerman and Uzoegwu, 2010).

Barbituates
Drug overview
Barbituates are a class of sedative–hypnotic and anticonvulsive drugs. Examples include pheno-barbital, pentobarbital, thiopental, butalbital, secobarbital, chloral hydrate, zolpidem, and others drugs that have mixed properties. Serum concentration levels can be measured for certain barbiturates. Tolerance can develop over time with multiple drug ingestions. Barbiturates are used to treat seizures, anxiety, withdrawal symptoms, musculoskeletal disorders, and for anesthesia. Withdrawal symptoms with abstinence may be present after chronic use. Chronic toxicity can develop with insidious signs and symptoms such as confusion, sedation, nystagmus, and ataxia.

Most barbiturates work to either increase inhibitory tone or decrease excitatory tone. They may be classified as either short- or long-acting. They may also be classified as anticonvulsant, sedative–hypnotic, or anesthetic. Barbiturates bind to barbiturate receptors in the CNS. This receptor is part of the GABA-A receptor complex. Binding on this receptor facilitates GABA neurotransmission, causing CNS depression. GI absorption is rapid and effects depend on the lipid solubility of the substance. Protein binding may be extensive for some drug forms and drugs such as chloral hydrate may produce active metabolites and prolonged elimination. Most drugs are metabolized in the liver, except baclofen and chloral hydrate, which are renally excreted.

Symptoms of overdose
Signs and symptoms of CNS depression are common. Coma can occur with thermoregulatory depression in the brain stem which can cause apnea, hypothermia, and shock. Respiratory depression and hypotension can occur. Signs and symptoms of depressed myocardial activity and skeletal muscle weakness are common. Symptoms may be highly variable depending on the barbiturate ingested.

Diagnostic testing and monitoring
Drug screening is recommended for barbiturates or specific substances ingested. Often drug levels must be sent to outside laboratories and may take up to 4–6 days to obtain results. Other testing should include CBC, complete metabolic panel, blood glucose monitoring, end–tidal CO_2 monitoring, ABGs, and ECG monitoring. Ventilation may be needed along with IV access and crystalloid support for hypotension.

Antidotes/binding agents/treatments
Care is supportive. Charcoal may be beneficial with acute ingestion within 1–2 h but is of little benefit with chronic ingestion. Vasoactive drugs can be used if hypotension is present and does not respond to fluid resuscitation. Naloxone may reverse CNS depression in patients who have valproic acid overdose who are not opioid-tolerant. To enhance elimination of long-acting barbiturates, infusion of sodium bicarbonate can be used to alkalinize the urine to a pH between 7.5 and 8.0. Infusion of 1–2 mEq/kg as a bolus followed by an infusion of 1 l of D5W with 2–3 ampules of sodium bicarbonate at 75–100 cc/h can be given. Hemodialysis is not indicated unless severe phenobarbital overdose is present with multisystem organ failure and failure to respond to other conventional therapies.

> **Clinical Pearls**
>
> Most barbituates are usually detected in the urine for less than 2 days, but up to a week for phenobarbital. Chloral hydrate overdose impairs myocardial contractility, shortens the cardiac refractory period, and sensitizes the myocardium to catecholamines. This can cause a variety of cardiac arrhythmias such as atrial fibrillation, ventricular tachycardias, and torsades de pointes. Beta blockers are the drugs of choice for this agent. Overdose with Ambien can produce drowsiness but coma and respiratory failure are uncommon.

Hallucinogens
Drug overview
Hallucinogens include LSD and "magic mushrooms." Effects and treatment are similar to PCP intoxication. LSD is usually sold in single or double squares, blotter paper, gelatin squares, or other residue powder. Typical doses range from 25 to 300 μg and massive ingestion can lead to life-threatening consequences. Lysergamides are also found in morning glory seeds and several hundred seeds are required for a hallucinogenic

effect. Magic mushrooms contain psilocybin. These have psychotropic properties similar to LSD. Magic mushrooms originate in the United States from the use by North American Indians in religious ceremonies. They can be grown or ordered over the Internet. Their chemical structure is very similar to that of LSD and serotonin. Symptoms of intoxication usually occur within 30–60 min of ingestion (Meehan, Bryant, and Aks, 2010). Symptoms include a feeling of euphoria, agitation, disorientation, and hallucinations. Bradycardia and hyperthermia may occur. Symptoms are usually self-limiting. Care is similar to LSD intoxication.

Symptoms of overdose

Patients rarely present with LSD/mushroom intoxication but can have auditory and visual hallucinations along with the symptoms described earlier. Symptoms generally occur within 30 min of ingestion. Effects can last up to 12 h and LSD may be coingested with other toxins. Patients can also develop hypertension, tachycardia, and hyperthermia. Mild methemoglobinemia may be seen with magic mushrooms. Doses in excess of 14 000 μg can produce life-threatening hyperthermia, seizures, coagulopathy, and respiratory arrest (Meehan, Bryant, and Aks, 2010).

Monitoring and treatment

Care is supportive and there is no specific antidote. CBC, complete metabolic panel, CPK levels, and glucose monitoring should be completed. ECG monitoring is advised in cases of large overdose. Hyponatremia may be present due to extreme dehydration. IV crystalloids should be given in large doses for extreme hyperthermia, dehydration, or rhabdomyolysis. Standard drug testing does not detect most hallucinogenics.

Clinical Pearls

Salvia divinorum has became a popular hallucinogenic over the last 5–6 years. It is a perennial herb found in the Sierra Mazatec area of Mexico. It acts as a kappa opioid and serotonergic agonist along with glutamate antagonism (Ghosh and Ghosh, 2010). It can be easily purchased over the Internet and is usually smoked or taken orally. Overdose is not common but it can be frequently coingested with other drugs as a hallucinogenic.

Club drugs/date rape drugs
Drug overview

Ecstasy or MDMA, gamma hydroxybutyrate (GHB), Rohypnol (see Section "Benzodiazepines"), ketamine, and DMX are a general group of drugs that are used to facilitate rape or are used recreationally in urban and suburban areas by young adults and teenagers. Ecstasy was patented in 1914 by Merck Pharmaceuticals as an appetite suppressant, but was later studied as a psychotherapeutic drug (DeMaria and Weinkauf, 2011). Ecstasy structurally resembles mescaline and amphetamines.

Drug-facilitated rape should be suspected in any person who appears intoxicated and confused who also has amnesia and may be partially clothed or unclothed. Any person who is admitted to the hospital and has been found unresponsive in suspicious circumstances should have a toxicology screen done and if criminal action has been committed or is suspected, extra blood should be drawn for more extensive toxicology. Rape kits may also need to be completed. Most state rape kits now include blood work for toxicology to rule out drug-facilitated sexual assault. If in doubt, err on the side of caution and draw and process the kit. If the patient wakes up and remembers that nothing happened, the kit does not have to be processed. Most states allow submission of the kit with a control number for patients who want to submit anonymously. Ingestion results in signs and symptoms of confusion, intoxication, slurred speech, amnesia, unsteady gait, high fever, tachycardia, euphoria, and high-risk behaviors. Ecstasy is an amphetamine-MDMA used commonly at clubs and is usually taken in conjunction with alcohol. Ecstasy is usually not physically addictive.

Symptoms of overdose

Effects are generally seen within 30 min and last up to 8 h. Use of MDMA produces feelings of euphoria, and increases energy and psychomotor drive. It causes an increased positive mood and sense of closeness with others. Adverse effects include anxiety and thought disorders, hypertension, increased myocardial oxygen demand, jaw clenching, high-risk sexual behavior, tachyarrhythmias, seizures, and hyperthermia with acute dehydration.

Myocardial infarction and dilated cardiomyopathy has been reported (DeMaria and Weinkauf, 2011). Hyponatremia is common due to acute water intoxication from excessive thirst. Increased antidiuretic hormone secretion from MDMA central effects may worsen hyponatremia. Neurotoxicity has been reported. There have been reported cases of liver failure and cerebral hemorrhage. Long-term use can cause chronic psychosis in at-risk individuals and possible neurotoxicity (Britt and McCance-Katz, 2005).

Diagnostic testing and monitoring

Testing should include CBC, serum metabolic panel, CPK levels, and ECG monitoring. IV hydration with crystalloids should be given to correct dehydration. Standard drug toxicology should be done for coingestion along with alcohol testing. MDMA is not detected in regular drug screens unless specifically tested for; contact the laboratory for specific drug testing coverage.

Antidotes/binding agents/treatments

Care is supportive. Seizures should be treated with benzodiazepines. Rhabdomyolysis is common in cases of extreme hyperthermia and internal cooling devices may be needed. If acute pill ingestion occurred within 1–2 h, treatment with activated charcoal in 1 g/kg dose may be given. The maximum dose is 50 g. There is no specific antidote or binding agent. In causes of extreme hyperthermia and rhabdomyolysis, dantrolene has been used. Dantrolene is a muscle relaxant that depresses excitation and contraction coupling in skeletal muscles by binding ryanodine receptors and

---

Clinical Pearls

Most use of ecstasy is consumed at RAVEs, which are large-scale dance parties generally held in urban areas. There is also a higher likelihood of polysubstance use at these events. Most common coingestions are with GHB, ketamine, and flunitrazepam. Common names for ecstasy are XTC, Adam, X, and E. Ecstasy is commonly combined with Viagra because of its effect that can cause erectile dysfunction. Viagra may be abused by the gay population and may lead to seropositive human immunodeficiency virus (HIV) results due to unsafe sexual practices (Lessenger and Feinberg, 2008).

---

decreasing intracellular calcium concentration (Hall and Henry, 2006).

Ketamine
Drug overview

Ketamine produces symptoms similar to PCP when it is abused. It can be used orally, intravenously, nasally, or by inhalation. It can be combined with other drugs. It has a rapid onset and due to the hallucinogenic effects it is difficult for the user to resist the attacker if this is used as a date rape drug. It generally produces loss of pain perception with little to no depression of airway reflexes or ventilation. Ketamine is not physically addictive. It is used mostly by anesthesiologists for children because of its analgesic role (Demaria and Weinkauf, 2011). It is also commonly used in veterinary medicine. Ketamine abuse has risen over the last decade and is commonly combined with MDMA.

Ketamine is an NMDA receptor agonist. This causes noncompetitive antagonism of glutamate in the CNS. Ketamine binds to the same receptor site as PCP located on the calcium channel, leading to a blockage of calcium flow. This decreased neurotransmission causes altered perception, memory, and cognition. Blockage of the NDMA receptor causes feelings of relaxation at low doses and acute dissociative states and phychosis with visual hallucinations at higher doses. Effects of ketamine generally last for 1–3 h, but depending on the amount of the overdose, effects can be seen for up to 14 h (DeMaria and Weinkauf, 2011). Ketamine is eliminated hepatically with small amounts excreted by the gastric and renal systems. Usual therapeutic doses are 1–5 mg/kg IV. Recreational doses are usually much higher with inhalation doses of 10–250 mg, oral doses of 40–450 mg, and intramuscular (IM) doses of 10–100 mg. These higher dosages are taken to try to reach a psychic state known as the "K-hole" (Britt and McCance-Katz, 2005).

Symptoms of overdose

Vertical and horizontal nystagmus is a key feature of intoxication that helps to distinguish ketamine use from other drugs. Severe agitation and psychosis may also occur (DeMaria and Weinkauf, 2011). It may be necessary to intubate and sedate patients using a benzodiazapine to be able to control aggressive behavior. Use of Haldol may be necessary depending on the degree of psychosis. Haldol can decrease the seizure threshold. Polydrug use also needs to be considered as most overdoses with ketamine occur in young adults who are experimenting with drug use. Patients may have tonic–clonic movements or seizures. Because the sympathomimetic system is triggered, hypertension, tachycardia, and arrhythmias are common. Ketamine has generally no effects on the renal or hepatic system.

Diagnostic testing and monitoring
Care is supportive with maintenance of airway, breathing, and circulation. Patients may require ICU level of care to manage their airway, agitation, and psychosis. CBC, CPK levels, extended metabolic panel, and ABGs should be completed. Continuous ECG monitoring should be done. Hyperthermia and rhabdomyolysis may occur. General testing is not available for ketamine levels. Aggressive hydration with crystalloids may be needed.

Antidotes/binding agents/treatments
There is no specific binding agent or treatment. For oral ingestion, charcoal can be given within the first hour. Dialysis or use of bicarbonate is not helpful.

> **Clinical Pearls**
>
> Always run routine drug, alcohol, and other levels on patients with signs and symptoms of drug toxicity. In patients with ketamine overdose, the agitated behavior may fluctuate between psychosis and catatonia.

Fake marijuana
Drug overview
Use of synthetic marijuana has become increasingly popular among teens in recent years. Synthetic marijuana is usually sold as incense and referred to as K2, Spice, Genie, smoke, skunk, and zohai (Korioth, 2011). It is commonly sold in retail shops and over the Internet. It is a smokable product and promoted as a cannabis alternative that is not detectable on conventional drug screens. There have been some reports of severe effects of these drugs depending on what they contain. As of August 2010, there were 1057 reports of synthetic cannabinoid toxicity across the United States (Wells and Ott, 2011). Synthetic canniboids may contain such chemical compounds as JWH-, CP-, and HU- along with oleamide, a fatty acid with cannabinoid-like activity (Every-Palmer, 2011). The primary effect of these agents is hallucinations, anxiety, and psychosis and they tend to cause tachycardia and increased blood pressure. This herbal cocktail can consist of canavalia rosea, clematis nuciferia, heima salicfolia, and ledum palustre. When smoked, they produce an intoxicating effect on the brain very similar to marijuana. Many of these substances have been banned, but as soon as they are, more chemically synthetic compounds are produced and marketed. Ingestion of these substances is detected from history as there is no standardized drug testing (Ernst et al., 2011).

Symptoms
Intoxication may be seen in the acute hospital settings and can cause significant bradycardia, psychomotor agitation, violence, and hallucinations. Four agents may be used in the making of Illy and they are marijuana (THC), phencyclidine, formaldehyde, and embalming fluid (ethyl alcohol). Embalming fluid may contain methanol, formaldehyde, ethanol, or ethyl alcohol. Use of Illy or "wet" is popular among teens and gangs because the marijuana joints burn more slowly, prolonging the level of intoxication. Drugs levels may come back positive for PCP and marijuana.

Diagnostic testing
There is no specific drug test for Illy and monitoring is based on self-reporting. Symptoms include psychomotor hyperactivity, hallucinations, and aggressive behavior. Signs and symptoms clear after 24–36h depending on the drugs used. Care is supportive with monitoring of ECG and vital signs and volume resuscitation. CBC and extended metabolic panel should be done. ABGs will determine if significant metabolic acidosis is present. Treatment of agitation can be managed with

the use of benzodiazepines or Haldol (Modesto-Lowe and Petry, 2001).

Antidote

There is no test or antidote available. Care is supportive.

> ### Clinical Pearls
>
> Illy may be a common drug used with those who have gang affiliations. Patients will usually test positive for marijuana and may be positive for PCP. Inhalation of formaldehyde can cause acute onset of respiratory and mucosal irritation with difficulty in swallowing and breathing and metabolic acidosis may or may not be present due to the use of embalming fluid derivatives.

Dextromethorphan

Drug overview

This is a medicine that is used to suppress cough. DMX overdose occurs when someone accidentally or intentionally takes more than the recommended amount. DMX is commonly abused by 10th–12th graders. DMX is a synthetically produced substance that is chemically related to codeine, though it is not an opiate. Most users of DMX ingest the drug orally, although some snort the powdered form of the drug. Some abusers ingest 250–1500 mg in a single dosage, far more than the recommended therapeutic dose of 10–20 mg every 4 h (Intelligence Bulletin: Dextromethorphan, n.d.).

DMX is classified as a nonopiod tussive, the cytochrome P450, CYP2D6 isoenzyme is responsible for the conversion of DMX to dextrorphan; and P450 CYP3A4 and CYP3A5 isoenzymes are responsible for converting DMX to 3-methoxymorphinan and 3-hydroxymorphinan. Potential inhibitors of these isoenzymes could decrease the rate of DMX elimination if administered concurrently, while potential inducers could increase the rate of elimination (Falck *et al.*, 2006).

OTC products that contain DMX often contain other ingredients such as acetaminophen, chlorpheniramine, and guaifenesin. Large dosages of acetaminophen can cause liver damage. Large dosages of chlorpheniramine can cause tachyarrhythmias, ataxia, seizures, and coma, and large dosages of guaifenesin can cause vomiting. First-time users may decide not to abuse DXM if they experience negative side effects such as vomiting, which can be commonly associated with the other ingredients contained in OTC DXM medications. DXM abusers can "robo shake," which is a practice where they drink a large amount of DXM and then force themselves to vomit, so they absorb enough DXM through the stomach lining to get high while getting rid of the other ingredients. More experienced abusers use a chemical procedure to extract the DXM from the other ingredients contained in cough syrups to avoid such side effects. This procedure cannot be used on DXM products sold in nonliquid form. There are also reports that DMX is used in combination with Heroin to enhance the effects of the drug (Intelligence Bulletin: Dextromethorphan, n.d.).

Symptoms of overdose

Hallucinations, euphoria, altered state of consciousness, seizures, syncope, tachycardia, mydriasis, hypertension, vomiting, and dissociation to events are typically seen in overdose. Withdrawal can also occur with abuse of DMX. Life-threatening effects can occur at higher dosages including respiratory depression. Most moderate overdosages resolve spontaneously without serious events but 5% of those with European ethnicity lack the ability to metabolize the drug normally, which can lead to rapid, toxic levels secondary to decreased metabolism and elimination. Symptoms can be similar to PCP intoxication (Lessenger and Feinberg, 2008). DMX can inhibit serotonin reuptake, which can lead to serotonin syndrome. Symptoms can generally occur at doses higher than 10 mg/kg.

Diagnostic testing and monitoring

Blood and urine tests can be done to detect the drug. Tests are usually sent out from hospitals and are not usually included on a standard drug screen. Care of DMX overdose is supportive, consisting of IV fluids and support of the airway. Monitoring and testing for concommitant drug use and treatment is needed.

Antidotes

No antidote is available.

Clinical Pearls

DXM use can cause false positives for PCP on drug screens. DMX can inhibit serotonin reuptake at the 5-HTA receptors and can lead to serotonin syndrome, especially when other SSRIs are used (Neerman and Uzoegwu, 2010).

Bath salts

Drug overview

Bath salts are a newer form of chemically engineered "designer drugs" that have been popular in Europe for a number of years and are now being seen in the United States. Poison Control Centers in the United States reported 6138 calls in 2011 related to bath salt exposure (American Association of Poison Control Centers, 2012). These chemical compounds are usually substances that contain any of the following substances in various combinations with other additives that are frequently changing: mephedrone, synthetic cathinone, methylone, methylenedioxypyrovalerone (MDPV), methedrone, and fluoromethcathinone. Cathinone is a naturally occurring beta-ketone amphetamine from the *Catha edulis* plant (Prosser and Nelson, 2011).

Synthetic cathinones are derivatives of these drugs. These drugs produce amphetamine-like effects and are also able to modulate serotonin levels, which causes psychotic effects. They are frequently sold on the Internet and advertised as bath salts. They are sold under names such as Ivory Wave, Vanilla Sky, Snow, and Hurricane (Smith, Cardile, and Miller, 2011). Cathinones are similar in structure to ecstasy. Drugs can be snorted, smoked, taken orally or rectally, and injected.

Symptoms of overdose/use

Bath salts are commonly coingested with other drug substances such as marijuana, cocaine, alcohol, or opiates. Effects of the synthetic cathinones include increased libido but inability to perform, increased energy, and a feeling of euphoria. Adverse and overdose symptoms include psychotic behavior, aggression, increased agitation and strength, hallucinations, nausea, vomiting, diaphoresis, high fever, and signs and symptoms affecting the cardiac, neurological, and psychiatric systems. Acute lung injury and pulmonary edema have also been reported. The most common symptom is agitation to severe psychosis that requires extreme chemical sedation and restraint. Other cardiovascular symptoms include acute myocardial infarction, syncope, and arrhythmias. Symptoms reported to two regional Poison Control Centers in 2009 and 2010 included agitation, combative behavior, tachycardia, hallucinations, paranoia, confusion, chest pain, myoclonus, hypertension, mydriasis, CPK elevations, hypokalemia, and blurred vision (Spiller *et al.*, 2011). Symptoms may mimic a sympathomimetic toxidrome with associated neurological symptoms.

Diagnostic testing and monitoring

There is no available standard drug toxicology test or antidote. Testing is done by using gas spectrometry or liquid chromatography mass spectrometry techniques and can be measured in blood, urine, hair, and stomach contents (Prosser and Nelson, 2011). Patients should have CBC, extended chemistries, CPK, ABGs, chest X-ray, and cardiac enzymes and continuous ECG monitoring.

Antidotes/binding agents/treatments

Treatment is supportive and focused on maintaining airway, breathing, and circulation. For hyperthermia, use of active hypothermic cooling may be required. Seizures and agitation can be treated with benzodiazepines. If psychosis agitation and aggression are profound, use of intubation with chemical paralysis may be needed. IV crystalloids should be given to initially manage hypotension with use of inotropic agents after adequate volume resuscitation. Use of propofol may be needed. Seizures can be treated with Dilantin and Keppra. Information on withdrawal and addiction is evolving as not much is known about this designer class of synthetic cathinone drugs. There have been reports of anxiety and depression and reports of up to 50% of users who felt it was addictive (Prosser and Nelson, 2011).

> **Clinical Pearls**
>
> Bath salts are an evolving area of research and most information is available as case reports and antidotal evidence. Ingestion of this substance should be considered in areas where college age and teenage populations are numerous or when patients present with behavior that is not reflective on drug screens. Some evidence exists that the psychotic behavior is extreme and patients are uncontrollable, placing EMS and health-care providers at risk of significant injury. All care and precautions should be maintained. Urine also has a characteristic "fishy odor," which has not been explained but may be due to mephedrone use.

Skeletal muscle relaxants
Drug overview
Skeletal muscle relaxants (SMRs) such as Soma (carisoprodol), Flexeril (cyclobenzaprine), and Lioresol (baclofen) are drugs used to treat muscle spasm and spinal dystonia and dysreflexia. They act as simple sedative–hypnotic agents that produce skeletal muscle relaxation indirectly. Abuse of muscle relaxants frequently occurs in combination with other drugs. Soma is frequently used in large doses as a sexual stimulant when taken with alcohol. Soma abuse can lead to tolerance, dependence, and withdrawal. Phenobarbital has been used successfully in Soma withdrawal (Boothby, Doering, and Hatton, 2003).

All muscle relaxants do not share the same mechanism of action or molecular structure. What they have in common is a shared centrally acting process that effectively depresses postsynaptic reflexes, monosynaptic reflexes, and gross motor activity. Soma is converted in the body to meprobamate (Equanil), which is considered a Schedule IV controlled substance (Boothby, Doering, and Hatton, 2003). Equanil is a carbonate derivative with tranquilizer properties that has largely been replaced by benzodiazepines. It is highly addictive. Soma is considered a Schedule IV controlled substance in some states but not at the federal level. Soma is frequently obtained over the Internet from pharmacies in Mexico and is often coingested with other drugs such as alcohol and codeine. Abusers of Soma and Vicodin state that the effects of this drug

combination are similar to Heroin (Boothby, Doering, and Hatton, 2003).

Flexeril is similar in structure to amitriptyline but does not cause the same effects as TCAs such as widened QRS and ventricular arrhythmias (Bebarta et al., 2011). Flexeril has antihistamine, anticholinergic, and sedative properties and accounts for 30% of all muscle relaxant overdoses (Bebarta et al., 2011). There have been case reports of the use of Flexeril with SSRIs precipitating serotonin syndrome. Flexeril is a weak inhibitor of presynaptic norepinephrine and serotonin, and any substance with proserotonergic properties can precipitate this syndrome (Day and Jeanmonod, 2008). Toxic doses with anticholinergic symptoms occur at doses of more than 100 mg and can cause significant rhabdomyolysis (Chabria, 2006).

Baclofen is an agonist at the GABA (B) receptor. Symptoms of overdose can produce CNS depression and respiratory depression. Seizure-like activity and paradoxical muscle hypertonicity have been reported. Hallucinations, seizures, and hyperthermia have been reported with withdrawal from baclofen. The toxic dose of SMR varies depending on drug tolerance and dependency. Overdose can also depend on coingestion of other drugs such as sedatives and alcohol.

Symptoms of overdose
Symptoms vary depending on the SMR used. All typically cause altered mental status and result in CNS depression. Most cause muscle hyperreflexia. Hypotension can also occur. Flexeril can cause anticholinergic signs and symptoms. Soma can cause muscle rigidity and hyperreflexia. Baclofen has caused coma, respiratory depression, bradycardia, and seizure-like activity.

Diagnostic testing and monitoring
Drugs can be detected on comprehensive toxicology urine screening. CBC, extended metabolic panel, CPK levels, standard drug toxicology tests, ethanol, ASA, and Tylenol levels should be completed. ECG monitoring and monitoring of the airway and ventilation status should be done. Intubation and ventilation may be needed.

Antidotes/binding agents/treatments

There is no specific antidote or binding agent. Activated charcoal can be given within 1 h of ingestion. Because of extensive tissue distribution of these drugs, dialysis and hemoperfusion are not effective. Treatment is supportive with maintenance of airway and support of blood pressure with crystalloids. Inotropic support may be needed. Hypotension usually responds to IV crystalloids but use of vasopressors such has norepinephrine may be needed. Dopamine is very effective and has an inotropic effect on the incidence of bradycardia and hypotension due to its chronotropic effects on the heart.

Clinical Pearls

Be aware that there are also implanted intrathecal pumps that contain baclofen which can malfunction or catheters can migrate from their postoperative position and cause inadequate or overinfusion of the drug with concurrent signs and symptoms of toxicity.

Psychiatric drugs

Drug overview

Drugs such as SSRIs, SSIs, monoamine oxidase inhibitors (MAOI/MAO), lithium, and neuroleptics may be used as agents of overdose. Most psychiatric drugs produce signs and symptoms that can affect the neurological system. Serotonin syndrome is caused from excessive 5-hydroxytryptamine stimulation. It can be caused by overdose, overuse, or interactions between certain drug groups. MAOIs used in combination with drugs such as meperidine, DMX, SSRIs, and ecstacy can predispose patients to the development of severe serotonin syndrome (Boyer and Shannon, 2005). Symptoms include altered mental status such as coma, delirium, and agitation. Autonomic dysfunction is common and can include hyperthermia, flushing, diaphoresis, tachycardia, and mydriasis. Patients may also exhibit muscular rigidity, tremors, and seizures. The diagnosis of serotonin syndrome or toxicity can be very confusing and generally accepted criteria from toxicologists include Sternbach's serotonin toxicity criteria or Hunter's criteria. Hunter's has been shown to be more sensitive and specific than Sternbach's criteria (Dunkley et al., 2003). Hunter's decision rules for diagnosing serotonin toxicity involve the use of well-defined diagnostic criteria. The single most important is clonus, either spontaneously inducible or ocular. Other signs and symptoms include agitation, diaphoresis, tremor, hyperreflexia, hypertonia, and fever (Dunkley et al., 2003) (see Table 13.2).

The difference between serotonin syndrome and neuroleptic malignant syndrome (NMS) can usually be made by physical examination and use of Hunter's criteria. NMS is a hypodopaminergic state where bradykinesis results in immobilization, stupor, akinesia, "lead pipe rigidity," fever, and autonomic instability. It is unlikely to be dose-related, and is rare in occurrences of overdoses (Gillman, 2011). Serotonin syndrome, on the other hand, may be related to dosage or multiple SSIs/SSRIs that have been overdosed or prescribed. The excessive CNS serotonergic activity is caused by increased 5-HT production from tryptophan, increased reuptake inhibition from SSRIs and cyclic antidepressants, increased presynaptic release from sympathomimetics, receptor agonism by tryptans, lithium, L-dopa, and bromocryptine, and inhibited metabolism by MAOIs (Brush, 2005).

Selective serotonin reuptake inhibitors

Drug overview

This category includes drugs whose mechanism of action is to inhibit the reuptake of 5-HT resulting in variable effects on other neurotransmitters. Newer SSRIs are able to inhibit the reuptake of both norepinephrine and serotonin.

Symptoms

Patients usually present with symptoms 6–24 h after a medication change or addition. Common medications that are given for various medical disorders such as Flexeril, fentanyl, Ultram, Zofran, Reglan, Tegretol, Zyvox, and Demerol have also been indicated in serotonin syndrome (Ables and Nagubilli, 2010). SSRIs are safer and better tolerated than MAO and cyclic antidepressants. The basic action is to modulate the reuptake of the neurotransmitter

Table 13.2 Drug-induced hyperthermia syndromes.

	Neuroleptic malignant syndrome	Serotonin syndrome	Sympathomimetic syndrome	Anticholinergic syndrome	Malignant hyperthermia
Cause	Use of neuroleptic drugs that block dopamine	Use of serotonergic drugs/ agonist drugs	Drugs that alter levels of norepinephrine, dopamine, and 5-HT by enhancing or inhibiting	Blockage of both central and peripheral muscarinic acetylcholine receptors	Genetic rare autosomal-dominant disorder of skeletal muscles
Drugs	Exposure to antipsychotic drugs Other drugs: prochlorperazine, metoclopramide, and promethazine	Exposure to SSRIs, MAOs, SNRIs, and TCAs. Other common drugs: tramadol, linezolid, fentanyl, lithium, dextromethorphan St John's wart Bath salts (synthetic canthinone derivatives), ecstasy, and ondansetron	Exposure to amphetamines, methamphetamines, cocaine, ecstasy, and MAOs	Exposure to anticholinergic activity drugs, TCAs, other common drugs, atropine, antiparkinsonian drugs, scopolamine, neuroleptics, and alkaloid drugs	Exposure to inhalation anesthetic agents such as Halothane, Sevoflurane, and Desflurane and/ or depolarizing neuromuscular blocking agents such as Succinylcholine
General symptoms	Altered mental status, hyperthermia, elevated CPK, elevated transaminases, hypertension, tachycardia, cardiac dysrhythmias, incontinence, abnormal involuntary movements, leukocytosis Rhabdomyolysis Low serum iron levels	Altered mental status, hyperthermia, elevated CPK, elevated transaminases, hypertension, tachycardia, cardiac dysrhythmias, incontinence, abnormal involuntary movements, leukocytosis mydriasis, nystagmus, shivering, and rhabdomyolysis Severe form: metabolic acidosis, coma, multisystem organ failure, disseminated intravascular coagulation, and cardiac arrest	Hyperthermia, psychomotor agitation, altered mental status, hallucinations, panic, electrolyte disturbances, elevated CPK, seizures, rhabdomyolysis, hypoxia, myocardial infarction, and arrhythmias Severe forms: status epilepticus, coma, and death	Altered mental status, inability to sweat, hyperthermia, dry mouth, mydriasis, urinary retention, sinus tachycardia, tremor, hallucinations, agitation, or muteness Severe forms: coma, convulsions, and death	Early signs: cardiac arrhythmias, tachycardia, tachypnea, muscular rigidity first in the masseter muscles (Musselman and Saely, 2013) Late signs: malignant hyperthermia, muscular rigidity, and metabolic acidosis
Muscular symptoms	Muscular rigidity is an early symptom (described as lead-pipe rigidity)	Tremor, hyperreflexia, and hypertonia are symptoms; usually more pronounced in lower extremities versus upper Rigidity is a terminal event	Psychomotor excitability	Absence of muscular rigidity	Progression of muscular rigidity that starts in the face and progresses

Onset	Slow onset and progression (24h to days)	Rapid onset and progression with overdose or addition of agonist agents (minutes to within 24h)	Varying onset and progression depending on dosages and agents	Varying onset and progression depending on dosages and agents	Minutes to hours after receiving offending anesthetic agents
Clonus	No clonus	Spontaneous or inducible myoclonus/ocular clonus/ankle clonus	No clonus	Myoclonus	No clonus
Treatment	Discontinue neuroleptics Supportive care: core temperature monitoring external cooling, IV fluids, antipyretics, benzodiazepines	Discontinue serotonergic agent Supportive care: core temperature monitoring external cooling, IV fluids, antipyretics are usually not effective, benzodiazepines	Discontinue offending agent Supportive care: rapid aggressive cooling by internal or external devices	Discontinue offending agent Supportive care: external cooling devices	Discontinue offending agent Supportive care: hyperventilation with 100% oxygen and anesthesia should be continued with opioids, propofol benzodiazepines, and non-depolarizing neuromuscular blockers
			Core temperature monitoring , IV fluids, antipyretics, and benzodiazepines	Core temperature monitoring , IV fluids, antipyretics, and benzodiazepines	External cooling devices, core temperature monitoring , IV fluids, antipyretics
		In extreme cases, non-depolarizing paralytic agents and mechanical ventilation may be needed	In extreme cases, non-depolarizing paralytic agents and/or barbiturates with mechanical ventilation may be needed		
	Blood work: CBC, electrolytes, CPK, iron levels, cardiac monitoring	Blood work: CBC, electrolytes, CPK, ABGs, cardiac monitoring	Blood work: CBC, electrolytes, CPK, troponin I levels, ABGs, cardiac monitoring	Blood work: CBC, electrolytes, CPK, ABGs, cardiac monitoring	Blood work: CBC, electrolytes, CPK, ABGs, cardiac monitoring
	Bromocriptine, dantrolene, and amantadine have been used for treatment in severe cases	Cyproheptadine hydrochloride, an antihistamine that blocks 5-HT, can be administered for severe cases	Dantrolene has been used in ecstasy overdose. Avoid use of B-blocking drugs in cocaine overdose	In cases that are severe and unresponsive to supportive care, physostigmine can be given to resolve anticholinergic symptoms	Dantrolene IVP followed by infusion
		Bromocriptine and dantrolene should not be used			

Adapted from Dunkley et al. (2003); McAllen (2010), Musselman and Saely (2013); and Sternbach (1991).

serotonin. Common drugs that are classified as SSRIs are Celexa, Lexapro, Prozac, Trazodone, and Venlafaxine. The risk of developing serotonin syndrome occurs when these drugs are used in combination with each other or with other MAOIs such as Nardil, isocarboxazid, and Furoxone. St John's wart, a popular herbal, also partially acts as an MAOI.

Diagnostic testing and monitoring

Admission to a critical care unit is necessary. General laboratory values should include CBC and extended metabolic panel. Cardiac monitoring and daily 12-lead ECG testing is recommended until resolution of symptoms occurs. If CNS depression or fever is present, a chest X-ray and CPK level should be done with particular attention to symptoms of serotonin syndrome. Patients should be examined for the presence of clonus. Drug levels are not readily available and are not useful in the management of overdose. Frequent monitoring of the QT and QTc interval should be done. Patients may have autonomic instability and if hypertension is present, it is best managed with a short-acting IV infusion of Esmolol (Eyer and Ziker, 2007).

Antidotes/binding agents/treatments

Withdrawal of the offending medication is necessary. Activated charcoal can be given if overdose is within the first couple of hours of ingestion. Treatment is supportive using advanced life support measures if needed. Benzodiazepines should be given to manage seizures. Hypotension should be managed with IV crystalloid infusion; if the patient does not respond to adequate volume resuscitation, vasopressors may be needed. If shock states persist, intra-aortic balloon pumping may be needed to support cardiac function. Use of paralytic agents may be needed to manage muscular rigidity and tremors. External or internal cooling devices may be needed to manage fever. If any sustained-release preparations were ingested, whole-bowel irrigation should be employed. Cyproheptadine has been used as an antidote in case reports. Cyproheptadine is an antihistamine with both anticholinergic and antiserotonergic properties, and has mitigated symptoms in moderate

to severe forms of serotonin syndrome. Dosage recommendations are 12 mg initially followed by an additional 2 mg every 2 h for persistant symptoms. A maintainence dose of 8 mg every 6 h can be administered if needed. Urinary retention is a common side effect (Ables and Nagubilli, 2010). Chlorpromazine has also been used and the starting dose is 50–100 mg IM (Eyer and Ziker, 2007).

> **Clinical Pearls**
>
> Citalopram and escitalopram can cause wide complex tachycardias. All SSRIs have various half-lives, the most common being one day. The SSRI Fluoxetine has a half-life of up to 4 days. Some of the SSRIs affect cytochrome (CYP450), and coingestion of other drugs that affect this enzyme should be considered. There have been many case reports of interactions with citalopram (Celexa) and fluconazole. Fluconazole inhibits CYP2C19 and citalopram is a substrate of 2C19. Inhibition of its metabolism can precipitate serotonin toxicity (Levin et al., 2008).

Monoamine oxidase inhibitors
Drug overview

This drug class is used to treat severe depression. Serious toxicity can occur with this class of drugs either from overdose or interactions between the drug and certain food groups. MAOIs are intracellular enzymes that break down and inactivate monoamine. Monoamine is responsible for the interruption of catecholamines within the neurons in the brain. MAOIs are also found in the liver and intestinal system, where they metabolize tyramine and prevent its entry into the systemic circulation. Serious toxicity results from the excessive release of neuronal stores of vasoactive amines, the inhibition of metabolism of catecholamines, interaction with certain drugs, or release and absorption of large amounts of dietary tyramine, which causes release of catecholamines from neurons. There are multiple interactions between MAO/MAOIs and other drug classes. Significant interactions exist between many SSRIs, tramadol, demeral, DMX, and amphetamines. Food interactions exist with beer, red wine, chesses, fava beans, yeasts, smoked, pickled, or aged meats, snails, and chicken liver (see Tables 13.3 and 13.4).

Table 13.3 MAO/MAOI drug interactions.

Amphetamines	Buspirone	Cocaine	Dextromethorphan	Ephedrine
Fluvoxamine, fluoxetine	LDS	Imipramine Amitryptyline	Meperidine, methadone	Tramadol
Methyldopa	Paroxetine	Phenylephrine	Sertraline	Venlafaxine
Tryptophan	Reserpine and related compounds	Terbutaline (no longer available in the United States)	Norepinephrine	Epinephrine
Tyramine-containing foods and drugs				
Albuterol	Dopamine	Ketamine	Isoproterenol Hydrochloride	Isoetharine
Methylphenidate	Pseudoephedrine	Salmeterol	Phentermine	Pemoline

Adapted from Olson (2012) and Wimbiscus *et al.* (2010).

Table 13.4 MAO/MAOI food interactions.

Red wine	Aged cheeses	Sauerkraut	Soybean curd	Soy sauce
Tap beers	Aged meats Cured meats	Snails	Concentrated yeast	Broad bean pods
Dry sausages	Spoiled or bacteria-contaminated meats	Pickled herring	Chicken liver	Fava beans

Adapted from Olson (2012) and Wimbiscus *et al.* (2010).

Symptoms of overdose

Symptoms are usually delayed for up to 12 h and symptoms and death can occur days after overdose. Most symptoms of acute intoxication are neurological manifestations related to CNS hyperactivity. These develop from excessive concentrations of catecholamines at the nerve terminals. Patients may experience headache, agitation, hypertension, tachypnea, hyperthermia, nystagmus seizures, muscular rigidity, myoclonus, coma, and mydriasis. As poisoning becomes severe, hypotension, bradycardia, and asystole can occur, resulting from depletion of cathecholamines at nerve terminals. Late effects of toxicity may include rhabdomyolysis, disseminated intravascular coagulation, pulmonary edema, and myoglobinuric renal failure.

Diagnostic testing and monitoring

ECG monitoring for a minimum of 24 h in critical care is needed. CBC and complete metabolic panel along with serial 12-lead ECGs, ABGs, and CPK levels are recommended.

Antidotes

Activated charcoal is given if ingestion has occurred within 1–2 h. Initiate other supportive care such as maintenance of the airway, treatment with benzodiazepines for seizures, and crystalloid IV fluid administration for hypotension. Severe hypertension is initially treated with a short-acting titratable drug such as nitroprusside. Because hypertension can be quickly followed by hypotension, longer agents should not be used. Beta blockers should be avoided because they may cause unopposed alpha stimulation and elevated blood pressure. If patients develop reflex bradycardia, avoid the use of atropine as it can also cause dangerously high hypertension. Hemodialysis is not effective in MAO/MAOI toxicity because these are highly protein-bound medications.

Clinical Pearls

Amphetamines may show up as positive on a drug screen for tranylcypromine and selegiline because they are structurally similar and metabolized into amphetamines and methampetamines.

Lithium
Drug overview

Lithium is a drug used in psychiatric medicine to treat bipolar and unipolar depression. Therapeutic serum concentrations are 0.8–1.25 mEq/l. It is available in both immediate and sustained-release forms.

Lithium competes with NA+ for ion transport. It enhances serotonin and acetylcholine effects and acts as an inhibitory second messenger via inositol phosphates. With toxic levels it suppresses neural excitation and synaptic transmission. Toxicity depends on chronic or acute ingestion. Chronic toxicity is usually from decreased renal clearance and acute toxicity occurs with deliberate or accidental overdose. Absorption occurs within 1–6 h for immediate release and is prolonged for up to 48 h in sustained-release forms. The half-life is usually 24 h but can be prolonged for up to 48 h. Acute ingestion of 20–30, 300 mg tablets would likely cause serious toxicity. Ninety-five percent of lithium is cleared by the kidney. Renal tubular reabsorption is increased in sodium-depleted and dehydrated states.

Symptom of overdose

Most symptoms of acute intoxication consist of neurological manifestations and GI symptoms. Mild toxicity (levels <1.5 mEq/l) usually presents with nausea, vomiting, lethargy, fine tremors, and memory impairment. Moderate toxicity (levels of 1.5–3.0 mEq/l) usually presents with confusion, agitation, hyperreflexia, hypertension, tachycardia, ataxia, nystagmus, extrapyramidal symptoms, and dysarthria. Severe toxicity (levels >3.0 mEq/l) results in bradycardia, seizure, coma, hypotension, and hyperthermia. Lithium levels do not always correlate with clinical toxicity because of their slow distribution. After initial early ingestion, an elevated level that would correlate with toxicity but no symptoms may be seen because of measurement before final tissue distribution. Nonspecific ECG changes can also occur including U waves, flat, biphasic, or inverted T waves, and sinus, junctional, or atrioventricular (AV) nodal blocks. Leukocytosis may also develop. Nephrogenic diabetes insipidus with dilute urine, hypernatremia, and elevated blood urea nitrogen (BUN) and creatinine is also common.

Diagnostic testing and monitoring

Lithium levels should be measured every 2–4 h until peak levels are seen. Monitoring of CBC and complete metabolic panel should be done daily until levels are trending down. Continuous ECG monitoring is needed until lithium levels have normalized.

Antidotes/binding agents/treatments

There is no specific drug antidote. Treatment depends on symptoms and lithium blood levels. Activated charcoal can be given within the first 1–2 h of acute ingestion but is ineffective in chronic toxicity. Whole-bowel irrigation should be used for sustained-release toxicity. Maintain a patent airway in patients who are obtunded. If dehydration is present, crystalloid fluids are administered with 1–2 l of normal saline followed by 0.45% normal saline. Monitor serum metabolic panel to manage fluid balance. Loop diuretics or mannitol are not recommended as initially they may increase lithium excretion but if the patient becomes water- or salt-depleted, lithium reabsorption will increase and toxicity will worsen. Lithium is a small ion, is not protein-bound, and has a small apparent volume of distribution and is able to be removed by dialysis. Dialysis is indicated for a patient with severe neurological symptoms and two consecutive lithium levels greater than 4.0 mEq/l. There should be no history of previous acute lithium toxicity. Dialysis can also be considered in patients who would not be able to handle adequate fluid replacement such as patients with heart failure, edematous states, and pulmonary edema. Lithium levels should be redrawn 6 h after dialysis as lithium is only removed from the plasma during dialysis. Once lithium from the intracellular space equilibrates with the

---

Clinical Pearls

Benzodiazepines should be given for seizures. Volume replacement should target a goal of 1–3 ml/kg of urine output per hour. If hyperthermia is present, cooling measures should be started. Although charcoal is usually ineffective, many lithium overdoses contain coingestion so it should be considered. Dialysis may also be effective in acute or chronic intoxication but generally is not useful in chronic toxicity.

serum, a higher level may occur. If the level is high or severe and symptoms persist, the patient should have dialysis repeated.

Neuroleptics
Drug overview
Neuroleptics are drugs that are used for treatment of a variety of psychological disorders. Psychotic disorders are thought to occur from an excess of dopamine in certain areas of the brain. Nondopamine receptors are also thought to be involved. These drugs are used to treat agitation, hallucinations, and acute delirium. Drugs in this class are agents that contain antipsychotic properties and extrapyramidal symptoms (EPS). EPS are thought to arise secondary to excess dopamine blockade, which leads to tremor, rigidity, and other parkinsonian effects. Effects can also occur in the endocrine system and can cause sexual dysfunction. These drugs can also cause akathisia, which is an inner feeling of the need to be in constant motion. Patients are compelled to constantly move or rock themselves. The cause of NMS is thought to be secondary to dopamine deficiency. Excess serotonin has been shown to cause dopamine deficiency. Usually NMS presents over the course of several days and always presents with fever.

Neuroleptic agents are dopamine receptor antagonists. They may block four different pathways for dopamine. Symptoms of overdose will depend on which drug is used and which pathway it has blocked. The primary mechanism of action of these drugs is postsynaptic blockade of the D-2 receptor but some also have H1 receptor blockade, peripheral alpha receptor blockade, or muscarinic receptor blockade. Neuroleptics may be classified as older typical agents. These usually carry more of a risk of EPS and seizures (Hedges, Jeppson, and Whitehead, 2003). Newer atypical agents generally have fewer EPS. Low-potency medications can cause more sedation, anti-acetylcholine (ACH), and orthostatic hypotension. High-potency medications can cause more EPS.

Symptoms of overdose
Side effects of toxicity may include hypotension, prolonged QT interval, tachycardia, and dry mucous membrane. Depending on the drug ingested, symptoms are varied but most include the CNS and cardiovascular system. Dystonic reactions, parkinsonism symptoms, seizures, hypotension, cardiac arrhythmias, hypo- or hyperthermia, and decreased GI motility can occur. Symptoms of anticholinergic toxidrome for some drugs may be seen.

Diagnostic testing and monitoring
Patients should be admitted to a critical care unit. Continuous ECG monitoring and airway protection may be needed depending on altered mental status symptoms. Drug levels are generally not available. CBC, ABGs, and complete metabolic profile should be obtained, and drug toxicity panels should be ordered to rule out coingestions.

Antidotes/binding agents/treatments
Recognition of NMS is important so treatment is not delayed. Care is supportive and there is no specific antidote. Because neuroleptics tend to lower the seizure threshold, seizures may be common and respond well to benzodiazapams. Hypotension is best treated with IV crystalloids and pure alpha agonists such as norepinephrine and phenylephrine. Use of mixed beta and alpha adrenergic agents such as epinephrine and dopamine should be avoided as they can worsen hypotension through vasodilation from unopposed beta stimulation. Hemodialysis is not effective due to the large volume of distribution and high protein binding. Dantrolene and bromocriptine have also been used to relax skeletal muscles and treat parkinsonism symptoms from abrupt discontinuation of dopamine-stimulating medications but their use remains controversial (McAllen and Schwartz, 2010).

Clinical Pearls

Common dystonic reactions include oculogyric crisis, which is an upward-gaze paralysis, torticolosis, retrocollis, scoliosis, and abdominal wall spasms. Dystonic reactions usually occur within 4–60 days but can occur immediately after dosing of the offending drug. Treatment of dystonic reactions or EPS is fairly simple. Treatment consists of the use of benzodiazapines and anticholinergic drugs. Doses for Benadryl should be 50–100 mg or 1–2 mg/kg. Ativan 1–2 mg IVP and Cogentin 1–2 mg IM or 1–4 mg/po may be used. Avoid all class 1A antiarrhythmics as these can prolong the QT interval and exacerbate arrhythmias.

Tricyclic antidepressants
Drug overview

Cyclic antidepressants are drugs used to treat depression. Poison Control Centers in the United States report TCAs as the third most reported type of poisoning. The most common TCAs reported in overdose are amitriptyline, dosulepin, and imipramine (Howell and Chauhan, 2010). TCAs work by inhibiting the reuptake of the transmitter's serotonin, norepinephrine, and dopamine, resulting in greater availability of these transmitters at the synapse. They generally have a low therapeutic index and serious overdose can happen with less than 10 times the therapeutic dose. TCAs also have secondary effects. They inhibit fast sodium channels in the myocardium, which can cause widened QRS and inhibit calcium entry into the myocardial cells, decreasing cardiac contractility. They also inhibit cholinergic responses and produce classic anticholinergic toxicity. Inhibition of the alpha-adrenergic receptors may occur, causing peripheral vasodilation.

Common drugs include amitriptyline, doxepin, imipramine, and Flexeril. Tricyclic toxicity generally affects the cardiac system and CNS. Anticholinergic effects of these drugs delay gastric emptying so that absorption is slow and erratic. Onset of action may be as quick as 30 min. Peak concentrations occur within 2–6 h after ingestion. Many have active metabolites. They are extensively bound to plasma proteins and body tissues, resulting in large volumes of distribution and long half-lives. Elimination is variable and may be between 8 and 30 h. Some are available in sustained-release form and can have significant delayed peak serum concentrations. The general toxic dose is 10–20 mg/kg. They are metabolized by the liver.

Symptoms of overdose

Symptoms include anticholinergic effects, cardiac arrhythmias, and QRS prolongation greater than 0.10–0.12 s, hypotension secondary to venous dilation and myocardial depression, and seizures that may be persistent and lead to status epilepticus. QRS prolongation is the single most important indicator of toxicity. Patients can deteriorate rapidly. Most toxic responses to tricyclic overdose occur within the first 6 h.

Diagnostic testing and monitoring

Overdose should be suspected in any patient presenting with lethargy, coma, seizures, and QRS prolongation greater than 0.12 s in the limb leads. Patients should be monitored in a critical care unit. Serial 12-lead ECGs should be done on admission and hourly for the first 6 h. Standard drug screens should be used to rule out coingestions. Decontamination with activated charcoal should be done with ingestions that have occurred within 1 h. CBC, comprehensive metabolic panel, ABGs, and CPK levels should be drawn. Patients who are given bicarbonate or placed on a bicarbonate drip need serial ABGs monitored. Death from toxicity usually occurs within a few hours of overdose and results from ventricular fibrillation, intractable cardiac arrhythmias, cardiogenic shock, seizures, and hyperthermia. Development of bradyarrhythmias is a very ominous finding. Monitoring the QRS interval is a much more reliable measure of toxicity than TCA laboratory assays.

Antidotes/binding agents/treatments

Charcoal can be administered within the first hour of ingestion. If QRS prolongation is present, sodium bicarbonate should be administered. The mechanism of action is thought to be a combination of sodium load along with serum alkalization, which negates the fast sodium channel inhibition in the myocardium. Alkalization of the serum can also cause increases in plasma protein binding of the drug. Sodium bicarbonate dose is usually 1–2 mEq IVP until the QRS narrows to normal limits or serum pH is 7.50–7.55. An IV infusion can then be given of 3 amps of sodium bicarbonate in 1 liter of D5W administered at 75–150 cc/h for 6 h. Use of antiarrhythmic drugs class IA and IC, which block sodium channels, is contraindicated. Class III antiarrhythmics such as amiodarone and bretylium are also contraindicated. Lidocaine, a class IB, can be used safely in refractory arrhythmias. Physostigmine is not helpful to manage anticholinergic symptoms and has been shown to precipitate seizures and can also cause asystole (Kerr, McGuffie, and Wilkie, 2001). Seizures should be treated with benzodiazepines and if intractable seizures are present, the use of phenobarbital is useful. Phenytoin can also be used as it is a class IB antiarrhythmic. Intubation and ventilation may be needed with altered mental states or cardiogenic shock states. Hypotension should be treated with IV crystalloid infusions of normal saline with the use of inotropic drugs such as dopamine or norepinephrine if needed.

Clinical Pearls

There are new therapies being developed in antibody fragment (Fab) therapies for TCA overdose. Fab therapies have a high binding capacity for the toxin and work like Digibind in digoxin overdose. The procedure for antibody isolation is very complex and expensive to develop and so far has required large amounts of Fab. There have been cases of small human studies with mild TCA overdose that have shown success using this therapy but it is not yet approved for use in the United States and studies are continuing (Howell and Chauhan, 2010). There have also been several case reports that have used ILE therapy in TCA overdose that is unresponsive to standard toxicology treatment (Roberts, 2010).

Carbon monoxide
Drug overview
Poisoning from carbon monoxide (CO) is a common problem accounting for approximately 50 000 emergency department visits each year in the United States, more commonly seen in the fall and winter (Ruth-Sahd, Zulkosky, and Fetter, 2011). Causes of CO poisoning include exposure or use of improperly ventilated fuels or impaired furnace functions, industrial chemicals such as paint stripper, or exhaust fumes. CO is a colorless, odorless gas that exerts a pathological effect on the body through a variety of mechanisms and causes approximately 2700 deaths annually according to the Centers for Disease Control. Mortality of patients treated in a hospital setting is 3% and significant mortality correlates with fire as a source of CO_2, loss of consciousness, carboxyhemoglobin level, arterial pH, and presence of endotracheal intubation during hyperbaric treatment (Hampson and Hauff, 2008).

Pharmacology
CO poisoning leads to impairment in oxygen delivery and utilization of oxygen by the body. Impairment of oxygen delivery causes an oxidant stress injury. High-affinity CO binds to hemoglobin, resulting in high levels of carboxyhemoglobin. This causes decreased oxygen-carrying capacity from the displacement of hemoglobin and causes a shift to the left on the oxyhemoglobin dissociation curve. CO increases levels of cystosolic heme, which leads to oxidative stress. The binding of platelet heme protein and cytochrome *c* oxidase interrupts cellular respiration, which induces a stress response and activates hypoxic inducible factor. Acute inflammation occurs through a variety of mechanisms and pathways and results in both neurological and cardiac injury (Weaver, 2009). Organs with high metabolic demands such as the heart and brain are the most affected by CO toxicity.

Symptoms
Symptoms of acute poisoning are vague and nonspecific. They can include muscle aches and tenderness, fatigue, headaches, and dizziness, similar to viral infection symptoms. Severe exposure to CO can result in loss of consciousness, seizures, cardiac arrest, pulmonary edema, myocardial infarction from angina, and death. Symptoms of chronic poisoning may differ from acute poisoning and may include memory deficits, fatigue, polycythemia, neuropathy, and difficulty with concentration. Levels greater than 3% in nonsmokers and greater than 10% in smokers are considered positive for exposure. The level generally does not correlate with symptoms or duration of exposure (Weaver, 2009). Later adverse outcomes may not be related to actual levels but more to inflammatory effects at the cellular level. Long-term effects can include motor and gait disturbances, hearing and vestibular abnormalities, and peripheral neuropathies. Patients can also develop CO-induced delayed neuropsychiatric syndrome, which develops after injury and apparent recovery and includes declining cognitive functioning, dementia, development of parkinsonism, and personality changes. Most of these symptoms may resolve within a year after recovery.

Diagnostic testing and monitoring
Monitoring should include neurological testing, CBC, extended chemistries, serial ABGs, and serum carboxyhemoglobin (CO-Hgb) testing.

The use of a co-oximeter is preferred to routine blood gas analyzers, which only measure oxyhemoglobin. A co-oximeter measures different levels of normal and abnormal hemoglobins as opposed to calculated values of carboxyhemoglobin. In cases of severe CO poisoning, lactic acidosis and anion gap metabolic acidosis may be present. Pulse oximetry is frequently inaccurate and may be falsely elevated in cases of significant poisoning. If severe coma from poisoning is present, head CT scanning may be necessary to identify severe hypoxia or ischemic cellular damage. Bilateral globus pallidus low-density lesions have been reported in severe posionings and may not be present until several days after exposure. Patients may also have symmetric white matter lesions on magnitic resonance imaging (MRI) (Kao and Nanagas, 2004). ECG and cardiac isoenzymes should also be performed to assess for any ischemic changes in cardiac rhythm. Patients with a history of myocardial disease are more susceptible to myocardial injury.

Antidotes/binding agents/treatments

Supportive care, high-flow supplemental oxygen for treatment of hypoxia, and accelerated removal of CO are urgent treatments. Use of a 100% non-rebreather oxygen mask or intubation with 100% oxygen until carboxyhemoglobin levels are less than 5% is recommended (Weaver, 2009). Abnormal vital signs should be treated aggressively. In cases of cardiac instability, standard therapy with antiarrhythmics, ASA, and nitrates is effective. In cases of severe poisoning with neurological deficits, seizures, and cardiac dysrhythmias, the use of a hyperbaric oxygen chamber may be needed and has been shown to reduce adverse neurological outcomes (Kao and Nanagas, 2004). The use of hyperbaric oxygen remains controversial (Weaver, 2009).

Clinical Pearls

In cases of deliberate CO poisoning, coingestions of other substances must be ruled out. Long-term chronic exposure to CO can causes symptoms of chronic fatigue, memory deficits, neuropathy, polycythemia, recurrent infections, and vertigo. Symptoms such as headache, neurological problems, and memory deficits may persist after treatment for up to 6 weeks and beyond (Weaver, 2009).

Hydrocarbons and toxic inhalants
Drug overview

These are substances that usually have mind-altering effects when inhaled. They are used by individuals to "get high." The practice of using inhalents is referred to as huffing, sniffing, or bagging. Huffing is the wetting of cloths and directly breathing in and out, sniffing is direct use out of the container, and bagging is discharging the toxin into a bag and inhaling. Inhalation provides effects of euphoria (Simlai and Khess, 2008). Some common toxic inhalants used are white out, toluene (methylbenzene) paint stripper, glue, benzene, Freon (fluorocarbons), nitrates (for sexual vasodilator effects), and felt tip marking pens. Individuals who experiment with toxic inhalants are usually adolestants, professional adults who have access to inhalants, and homosexual groups. National Poison Data System (NPDS) collects data in real time from 60 US Poison Control Centers. The prevalence of inhalant use decreased by 33% from 1993 to 2008 and the highest use was observed in the 12–17-year-old age group, with peak ages of 14–15 years. Males comprised 73.5% of cases where gender was known. The highest prevalence was seen in western mountain states and West Virginia. Common toxins include gasoline, propellants, and paint. Butane, propane, and air fresheners had the highest fatalities (Marsolek, White, and Litovitz, 2010).

Pharmacology

Volatile substance abuse can sensitize the myocardium to endogenous cathecolamines and predispose individuals to ventricular arrhythmias and asystole. They are highly lipid-soluble and take seconds to have an effect. Bagging offers the highest concentration and most effects. Pharmacology of inhalants will vary by the substance inhaled. Most acute effects last less than 2 h but permanent CNS effects can be seen with chronic use. Generally, acute high-level exposures to volatile substances are usually reversible while chronic exposures carry the risk of permanent disability (Iqbal, 2001). Metabolic processes for toxic effects vary and depend on the substances inhaled and cellular damage and effect. Toluene amounts as small as 15–20 ml have been reported to cause significant toxicity.

Diagnostic testing and monitoring

Diagnosis is usually made by history of inhalation, either deliberate or accidental. Depending on organ system involvement, signs, and symptoms, patients may need to be monitored in a critical care unit. ECG monitoring and oxygen saturation monitoring should be conducted continuously. Standard drug panels, CBC, electrolytes, CPK, ABG, and LFTs should be drawn and monitored based on symptoms of organ toxicity. A chest radiograph should also be obtained to rule out pulmonary toxicity due to aspiration or inhalation injury.

Signs and symptoms

Common symptoms involving toxic inhalant use are euphoric actions, ataxia, slurred speech, various altered mental status, GI effects such as nausea and vomiting, and respiratory difficulty. Organs that are particularly vulnerable to inhalents are the kidneys, with distal tubular acidosis often found. Respiratory symptoms include acute respiratory distress syndrome and aspiration. Hepatic system effects include liver necrosis, and cardiovascular system effects can include arrhythmias and cardiac arrest. Toxic inhalant use can also cause rhabdomyolysis and many hematological derangements. Toluene use has been linked to leukoencephalopathy, brain stem abnormalities, cranial neuropathies, and cerebellar syndrome (Filley and Kleinschmidt-DeMasters, 2001). Hexacarbons, which are present in glue and solvents, can cause toxic neuropathies that usually recover slowly over many months (Morrison and Chaudhry, 2012).

Antidotes/treatment

Care is supportive. In accidental inhalation, the patient should be removed from exposure. Remove all contaminated clothing items and wash all exposed skin with soap and water. Irrigate eyes with water or saline. If coma and bronchospasm occur, protect airway and administer bronchodilators. If cardiac arrhythmias occur, sympathomimetics drugs such as epinephrine can worsen symptoms. Beta blockers such as propanolol or esmolol are recommended.

> **Clinical Pearls**
>
> Toluene, which is present in glue, paint, and solvents, is a common agent of abuse, readily available and cheap. It is a known neurotoxin and in chronic users usually produces extensive cerebellar dysfunction and gait ataxia, which is usually permanent. It has been postulated that a genetic link to concentrations of P450 enzymes that are present in the body and vulnerability to permanent disabilities with use of inhalants may be due to the bioactivation of the metabolic processes involved to detoxify inhalants (Iqbal, 2001).

Cardiac medications
Drug overview

Beta blockers, calcium channel blockers, nitrates, and digoxin are cardiac medications that may result in overdoses.

a. **Beta blockers**—examples include Coreg, metropolol, and labetalol. These drugs are generally prescribed for hypertension, dysrhythmias, angina, vasovagal syndrome, migraines, and panic disorders. They can also be used for the treatment of thyrotoxicosis. Beta blockers work by blocking β-adrenergic receptors of the peripheral nervous system. They inhibit binding of epinephrine and norepinephrine to G- protein β-adrenergic receptors in the heart, kidney, and eyes, which are β1 receptors. They also inhibit β2 receptors present in blood vessels, bronchioles, liver, and pancreas. They may also bind to the β receptors and activate phosphodiesterase, which increases cyclic adenosine monophosphate (cAMP). Beta blockers may be cardioselective and may only block β1 receptors, may have sodium channel blocking, or have membrane stabilizing effects and antiarrhythmic effects. The half-life of certain types of beta blockers can be severely prolonged based on the patient's hepatic and renal clearance. Some beta blockers may be more lipophilic, such as propranolol, which crosses fatty cell membranes and affects the blood–brain barrier more readily. This can produce more CNS symptoms in overdose such as seizures and coma (see Table 13.5).

Table 13.5 Overdose of beta blockers: effects and treatment.

Name	Receptor site: β1 or β2	Lipid solubility	Half-life	Elimination	Major cardiovascular effects with overdose	Specific treatment
Metoprolol	β 1	High	3–4 h	Hepatic	Bradycardia, hypotension Hypoglycemia	Glucagon for bradycardia and hypotension Pacemaker Intra-aortic balloon pump for refractory CV compromise
Atenolol	β1	Low	6–9 h	Renal	Bradycardia Hypotension	Glucagon Dialysis may be useful
Carvedilol	β1, β2, and a1	High	6–10 h	Hepatic	Coma, seizures, bradycardia, hypotension	Glucagon
Nadolol	β1 and β2	Low	14–24 h	Renal	AV blocks, congestive heart failure	Dialysis may be useful
Labetalol	β1 and β2	Low	3–6 h	Hepatic	Hypotension, bradycardia	Glucagon
Sotalol	β1 and β2	Low	5–12 h	Renal	Delayed and prolonged Toxicity Hypotension, tachycardia Ventricular tachyarrhythmias Prolongs QT interval	Magnesium, lidocaine, cardiac pacing Dialysis may be useful
Esmolol	β1	Low	15 min		Hypotension Bradycardia	Dialysis may be useful
Acebutolol	β1	Moderate	3–6 h	Renal	Beta agonist effects may have sympathomimetic activity Seizures	
Betaxolol	β1	Low	14–22 h	Hepatic		Dialysis may be useful
Propanolol	β1 and β2	High	3–5 h	Hepatic	Coma, seizures, bradycardia	
Clonidine	Central acting alpha adrenergic agonist		6–24 h	Hepatic	CNS depression, coma Miosis, bradycardia Hypotension	Naloxone 0.1 mg IV q 30–60 s to dose of 0.5 mg, may need drip Atropine, vasopressors

Note: IV calcium, glucose, high-dose insulin and potassium therapy can be considered for refractory hypotension in beta blocker overdose/calcium channel overdose. May also consider intravenous lipid emulsion (ILE) for refractory treatment of symptoms with cardiovascular collapse (Cave, 2011). Consult with local Poison Control Center.

Beta blocker symptoms of overdose. Generally, symptoms occur within 20 min to 1 h. Most effects are seen within 6 h except with time-released formulas and Sotolol, whose effects can be seen for days. These effects include hypotension, hypoglycemia, seizures, and bradycardia. There can be various degrees of AV blocks and ventricular arrhythmias that can lead to cardiac arrest. Both CCBs and beta blockers typically cause prolongation of the PR interval and QRS prolongation.

Beta blocker diagnostic testing and monitoring. There are no specific tests available at the hospital for drug level testing in beta blocker overdose. Generally, toxic effects may be seen with two to three times the therapeutic range. Admission to critical care is needed.

Tests should include continuous ECG monitoring, serial 12-lead ECG, BP monitoring, and complete metabolic panel. Chest X-ray and serial ABGs may be necessary. Protection of the airway with intubation and ventilation may be needed in situations involving cardiogenic shock states. Beta 2 blockade can also cause increased airway resistance, especially in patients with lung disease. Frequent monitoring of blood glucose levels should be done due to hypoglycemia and hyperglycemia secondary to impaired glycogenolysis.

Beta blocker antidotes/binding agents/treatment. Charcoal and gastric lavage can be used if time of overdose is known and may be effective within the first hour. In sustained-release forms, repeated doses may be necessary.

Whole-bowel irrigation and cathartics for sustained-release forms may be used. Aggressive fluid hydration is recommended and airway protection may be needed if signs and symptoms of profound cardiac instability and shock occur. Be aware that there are many combination cardiac prescriptions so coingestion is common. For mild symptoms of bradycardia and hypotension, fluids and atropine may be all that are needed.

Glucagon is the treatment of choice for hypotension and bradycardia. Doses of 5–10 mg IV bolus are usually needed followed by 1–5 mg/h infusion. Calcium chloride IV can be given at a dose of 1 g of 10% solution or calcium gluconate 30 ml of a 10% solution can be administered. Infusion of calcium will increase inotropic effects of the heart. Catecholamines may be effective, but large doses may be needed. Drugs such as norephinephrine, dopamine, dobutamine, Isuprel, and epinephrine can all be effective. Keep in mind that these drugs can be proarrhythmic. Epinephrine may be used at doses of 1–4 µg/min. Sodium bicarbonate may be used for wide complex conduction defects caused by membrane-depressant effects at a dose of 1–2 mEq/kg. Heart rate may be refractory to atropine but it is safe to use. Aggressive fluid resuscitation is usually needed. Cardiac ultrasound may be useful. QT prolongation from Sotolol can be treated with magnesium, isoproterenol infusion, or pacemaker insertion and overdrive pacing. Cardiovascular instability unresponsive to standard therapy may need temporary transvenous pacemaker or intra-aortic balloon pumping therapy. Hypoglycemia is frequently seen most often in children and seizures should be treated with glucose.

Clinical Pearls—Beta Blocker

If intubation is needed, pretreatment with atropine should be considered to mitigate potential vagal-induced bradycardia (Anderson, 2007). Coreg and labetolol are known to cause significant hypotension due to their combined beta 1 blockade and vasodilating effects. Labatolol may also cause hyperkalemia in patients with renal failure due to the increase in insulin secretion from beta-adrenergic agents, which augments cellular potassium uptake (Anderson, 2007). Newer therapies involving IV calcium and high-dose insulin–glucose therapy have been used successfully.

---

b. **Calcium channel blockers.** CCBs are drugs most commonly prescribed to treat angina, atrial arrhythmias, and hypertension. They decrease myocardial oxygen demand and increase coronary blood flow. In 2008, the American Association of Poison Control Centers reported 10 398 exposures to CCBs resulting in 12 deaths and 63 major adverse outcomes (Horowitz, 2012). Overdose of CCB can result in arrhythmias and severe hypotension and shock, leading to ventricular fibrillation, asystole, and cardiac arrest. Patients who are asymptomatic are unlikely to develop symptoms if ingestion of immediate release is greater than 6 h from presentation, 18 h for modified release, and 24 h for sustained release (Baud *et al.*, 2007).

CCB pharmacology. CCBs inhibit the movement of calcium ions into the cells by interfering with the action of the voltage-gated calcium channels. As calcium enters into the cardiac myocytes, three results occur: negative inotropic, chronotropy, and dromotropy actions. These actions cause impaired impulse and conduction in the sinoatrial and AV nodes, which slows heart rate and may cause AV blocks.

CCB symptoms of overdose. Symptoms of overdose include varying forms of AV block and cardiovascular collapse, metabolic acidosis, and shock states. Hypotension and bradycardia are common. Patients with severe poisoning may present with heart rates less than 50 and systolic blood pressure less than 100. Hyperglycemia occurs from the inhibition of calcium-dependent insulin release. Other symptoms include nausea, vomiting, and lethargy.

CCB diagnostic testing and monitoring. Patients should be monitored in a critical care unit with continuous ECG monitoring for symptoms of hypotension, bradycardia, and AV blocks. Serial 12-lead ECGs should be performed. Clinical testing of blood levels for CCB is generally not available. Standard drug screens should be utilized to assess for coingestions. If patients are on digoxin or coumadin, digoxin levels and PT/INR should also be done. CBC and extended metabolic panel should be done. Patients on continuous insulin and glucose therapy should have Q1 hour fingerstick glucose levels. Hyperglycemia can occur as CCB inhibits release of insulin. For refractory shock, hemodynamic monitoring and ECG should be done (Baud *et al.*, 2007).

CCB antidotes/binding agents/treatment. Activated charcoal should be given if ingestion is within 1 h. Whole-bowel irrigation with Golytely 2 l/h should be used for extended-release formulas. Boluses of 1 g of calcium chloride every 15–20 min, for a total of four doses, or 1 g every 2–3 min can also be utilized if CCB toxicity is verified. Monitoring of ionized calcium levels should be utilized. Large doses up to 10 g may be needed. Calcium has a variable effect on hypotension but has a minimal effect on bradycardia. Avoid giving calcium to a patient with concomitant cardiac glycoside toxicity (digoxin) as fatal arrhythmias can develop. Initiate high insulin/glucose therapy early for severe CCB overdose. Administration of insulin 0.1–1 μ/kg/h with concurrent dextrose infusion of D10W or D25W may be warranted. Titration of both should be done to maintain normal serum glucose levels. This therapy has been shown to stabilize cardiac output by affecting myocardial function, catecholamine release, modulation of the inflammatory cascade, and cellular apoptosis. If patients are receiving this therapy, glucose monitoring should be performed every 20–30 min. Glucagon can be given at doses of 5–15 mg over 1–2 min for hypotension. Dosages can be repeated every 3–5 min. Response is usually seen within 1–3 min with peak effects at 5–7 min. Glucogen has a short half-life so if resolution of symptoms occurs, an infusion can be started at 2–10 mg/h in adults. Glucagon's therapeutic effects may decline over time due to loss of ability to increase cAMP levels and in some situations repeated boluses may be preferred (Anderson, 2007). Glucagon activates adenylate cyclase, which is independent of the B receptor. Atropine can be used for CCB overdose but is usually ineffective. IV crystalloids should be given for hypotension but frequently inotropic medications are needed. Dopamine works well for bradycardia and hypotension. Norepinephrine and vasopressin

may be needed for additional management of hypotension. Milrinone or Inocor, both of which are phosphodiesterase inhibitors, may be useful to support cardiac contractility. On initial infusion they can cause hypotension. Patients with refractory hypotension may need intra-aortic balloon pumping therapy. Patients with refractory bradycardia and high-grade AV blocks may require ventricular pacemaker insertion.

Clinical Pearls—CCB

Severe cardiac toxicity usually doesn't respond to single-dose therapy and usually requires multiple-drug combination modalities. There have been case reports of CCB overdose that have been successfully treated with Levosimendan (Teker *et al.*, 2010). Levosimendan is an inotropic drug that is a calcium sensitizer. It enhances cardiac contraction by improving the use of cytosolic calcium. Dosages used were an initial loading dose of 2 μg/kg followed by an infusion at 2 μg/kg/h and continued for 30 h. Patients had good responses to therapy. There have also been good results from intralipid infusions. For severe cardiovascular shock that is unresponsive to standard therapy, there have been case reports of the use of peripheral cardiopulmonary bypass to treat the diseased myocardium, along with continuous veno-venous hemofiltration (CVVH) and plasma exchange therapies (Baud *et al.*, 2007). Use of MARS has also been shown to be effective (DePont, 2007).

c. **Nitrates.** Nitrates and nitrites are drugs that produce venous dilation. They can also cause methemoglobinemia. Common drugs are nitroglycerin, isosorbide nitrates, amyl nitrate, sodium nitrate, and ammonium nitrate.

Nitrates pharmacology. Nitrates and nitrites cause venous smooth muscle relaxation at lower doses and can produce arterial dilation at higher doses. These effects can cause profound hypotension. Toxicity can be caused by inhalation, oral ingestion, and dermal absorption. Methemoglobinemia can also result in overdose, which converts hemoglobin to methemoglobin and decreases oxygen-carrying capacity and delivery to tissues.

Nitrates symptoms of overdose. Hypotension and tachycardia are common effects with ingestion. Cardiovascular side effects can include cyanosis, dysrhythmias, syncope, and myocardial infarction. Altered mental status can occur with seizures. Toxic doses are between 200 and 1200 mg of nitroglycerin-containing substances. Toxic dose of sodium nitrate is usually 1 g, and 10 cc of amyl nitrate can produce significant levels of methemoglobin. Nausea, vomiting, abdominal pain, and diarrhea can also occur. Headache is common. Dyspnea and decreased pulse oximetry can occur with methemoglobinemia.

Nitrates diagnostic testing and monitoring. Monitoring should include serum electrolytes and ABGs with co-oximeter because of inaccuracy of pulse oximetry due to methemoglobin. In cases of amyl nitrate toxicity, methemoglobin levels should be monitored. Levels less than 3% are nontoxic. Frequent monitoring should include CBC, chemistry panel, and ABGs. Arterial oxygen (PaO_2) and oxygen saturation levels may be normal despite significant hypoxia and methemoglobinemia.

Nitrates antidotes/binding agents/treatment. Gastric lavage and charcoal administration can be done in cases of overdose within 1 h. Treatment of cardiovascular effects is supportive with oxygen therapy, IV access, IV crystalloids, use of inotropic medications for hypotension not responding to fluids, and continuous ECG monitoring. In cases where methemoglobinemia develops, treatment with methylene blue may be needed. If significant CNS symptoms, hypoxia, or cardiac instability is present, administration of 1–2 mg/kg IV can be given over 5 min. Methemoglobin levels should be repeated and if they are still elevated and the patient remains symptomatic, the dose can be repeated at 0.5–1 mg/kg IV. Methemoglobin levels should continue to be monitored until decreasing levels are seen for at least 6 h. In patients with G-6-PD deficiency, hemolysis can occur and use of methylene blue is contraindicated.

Clinical Pearls—Nitrates

If indicated, use a vasopressor with less beta effects because of the increased sympathetic outflow with vasodilator toxicity and resulting tachycardia and increased myocardial contractility. For life-threatening methemoglobinemia that is not responding to methylene blue, exchange transfusion has been used.

---

d. Digitalis. Digitalis is a cardiac glycoside, derived from foxglove plant and is used for the treatment of systolic heart failure and rate control. Usually toxicity is caused from acute or accidental overdose or from other disease conditions such as acute renal failure, dehydration, and concurrent medications that potentiate digoxin, including paroxetine, rifampin, verapamil, diltiazem, tetracycline, and erythromycin.

Digitalis pharmacology/symptoms of overdose. Digoxin inhibits the sodium–potassium adenosine triphosphatase pump, which causes decreased atrial ventricular nodal conduction and increased cardiac contractility. It is absorbed in the serum over 6 h but patients become symptomatic once tissue levels increase and serum levels start to decrease. It is excreted renally. Symptoms of overdose include AV block with bradycardia, junctional tachycardia, ventricular tachycardia and fibrillation, nausea, vomiting, CNS effects, hyperkalemia, and visual disturbances such as yellow-green halos.

Digitalis diagnostic testing and monitoring. Serum digoxin levels are considered toxic if greater than 2.0 ng/ml. However, levels will be falsely elevated within 6 h of dosing and may not clinically correlate with symptoms. Acute overdose symptoms usually occur after 6 h, and for patients on chronic doses, toxicity can occur up to 5 days later. Serious arrhythmias usually occur within 24 h. Drug levels should not be relied upon for diagnosis. Diagnosis should be based on history and symptomology as patients can be toxic at therapeutic doses and asymptomatic at high doses. Patients will need continuous ECG monitoring, serial electrolytes, 12-lead ECG monitoring, renal function, oxygen saturation, ABGs, and chest radiographs. If symptoms are severe, advanced life support measures should be instituted along with administration of Digibind. ECG changes seen with digoxin toxicity are sinoatrial nodal dysfunction, prolonged PR intervals, short QT interval, and sloping of the ST segment. Tachycardia or heart block can occur from the suppression of the sinoatrial node and increased automaticity with decreased conduction at the AV node.

Digitalis antidotes/binding agents/treatment. Charcoal can be used if time of overdose is known. Hydration in the setting of dehydration and acute kidney injury should be initiated with D5NS or normal saline infusion. Atropine is first-line therapy for bradyarrhythmias that are symptomatic. Indications for Digibind include cardiac instability with ventricular arrhythmias or severe heart block, hyperkalemia with potassium levels greater than 5 mEq/l, and digoxin levels greater then 15 ng/ml regardless of symptoms. Digibind is given at a dose based on the total body level of digoxin taken 6 h after ingestion. The general rule is that 38 mg of Digibind (one vial) will bind 0.5 mg of digoxin and 40 mg of Digifab (one vial) will bind 0.5 mg of digoxin. If cardiac instability and arrest are imminent, Digibind may be given as a bolus dose; otherwise, it should be infused over 30 min. Lidocaine is usually not effective for ventricular arrhythmias. Phenytoin is the drug of choice for ventricular arrhythmias due to increase in the ventricular fibrillation threshold and enhanced conduction through the AV node. IV magnesium can also be given to stabilize cardiac function. Chronic overdose symptoms may be different from acute toxicity with symptoms of nausea, vomiting, and anorexia. CNS effects are common as are yellow and green halos and other altered color perceptions. Levels may be therapeutic or only minimally elevated. If patients are on diuretics, hypokalemia and hypomagnesemia can induce toxicity.

Antiarrhythmic agents

These are agents that exert action on the heart and can be very toxic with life-threatening consequences in cases of overdose and toxicity. There are several classes of antiarrhythmic agents that are classified based on the Vaughan–Williams classification system. Type 1 drugs inhibit fast sodium channels and cause cardiac cell depolarization and impulse conduction abnormalities, depressing myocardial functioning and contractility. Type 1a and 1c also block potassium channels and toxicity creates problems with depolarization and conduction in the cardiac cycle. This frequently prolongs QT intervals. Drugs such as flecainide and propafenone are Type 1c cardiac drugs and can cause prolongation of the QRS complex in overdose. Type 1b drugs, such as phenytoin and lidocaine, block sodium channels but have no effect on the QRS complex. Class II drugs are generally classified as beta blockers and block beta-adrenergic receptors. Type III cardiac arrhythmic agents are potassium channel blockers such as bretylium and Sotolol. Prolongation of potassium channels causes increased duration of the action potential and prolongs the refractory period. Class IV antiarrhythmics are classified as CCBs and slow the influx of calcium through cellular calcium channels. They primarily act on vascular smooth muscle and the heart. All drugs in this section are widely distributed to body tissues. These drugs usually have a narrow therapeutic index and may show toxicity even at therapeutic doses. Ingestion of twice the recommended dose can produce significant toxicity except in the case of amiodarone, which has an extensive distribution to tissues.

a. **Potassium blockers.** Antiarrhythmic drugs that interfere with conduction through potassium channels include drugs such as amiodarone, bretylium, and sotolol.

Clinical Pearls—Digitalis

Common causes of digoxin toxicity outside of intentional overdose are dehydration and acute kidney injury. Usually with hydration and improvement of renal function, digoxin levels improve. If Digibind is given, trending the digoxin level is not accurate and will be abnormally high. Testing for a free level of digoxin may be helpful but this is usually a send-out test in most hospitals and the results may take several days. Avoid calcium as this may potentiate cardiac toxicty because digoxin increases intracellular calcium. Hyperkalemia should be treated with regular insulin, dextrose 50, hydration, and Kayexalate 15–30 g by mouth four times a day (each 1 g in exchange for 1 mEq of potassium). Reoccurance of toxicity may develop in patients with acute renal failure or on dialysis. Patients should have a renal consult and may need to have dialysis done in a timely fashion. Toads from the Bufonidae family also secrete a toxin from their glands in their skin, which contains cardiac glycoside properties, that is added to some natural medications from the Far East. This acts as an aphrodisiac. Some people also practice licking of these frogs to get high (Garg, Hippargi, and Gandhare, 2008). Digibind has not shown to be effective in these situations (Leitch, Lim, and Bora, 2000).

Pharmacology. Potassium blockers block potassium channels by prolonging action potentials and the refractory period, which in turn prolongs the QT interval.

Amiodarone possesses noncompetitive beta-adrenergic blocking effects, which are very similar to calcium channel blocking effects. Amiodarone can frequently cause bradyarrhythmias, negative inotropic effects, pulmonary fibrosis, and hyper/hypothyroidism. Amiodarone is a drug that is extensively distributed throughout the tissues and even massive single doses produce mild toxicity. It is an iodine-based compound that is similar in structure to thyroxine. Large doses can also cause iodine toxicity. Half-life can be up to 50 days.

Sotalol has beta-adrenergic properties along with Class III antiarrhythmic activity. Overdosages are usually dose-dependent and can cause Torsades de pointes and ventricular fibrillation. Significant QTc prolongation can occur. Absorption is generally 1–4 h but can be longer with sustained-release formulas. See Table 13.6 for drugs that cause QT prolongation. See also Chapter 4.

Symptoms of overdose. Symptoms depend on the specific drug and half-life. Symptoms can include QT/QTc prolongation, bradyarrhythmias, AV blocks, and hypotension. Cardiogenic shock can occur. Neurological symptoms can include altered mental status.

Diagnostic testing and monitoring. Diagnosis is based on history. There are no specific tests that can detect overdose. Depending on the agent ingested, drug levels may be available but treatment should not be delayed. Patients with suspected overdose of these substances should be admitted to a critical care unit with continuous ECG monitoring and frequent monitoring of QT and QTc intervals for a minimum of 24 h if toxicity is present. Serial 12-lead ECGs should be monitored. Supplemental oxygen, IV access, administration of IV crystalloids, and vasopressors may be needed. CBC, LFTs, and electrolyte monitoring with calcium and magnesium should be assessed. ABGs should be monitored. Thyroid panel may be useful with amiodarone ingestions. Frequent neurological monitoring for coma and seizures should also be done.

Antidotes/binding agents/treatment. In cases of overdose within 1 h, gastric lavage and charcoal can be used. Laxatives may be needed for sustained-release formulas. Protect airway, breathing, and circulation. For arrhythmias do not treat Type 1a, Type 1c, or Type IIIc overdose with Type 1a drugs (Olsen, 2005). Administration of sodium bicarbonate for hypotension, arrhythmia, and QRS prolongation at dosages of 1–2 mEq/kg is usually effective. Treat seizures with benzodiazepines.

Clinical Pearls—Antiarrhythmics

Dialysis or hemoperfusion is usually ineffective due to extensive tissue distribution.

---

b. **Sodium channel blockers** are Class IA, IB, and IC drugs. Class IA prolongs the QRS and QT intervals. Class IB agents shorten the action potential and have less effect on the fast sodium channels so there is little effect on the QRS, QT, and PR intervals. Class IC drugs decrease conduction and have potent sodium channel blockade, which increases the QRS interval more than the other Class 1 agents (Ling, 2001). These are drugs that block fast sodium channels. Examples of

Table 13.6 Drugs that cause prolonged QT interval (not all inclusive).

Arsenic	Droperidol	Organophosphates
Atypical antipsychiotics	Erythromycin	Phenothiazines*
Citalopram	Florides	Propoxyphene
Clarithromycin	Haloperidol	Scorpion or spider bite
Class Ia antidysrhythmics	Hypo Mg, K, CA	Tamoxifen
Class III antidysrhythmics	Lithium	Bactrim
Contrast injection	Octretide	Tricyclic antidepressaants

*Major phenothiazines causing QT prolongation are thioridazine and thiothixene.

Class IA drugs are Norpace, procainamide, and quinidine. Some examples of Class IB antiarrhythmics are Dilantin, lidocaine, mexiletine, and tocanide. Examples of Class IC are flecainide and propafenone.

Sodium channel blockers symptoms of overdose. General symptoms of overdose usually affect the cardiovascular system and include hypotension, bradycardia, widened QRS, Torsades de pointes, and prolongation of the QT interval. Class IC usually causes negative inotropic effects. Flecainide can also cause neutropenia, hypotension, AV blocks, and asystole due to the prolongation of the QRS and QT intervals. Lidocaine toxicity usually causes CNS symptoms, with confusion and agitation being the most common. Tocainide and mexiletine overdose can cause CNS alterations such as confusion, sedation, and coma.

Sodium channel blockers diagnostic testing and monitoring. Serum levels are available for most drugs in this class but treatment should not be delayed waiting for levels. Patients should be admitted to a critical care unit with continuous ECG monitoring and 12-lead serial ECG monitoring to assess for QRS prolongation and QTC prolongation.

Sodium channel blockers antidotes/binding agents/treatment. In cases of overdose within 1 h, gastric lavage and charcoal can be used. Laxatives may be needed for sustained-release formulas. Sodium bicarbonate infusion 1–2 mEq/kg IV is used in the setting of sodium channels overdose and QRS widening.

Clinical Pearls—Sodium Channel Blockers

Drugs such as cocaine, Benadryl, TCAs, phenothiazines, and Tegretol have sodium-blocking principles but are not classified as antidysrhythmics. Dialysis may be benefical in tocanide or flecainide overdose.

Toxic alcohols
Drug overview
These are substances that are toxic to all body systems and may be indicated in accidental and deliberate ingestion. Drugs discussed are ethylene glycol, propylene glycol, methanol, and isopropyl alcohol. Most of these alcohols cause profound metabolic and lactic acidosis. PG has a relatively low toxicity

and the most frequent cause seen in critical care is IV Ativan toxicity.

a. **Ethylene glycol** is a colorless, odorless, syrupy, sweet-tasting substance that is found in many household products such as antifreeze, detergents, deicing products, paints, hydraulic brake fluids, and other industrial fluids. Ethylene glycol becomes toxic after ingestion through its metabolites. Ingestion is often accidental but there have been many forensic science cases that have found deliberate poisoning attempts. The anion gap acidosis that is produced is due to the accumulation of glycolic, glyoxylic, and oxalic acid along with hydrogen ion titration from these. The formation of hippuric acid ensues and depletion of other cofactors for the tricarboxylic acid cycle results in an accumulation of lactic acid (Adler and Weening, 2006). Osmolar gap is usually increased first without acidosis, followed by evidence of toxic metabolites. Alcoholics have frequently ingested ethylene glycol substances as an alcohol substitute.

The toxic lethal dose in adults is around 100 ml or (1–1.5 ml/kg). The lethal blood level in untreated adults is 200 mg/dl. Peak levels occur 1–4 h after ingestion. It is widely distributed to the tissues. Blood levels usually do not correlate with the severity of illness. Three signs to look for when making this diagnosis are an elevated anion and osmolar gap, hypocalcemia, and urinary calcium oxalate crystals (Scalley *et al.*, 2002).

Ethylene glycol symptoms of overdose. Presentation is highly variable depending on amounts of ethylene glycol and time of ingestion. Anion gap acidosis with elevated osmolar gap is usually present but osmolar gap may be low in late presentation of ingestion where metabolites have already been processed by the kidney (Jammalamadaka and Raissi, 2010). Toxicity is usually fatal within 24–72 h if untreated. Toxicity may consist of three phases. The CNS phase consists of ataxia, confusion, nystagmus, seizures, myoclonic jerks, coma, and tetany from hypocalcemia. This usually occurs within the first 1–12 h after ingestion. GI complaints can occur in this phase. Ethylene is rapidly absorbed by the GI system and symptoms include nausea, vomiting, and abdominal pain. The second phase or cardiovascular phase usually occurs within 12–72 h post ingestion. Symptoms include hypertension, cardiac arrhythmias, tachycardia, respiratory difficulty, and hypothermia. Pneumonitis and ARDS have also occurred. Cardiac failure may also occur in cases of significant poisoning and shock. Phase 3 is the final phase with renal toxicity and failure. This can occur within 24–72 h after ingestion and patients develop flank pain and oliguric renal failure. The metabolite oxalate causes widespread tissue injury throughout the body and causes tubular damage in the kidney that may be permanent.

Ethylene glycol diagnostic testing and monitoring. Diagnosis is usually based on the history of ingestion. There is specific testing that should be done to check for toxic alcohol ingestion. Ethylene glycol, methanol, and PG levels should be drawn. Testing is usually done at large regional hospital centers and results are usually available in a matter of hours. If a strong suspicion of diagnosis exists, treatment should not be delayed while awaiting testing. Anion gap acidosis with osmolar gap is usually present. Oxalate or hippurate crystals may be present in the urine. Woods lamp testing can be performed. Antifreeze contains fluorescein, which gives it a yellow green color; urine may fluoresce with the use of a Woods lamp depending on the concentration and timing of ingestion. CBC, extended electrolytes, ABGs, serum osmolarity, drug toxicology panels, urinalysis, blood ketone levels, LFTs, lactic acid, and 12-lead ECG should be monitored every 4–6 h. ECG may show symptoms of hypocalcemia due to calcium oxalate crystals and prolonged QTC may occur. Hyperkalemia may occur in the setting of acute renal failure. Ethylene glycol levels should be sent every 12–24 h to monitor levels during fomepizide and dialysis treatments. In the setting of osmolar gap with alcohol ingestion, gap needs to be corrected for alcohol level. There are many online medical calculators that will do this.

Ethylene glycol antidotes/binding agents/ treatment. Airway and circulatory support is usually needed. Treat hypotension with crystalloids. Vasopressors may be needed in shock states. Electrolyte replacement may be indicated. Bicarbonate infusions may also be needed. Treat seizures with anticonvulsants. Fomepizole is the treatment of choice for ethylene glycol toxicity. Fomepizole is an inhibitor of alcohol dehydrogenase and prevents acidic ethylene glycol metabolites. The loading dose is 15 mg/kg followed by 10–15 mg/kg every 12 h for four doses. Fomepizole is continued until ethylene glycol levels are less than 20 mg/dl. If fomepizole is not available, ethanol infusion can be used. The dosage is 10% ethanol diluted in 5% dextrose and infused at 1.4–2 ml/kg/h after a loading dose of 8–10 ml/kg over 30 min. Ethanol is very toxic to the veins and central access may be needed. Hemodialysis can be used to remove ethylene glycol and its metabolites. Indications for use are severe metabolic acidosis with renal dysfunction and ethylene glycol levels greater than 25–50 mg/dl and continued until levels are less than 10 mg/ dl. Dosing of fomepizole needs to be adjusted when receiving dialysis.

Clinical Pearls—Ethylene Glycol

Many substances can elevate the anion or osmolar gap but only diabetic ketoacidosis (DKA), alcoholic ketoacidosis, ethylene glycol, and methanol elevate both. False positive levels of ethylene glycol can occur in patients who have high triglyceride levels and elevated levels of 2,3-butanediol, which may be present in chronic alcoholics and with ingestion of other glycols. In the setting of coingestion of alcohol and ethylene glycol, alcohol levels will be decreased. For differential diagnosis, think of the mnemonic "**METAL ACID GAP.**"

M—methanol, metformin
E—ethylene glycol
T—toluene (glue)
A—alcohol ketoacidosis
L—lactic acidosis
A—aspirin
C—carbon monoxide, cyanide
I—iron, Isoniazoid
D—DKA
G—generalized seizures
A—aminoglycoside agents
P—paraldehyde, phenformin

b. **Methanol drug overview.** This is a toxic alcohol that is clear, colorless, and has a slight alcoholic odor. It is generally found in industrial solvents, canned solid fuels (sternos), windshield washer fluid, glass cleaners, and octane boosters. Toxicity can occur through ingestion, inhalation (carburetor cleaner), and absorption through skin (Givens, Kalbfleisch, and Bryson, 2008). Methanol is rapidly absorbed through the GI system and symptoms of intoxication can occur within 1 h. Lethal dosages vary among patients but are usually between 30 and 240 ml. Peak blood levels usually occur 30–90 min after ingestion. Methanol converts to toxic formaldehyde and formate acid in the liver and causes metabolic acidosis. Formate acid is the cause of most of the serious effects of methanol toxicity including ocular edema and resulting blindness. Lactic acid occurs due to hypotension and tissue hypoxia from anaerobic glucose metabolism.

Methanol diagnostic testing and monitoring. Methanol drug levels should be obtained. Toxic levels are usually greater than 50 mg/dl and acidosis is usually present. Peak levels less that 20 mg/dl are usually asymptomatic. Levels greater than 150 mg/dl are usually fatal. Anion gap acidosis is present with osmolar gap. Laboratory monitoring and supportive measures are the same as ethylene glycol treatment.

Methanol symptoms of overdose. Early symptoms may include nausea, vomiting, and hemorrhagic gastritis. Vision deficits such as blurred vision or "snowfield blindness" (complaints of peering through a snowstorm) may occur. CNS effects are common with confusion and ataxia effects. Respiratory depression, seizures, and coma can occur. Hyperthermia or hypothermia can be present. Hyperemia and retinal edema may be present. Other symptoms are similar to ethylene glycol poisoning.

Methanol antidotes/binding agents/treatment. Treatment is the same as ethylene glycol. Fomepizole and dialysis should be initiated before visual disturbances occur. Mortality is 20% despite treatment and many patients are left with permanent ocular damage. Dialysis is usually indicted with ocular findings, severe electrolyte disturbances, and levels greater than 20 mg/dl.

Clinical Pearls—Methanol

When methanol is coingested with ethanol, ethanol inhibits conversion of toxic metabolites, which cause metabolic acidosis and thus an elevated osmolar gap may be present without an elevated anion gap.

c. **Isopropyl alcohol drug overview.** Isopropyl alcohol is usually found in substances such as rubbing alcohol, glues, nail polish remover, and in many industrial solvents. Toxic doses are usually 2–4 ml/kg. Isopropyl is an alcohol that, if ingested orally, causes significant CNS depression. Isopropyl is excreted in the urine unchanged and 50% is metabolized by the liver to acetone. Acetone is nontoxic and is readily excreted by the kidney. No toxic metabolites are produced. Metabolic acidosis should not occur unless there are signs and symptoms of poor perfusion and organ damage from hypotension.

Isopropyl alcohol symptoms of overdose. Symptoms are similar to alcohol ingestion but more severe as isopropyl is twice as potent. Symptoms generally affect the CNS with ataxia, slurred speech, coma, respiratory depression, or arrest. Hypotension and myocardial depression can occur from profound vasodilation. Gastritis and GI bleeding can also occur. Hypoglycemia and positive osmolar gap may also be present. Levels of more than 150 mg/dl usually cause coma and hypotension and levels over 200 mg/dl are not compatible with life. Maximal distribution occurs within 2 h (Jammalamadaka and Raissi, 2010).

Isopropyl alcohol diagnostic testing and monitoring. Treatment is supportive. Laboratory testing should consist of CBC, ETOH levels, extended chemistries, and ECG monitoring. Serum osmolarity and ABGs should be monitored. Support of the airway may be needed due to the respiratory effects of the isopropyl, and fluid resuscitation may be needed to support the circulatory system. Isopropyl levels can be drawn and are usually a send-out test with other toxic alcohols.

Isopropyl alcohol antidotes/binding agents. Charcoal is generally not effective due to rapid absorption of isopropyl by the GI tract. Overdose has frequently been seen in coingestions. There is no specific antidote.

d. **Propylene glycol drug overview.** PG is classified as an alcohol and is a viscous, colorless drug diluent that is used in various drug compounds to stabilize unstable drugs. IV solutions of lorazepam, valium, etomidate, nitroglycerin, trimethoprim, sulfamethoxazole, and Dilantin all contain various amounts of PG. Lorazepam has the highest concentration of PG per milliliter. Lorazapam vials, both 2 and 4 mg/ml, contain 0.8 ml (830 mg of PG) (Yaucher *et al.*, 2003). The World Health Organization recommends a maximum dose of 25 mg/kg/day of PG (Neale *et al.*, 2005). PG can cause adverse iatrogenic effects when administered in moderate to high doses and in some case reports has significant metabolic acidosis in minimal doses (4–6 mg/h) over short periods of time (Cawley, 2011).

Hydrophobic drugs are mixed with PG to stabilize them and produce liquid formulations for drug administration. Drug half-life varies from 1.4 h at low doses to 3.3 h at higher doses. Drug clearance decreases at higher doses and 45% of an administered dose is eliminated unchanged by the kidney. The remaining amount is metabolized by hepatic alcohol dehydrogenase, then to DL-lactaldehyde or methylglyoxal. This converts to DL-lactate and then to D-lactate. Because D-lactate clears slowly from the body, an excessive accumulation produces significant CNS symptoms from accumulation in the brain and elevated lactic acid levels in the blood. Patients with existing renal or hepatic dysfunction are at increased risk (Neale *et al.*, 2005).

Propylene glycol symptoms of overdose. PG has a relatively low toxicity. Patients have signs and symptoms of metabolic acidosis with positive anion and osmolar gap. Osmolar gaps higher than 10 can cause acute tubular necrosis in the kidney. Patients with renal insufficiency have a higher risk. Patients may have lactic acidosis.

Propylene glycol diagnostic testing and monitoring. PG levels can be sent for study. Elevated levels may not correlate with toxicity. If diagnosis is suspected, monitoring should include serial extended chemistries, serum osmolarity, and lactic acid until levels normalize.

Propylene glycol antidotes/binding agents/treatment. Discontinuation of PG-containing medications is recommended. Care is supportive. Sodium bicarbonate may be helpful. There is no indication for fomepizole. Dialysis may be helpful but is usually not indicated.

Anticholinergics/Cholinergics/Antihistamines (ACA)
Drug overview
Antihistamines are drugs that are usually found in OTC medications for motion sickness, cold, and allergy symptoms. Examples of H1 receptor antagonists include diphenhydramine. Loratadine is a newer nonsedating H1 blocker that is peripherally selective. Peripherally selective antihistamines have a lower affinity to alpha-adrenergic and cholinergic receptor sites and cause fewer symptoms of dry mouth, flushing, CNS depression, and tachycardia. Anticholinergic activity is present in drugs that contain antihistamines, antispasmodics, skeletal muscle relaxants, and TCAs. Specific plants may also contain anticholinergic alkaloids. There are many types of antihistamines (six structural classes) and anticholinergic drugs, which are impossible to cover in this brief summary. In the United States, calls to Poison Control Centers in 2008 accounted for 3.6% of exposures to H1 and H2 antihistamine antagonists. Diphenhydramine was the most common exposure (French and Tarabar, 2010).

Anticholinergic agents antagonize acetylcholine at central and muscarinic receptors. Inhibition of muscarinic receptors can lead to cardiac effects such as rapid or slow heart rate in the case of cholinergic agents. Glands that are most affected are exocrine glands (salivation and sweating). Smooth muscle is also affected. Antihistamines with H1 effects antagonize histamine at H1 receptor sites. First-generation H1 blockers (e.g., Benadryl) differ from second-generation H2 blockers (e.g., Zyrtec) in their neurotransmitter blockade in the CNS. H1 blockers block 50–90% of H1 receptors in the brain as opposed to 30% with Zyrtec (Simons, 2004). Certain H1 antagonists can also block fast sodium channels, which can cause cardiac conduction delays, dysrhythmias, and widening of the QRS. H2 antihistamines inhibit gastric acid secretion and usually do not produce toxic effects in overdose. The antihistamine drugs without anticholinergic effects are nonsedating. Loratadine (Claratin), a second-generation H1 blocker, is the most closely related to the anticholinergics. Diphenhydramine, a first-generation H1 blocker, has local anesthetic effects, depresses the CNS, and can cause sedation. It can also cause profound agitation and prolonged QRS at high doses. Rhabdomyolysis and acidosis have been reported from seizure activity. Dystonic reactions can occur. Absorption can be delayed with anticholinergic and antihistamine overdose due to the effect of decreased gastric motility. Cholinergics cause rapid gastric motility and the range of toxicity is variable based on the drug ingested. Generally, in antihistamine overdose, the toxic dose is three to five times the daily dose. Peak plasma effects can range from 3 to 24 h and metabolism occurs in the liver.

ACA symptoms of overdose
Diagnosis is based on the history of ingestion and symptoms of anticholinergic toxidrome, which include flushing, hyperthermia, dilated pupils, and various CNS symptoms ranging from anxiety and agitation to delirium. There is a broad range of differential diagnosis. Urinary retention and intestinal ileus can occur. Tachycardia, arrhythmias, hypertension, and cardiogenic shock have been reported and are more common in the antihistamines with prominent anticholinergic effects. Pulmonary edema can occur due to cardiovascular failure. Rhabdomyolysis has been reported with doxylamine ingestion of greater than 20 mg/kg.

ACA diagnostic testing and monitoring
Drug levels are generally not available. Monitoring of ECG, CBC, CPK, extended chemistries, LFTs, ABGs, and serial 12-lead ECGs should be conducted. CT scan of the head may be needed to rule out any other central process. Drug screenings should be done for coingestion of other substances.

ACA antidotes/binding agents/treatment
Care is supportive with maintenance of airway, breathing, and circulation. Activated charcoal and gastric lavage can be administered if within 1 h of ingestion. For profound CNS effects such as agitation, seizure, or coma, intubation may be necessary. IV crystalloid fluids should be administered and benzodiazepines given for any seizure activity and agitation. Physostigmine can be given as long as there are no cardiac abnormalities such as PR and QRS prolongation on ECG. Physostigmine is an acetylcholinesterase inhibitor that binds to acetylcholinesterase and reverses central and peripheral symptoms. It is indicated only with symptoms of single anticholinergic exposure, pronounced CNS effects that are unresponsive to benzodiazepines, seizures that are not responsive to other treatments, and absence of ECG changes to the PR and QRS complex. Dosage is 0.5–1 mg by slow IV infusion over 5 min; effects are usually seen within 3–5 min. A repeat dosage can be given within 10 min if needed to a total dose of up to 4 mg. For antihistamine toxicity with QRS prolongation, sodium bicarbonate can be used at 1–2 mEq/kg IV. Dialysis is not effective.

Clinical Pearls—ACA

Asians are much less sensitive to diphenhydramine (Benadryl) due to their increased acetylation to a nontoxic metabolite when overdose is present. The use of physostigmine should be avoided in patients with TCA overdose as it may cause asystole, AV blocks, and seizures.

Anticonvulsants
Drug overview
Anticonvulsants are a group of drugs that are used to treat seizures. They may also be used in chronic pain syndrome, migraines,

and bipolar disease. Anticonvulsants work by raising the seizure threshold. They function in the CNS by inhibiting or decreasing excitatory tone. Anticonvulsants such as gabapentin and levetiracetam have an unknown mechanism of action. Toxicity from anticonvulsants can be either acute or chronic.

In the CNS, glutamine is present as a neurotransmitter that produces excitation through sodium channels and the NMDA receptors. Sedation happens in the CNS through GABA neurotransmitters and receptors. Anticonvulsants generally work on these receptors. Some also block calcium channels.

Anticonvulsants symptoms of overdose

Diagnosis is usually based on history. Most anticonvulsants affect the CNS through sedation, lethargy, confusion, agitation, nystagmus, or ataxia. Coingestions with other drugs are common. Carbamazepine can cause cardiac dysrhythmias, respiratory depression, coma, and seizures at toxic levels greater than 16 μg/ml. The clinical picture of toxicity may not correlate with levels ingested (Yildiz et al., 2006). Lamotrigime can cause hypersensitivity reactions and multisystem organ failure (Wade et al., 2010). Phenytoin can cause cardiac arrhythmias. It is classified as a Class IB antidysrhythmic. Toxic cardiac doses have not been reported with oral dosage but have occurred with IV dosing. Hypotension, bradycardia, and cardiac arrest have occurred. Levetiracetam (Keppra) can cause significant agitation, aggression, and altered level of consciousness, which can lead to coma; intubation may be needed. Valproic acid can cause thrombocytopenia and metabolic acidosis with severe toxicity and has caused respiratory failure but most symptoms are mild. Toxic symptoms can occur in ingestions grater than 400 mg/kg (Isbister et al., 2003). Drug levels are available on certain drugs such as phenytoin, carbamazepine, valproic acid, and levetiracetam but may require send-outs to outside agencies. Elevated ammonia levels may also be present with valproic acid overdose but it generally does not produce hepatic toxicity or CNS symptoms.

Anticonvulsants diagnostic testing and monitoring

Patients should be admitted to critical care if signs and symptoms of CNS or cardiac toxicity are present. Depending on symptoms, agent used, and sustained-release formulas, monitoring may be needed for a minimum of 24 h. Drug levels should be drawn if testing is available. Coingestions should be considered and tested for. Continuous ECG monitoring, level of consciousness, CBC, extended electrolytes, LFTs, and ABGs should be monitored.

Anticonvulsants antidotes/ binding agents

There are no specific antidotes. Care is supportive. Administration of charcoal and gastric lavage may be used if ingestion is within 1 h. Whole-bowel irrigation may be needed with enteric forms of medications. Caution should be used in patients with active seizure disorders when lowering toxic levels so seizures are not precipitated. If seizures are precipitated, use of benzodiazepines should be the first-line therapy. Bicarbonate can be administered for severe metabolic acidosis.

Clinical Pearls—Anticonvulsants

There have been case reports in valproic acid overdose of the use of hemodialysis and high-volume hemofiltration (Licari et al., 2009). Hemodialysis has also been effective in gabapentin, levetiracetam, and topiramate overdose but is rarely needed and should be reserved for severe symptoms of hypotension and seizures with metabolic acidosis that is refractory to other supportive therapies. Acute carbamazepine overdose has also been treated with prolonged hemoperfusion and hemodialysis (Ozhasenekler et al., 2012; Peces et al., 2010). There have also been case reports of naloxone being effective in valproic acid overdose (Roberge and Francis, 2002).

Common toxidromes and treatments for poisoning conditions

A toxidrome is a word that describes a certain common group of symptoms related to a drug class. Generally, the label toxidrome is related to an overdose of this drug class. Symptoms are generally similar and use of the toxidrome facilitates rapid diagnosis and treatment for toxic overdose (Table 13.7).

Table 13.7 Common drug or toxin overdose and antidotes.

Drug	Antidote	Antidote dosages	Major overdose symptom
Acetaminophen	Mucomyst either IV or po	IV load with 150 mg/kg/15 min, followed with 50 mg/kg for 4 h, then 100 mg/kg for 16 h	Depends on stage of poisoning, initial SX are GI upset
Beta blocker Calcium channel blocker	Glucagon	5–15 mg IVP: may be followed by infusion if needed	Bradycardia and sinus blocks
	Calcium	High-dose calcium gluconate or chloride 1–3 g IV bolus, then 20–50 mg/kg/h	Hypotension
	High-dose insulin and glucose	High-dose insulin 0.5–1 u/kg/h with dextrose infusion	Cardiovascular collapse that can be fatal
	Consider ILE in refractory shock	Atropine 0.5–1 mg IVP	
Anticholinergics	Physostigmine	0.5–1 mg IV	HTN, tachycardia, urinary retention Psychomotor agitation/ delerium
Botulism	Botulism antitoxin	1–2 vials Need to obtain from specific state of federal agencies	Progressive symmetric descending paralysis
Iron	Deferoxamine indicated with shock and hemodynamic instability	Initial dose is 15 mg/kg/h, can titrate to 40 mg/kg/h Major side effect is hypotension	Symptoms depend on toxicity level
INH (isoniazid)	Vitamin B6 (Pyridoxine)	Usual dose: for each gram of INH ingested give gram of B6	Seizures
Arsenic/mercury	DMSA D-penicillamine		GI irritation/hemorrhage Cardiogenic shock
Tricyclics	Sodium bicarbonate IV magnesium for Torsade de pointes Experimental ILE therapy	D5W with 2–3 amps bicarbonate at 75–100 cc/h 1–2 g IVP	ECG changes, ORS widening, seizures
Opiates	Naloxone	0.4 mg IVP can be repeated every 2–4 min for a maximum dose of 2 mg	Respiratory depression, hypotension
Methotrexate	Folate, leucovorin calcium (give within 1 h of posioning)	Folic acid 15 mg po/IV q6 h until methotrexate level is nontoxic Leucovorin dose is equal to or greater than methotrexate dose given IV, further doses should be guided by methotrexate levels	GI/bone marrow hepatic and renal injury
Benzodiazepines	Flumazenil	0.1–0.2 mg IV to maximum of 2 mg	Sedation, seizures from withdrawal
Calcium channel blockers	Calcium gluconate	Patients may need large doses up to 10 g IV	Bradycardia, hypotension, hyperglcemia, and AV blocks
	Calcium cloride Glucagon Atropine	5–15 mg IVP 0.5–1 mg IV to maximum dose of 10 mg	
Cyanide	Amyl nitrate, sodium nitrate, thiosulfate	Cyanide antidote kit Goal is to obtain a methemoglobin level of 20–30% High-flow oxygen	Bradycardia, hypotension, agitation Cherry red skin
Methemoglobin-forming agents/ conditions	Methylene blue	1–2 mg/kg IV over 3–5 min, can repeat 1 mg/kg if symptoms not resolved	Cyanosis unresponsive to oxygen therapy Normal oxygen saturation Chocolate-colored blood
Organophosphates	Atropine, pralidoxime (2-PAM)	1 mg initially, then can be repeated to treat drying of oral secretions	Bradycardia, hypotension
Carbamates	Atropine	2-PAM 1–2 g IV, may repeat or start drip for continued muscle weakness	SLUDGE mnemonic

Table 13.7 (*Continued*)

Drug	Antidote	Antidote dosages	Major overdose symptom
Methanol	Ethanol, fomepizole, folate, leucovorin	Fomepizole 15 mg/kg loading dose, |then 10 mg/kg over 12 h × 4 doses, then 15 mg/kg over 12 h until methanol <20 mg/dl	Severe metabolic acidosis with organ failure
Ethylene glycol	Ethanol, fomepizole, pyridoxine	Folate and thiamine coadministration for cofactor support Folate 50–70 mg IV over 4 h × 24 h, then oral doses can be given until resolution of symptoms Thiamine 100 mg IV over 6 h for 2 days Pyridoxine 50 mg IV for 6 h for 2 days	
Lead	DMSA chelator/succimer	10 mg/kg or 350 mg/m² tid for 5 days then bid for 14 days	Anorexia, vomiting, abdominal pain, neurological symptoms
Coumadin	Vitamin K FFP	5–10 mg po/IV daily until INR normalizes	Bleeding
Heparin	Protamine 1 mg/100 units of heparin		Bleeding
Hypoglycemic agents, insulin	D50, dextrose	0.5–1 amp D50 IV repeated as needed for low blood sugar Infusion of dextrose/D50 IV Frequent blood glucose monitoring	Coma Hypoxic injury

Caution: ALWAYS check with Regional Poison Control Center for definitive treatment.

Anticholinergic toxidrome

Common with this toxidrome is the mnemonic "blind as a bat, mad as a hatter, red as a beet, dry as a bone, and hot as Hades or a hare." Common drugs that cause this toxidrome are antihistamines, TCAs, and ingestion of *Atropa belladonna*, antipsychotic antidepressants, Skeletal Muscle Relaxants (SMRs), jimson weed, amantadine, parasympatholytic medications, atropine, scopolamine, hyoscyamine, *Amanita muscaria* mushrooms, and antiparkinson medication (Kemmerer, 2007). Treatment is focused on managing symptoms such as decreasing fever and agitation. Anticholinergic toxicity is caused by agents that antagonize acetylcholine at peripheral muscarinic and central receptors. This causes inhibition at muscarinic receptors, which leads to symptoms of anticholinergic toxicity. Symptoms include hot flushes, dry skin, dilated pupils, rapid heart rates, agitation, confusion, anxiety, psychosis, constipation, urinary retention, and ileus. Symptoms can be delayed due to the effects on the gastric motility of this class of drugs and effects are often prolonged over 2–3 days. Diagnosis is based on the history of ingestion. Overdose requires monitoring in a critical care unit due to the extreme agitation and tachycardia. Treatment is supportive with IV crystalloids, continuous ECG monitoring, electrolytes, CBC, CPK, and ABG monitoring. Hyperthermia and rhabdomyolysis can occur and cooling and aggressive fluid management may be needed to prevent organ damage and acute kidney injury. Seizures and cardiac arrest can occur with tricyclic overdose and antihistamines. In extreme and severe toxicity such as hyperthermia, tachycardia, and delirium, a small dose of physostigmine 0.5–1 mg IV can be given. Physostigmine can cause AV blocks, asystole, and seizures, especially in tricyclic overdose (Reilly and Stawicki, 2008). Medications that should be avoided with this toxidrome include haloperidol, phenytoin, and Class IA, C, and III antiarrhythmics (Kemmerer, 2007).

Benzodiazepine toxidrome

Respiratory depression and altered mental status are common symptoms seen with this type of overdose. Vital signs are usually stable but hypotension can occur. Common drugs include Xanax, Ativan, and Klonopin. Altered mental status and coma are common and can range from mildly lethargic to deep coma states that require intubation to protect airway. Flumazenil can be used in acute benzodiazepine overdose. Dosages are 0.2 mg IVP with additional doses up to 1 mg given at 1 min intervals. Total dose should not exceed 3 mg/h.

Cholinergic toxidrome

This toxidrome is seen with drugs that directly stimulate cholinergic receptors or inhibit acetylcholinesterase. Remember the mnemonic "SLUDGE" (salivation, lacrimation, urination, defecation, gastric emesis) (Reilly and Stawicki, 2008). Symptoms vary depending on whether stimulation is at the muscarine, nicotinic, or central cholinergic receptor. Other symptoms include bradycardia, bronchospasm, seizures, and death. The most common drugs that cause signs and symptoms of cholinergic toxicity are organophosphates and certain mushrooms. Neostigmine, which is a drug that can be given to stimulate bowel function, can also cause these effects. The treatment of this toxidrome is usually supportive. The drug antidote is atropine, which reverses the muscarinic effects in organophosphate poisoning or the use of nerve gas agents. The dose of atropine is 2–6 mg IVP and can be escalated every 3–5 min until bronchospasm or wheezing stops. Atropine infusion may be needed for continuing symptoms. The hourly infusion rate is set at 20–30% of the total amount of atropine that is required to stabilize the patient. The infusion is maintained for 2–3 days with daily dose reductions of 25–33% (Reilly and Stawicki, 2008). Pralidoxime therapy may also be used in patients with signs and symptoms of organophosphate poisoning. It is specifically recommended for poisoning with carbamate. Pralidoxime reactivates cholinesterase after poisoning with an anticholinesterase agent. The recommended dose is 1–2 g IV over 30 min followed by a continuous infusion at 8 mg/kg/h in adults. This drug is especially useful for organophosphate poisoning that causes muscle paralysis.

Opioid toxidrome

These drugs bind to opioid receptors and cause CNS depression, bradycardia, hypotension, pinpoint pupils, decreased gastric motility, and constipation. Hypothermia is also common.

Narcan can be given for reversal. Clonidine overdose can sometimes be confused with opioid overdose because clonidine is an alpha 2 adrenergic agonist that causes G protein-mediated potassium efflux like Mu receptors, which cause hyperpolarization of neurons in the CNS. Both alpha agonists and Mu agonists cause pinpoint pupils, respiratory depression, and coma. Narcan can be given but the effect is not reliable in clonidine overdose.

Sympathomimetic toxidromes

This toxidrome is generally seen from an overdose of stimulant drugs. Signs and symptoms include diaphoresis, psychomotor agitation, hallucinations, dilated pupils, tremor, seizures, dysrhythmias, hypotension, hyperthermia (especially with MDMA, PCP, bath salts, and hallucinogens), fever, tachycardia, diaphoresis, and hypertension. Common drugs are theophylline, OTC decongestants, crack cocaine, cocaine, amphetamines, LSD, nicotine, ecstasy (MDMA), caffeine, PCP, and MAOI. Other drugs have sympathomimetic activity such as clonidine, certain decongestants, and herbals. This syndrome results from the release of or blocking of the reuptake of dopamine and norepinephrine, resulting in central and peripheral adrenergic hyperactivity from catecholamine release. Some sympathomimetics can also inhibit serotonin reuptake and norepinephrine (called SNRIs), which may cause adverse effects of hallucinations and extreme confusion with overdose or withdrawal. Examples of these drugs are Cymbalta, Effexor, and Pristiq. Drugs that have pure alpha or beta activity will produce varying symptoms.

Common cardiovascular symptoms are tachycardia, hypertension, tachypnea, and hyperthermia. Common neurological symptoms include agitation, psychomotor agitation, hyperreflexia, and seizures. Other effects include rhabdomyolysis, acute lung injury, and vasospasm of arteries with organ injury. Confusion can exist between this syndrome and anticholinergic poisoning. The main difference is the absence of diaphoresis in anticholinergic poisoning.

Management is supportive and geared toward treatment of the symptoms associated with this toxidrome. Large doses of benzodiazepines are needed to treat the neurological symptoms of muscular rigidity and cardiovascular stimulation. Cardioversion or adenosine is usually ineffective to treat supraventricular tachycardias resulting from sympathomimetic overdose. Beta blockers are more effective (Givens and O'Connell, 2007). Crystalloid fluid resuscitation and active cooling measures may be needed.

Rhabdomyolysis syndromes

Rhabdomyolysis is a clinical condition that is caused by leakage of intracellular myocytes from muscle damage injury. This injury causes excessive myoglobin to be released and ferrihemate and globulin to form at pH levels of 5.6. Ferrihemate causes a deterioration of kidney function by impairing renal tubular transport mechanisms and leads to tubular obstruction and cell death (Coco and Klasner, 2004). These injuries can be caused by drugs, alcohol, local muscle compression in coma, excessive muscular hyperactivity, rigidity, and seizures. Common drugs associated with elevated CPK levels and resulting in rhabdomyolysis are amphetamines and their derivatives, cocaine, clozapine, Zyprexa, lithium, MAOIs, phencyclidine, strychine, tetanus, and TCAs. Rhabdomyolysis from direct cellular toxicity can be caused by amatoxin-containing mushrooms, CO, colchicines, and ethylene glycol. Unknown mechanisms causing elevated CPK levels include barbiturates, chlorophenoxy herbicides, ethanol, gemfibrozil, hemlock, hyperthermia, statins, and trauma. Signs and symptoms include very high CPK levels, myalgias, swelling or tenderness over effected muscles signifying developing compartment syndrome hyperkalemia, hyponatremia, hypocalcemia, and decreased phosphorous levels.

Strychnine can also cause rhabdomyolysis; it has an alkaloid base, which can be found in rodent poison. It can also be found as an additive to cocaine or heroin. Strychnine causes increased neuronal rigidity, which can result generalized seizure activity and contraction of skeletal muscles. These muscle spasms may produce rhabdomyolosis, fever, or respiratory paralysis. Diagnosis is usually based on a history of ingestion. Specific levels can be measured in urine, blood, and bile, but generally may not be useful for toxic symptoms due to lack of correlation with levels. Treatment is supportive by maintaining airway. Symptoms of strychnine poisoning usually abate within several hours. Muscular rigidity is treated with benzodiazapines. Charcoal can be given within a couple of hours of ingestion of involved substances. Paralytic agents may be needed for severe muscle spasm and contraction. If compartment syndrome develops, surgical fasciotomy may be needed. Treatment with crystalloid fluids at rates of 200–300 cc/h to maintain urine output at 100 cc/h or greater is essential to prevent acute tubular necrosis. Treatment with mannitol and bicarbonate to increase urinary pH has shown to be effective in some patients with acute tubular necrosis but use of bicarbonate may potentiate an existing hypocalcemia (Coco and Klasner, 2004).

Treatment of hyperkalemia

The common treatment for hyperkalemia consists of giving 1– 2 amps (50–100 mEq) of sodium bicarbonate, 1 amp of calcium chloride IV, and 1 amp of D50 with 10 units of regular insulin IV. If the patient is able to take medications by mouth or has an intact GI system, Kayexalate can be given either by mouth, nasogastric tube, or rectally in doses of 15–30 g 1–4 times daily or until bowel movement occurs. The rectal dose is 30–50 g given as a retention enema every 6 h until stooling or resolution of hyperkalemia. **Remember!** Common arrhythmias are peaked T waves, but hyperkalemia alters the QRS complex, leading to bradycardia and AV blocks with later effects of hyperkalemia. These may respond to dopamine infusion and transcutanous pacing followed by transvenous pacing and acute dialysis. Isuprel has also been used. These treatments should be followed by urgent hemodialysis.

Packidrome

Packidrome is the unofficial term that describes mixed toxidromes. Body packers is a term applied to people who intentionally swallow packets of drugs that can contain cocaine or heroin. These packets can leak or burst and cause extreme toxicity. Abdominal X-rays and

CT scanning can be useful but may miss packages. Decontamination with charcoal can be useful and polyethylene glycol electrolyte lavage solution (PEG-ELS) has been used to decrease transit time. Emergent surgery with need for enterotomy may be required in case of packet rupture.

Alcohol withdrawal syndrome

Withdrawal from alcohol produces a hyperadrenergic state that is manifested by hyperexcitability, tremors, hallucinations, confusion, tachycardia, hypertension, and agitation. Tremors indicate mild to moderate withdrawal and generally occur within 6–8 h after last ethanol ingestion. Most seizures associated with alcohol withdrawal occur within 48–72 h of last ingested ethanol. Status epilecticus is a rare occurrence. The most severe form of ethanol withdrawal is called delirium tremens. This is usually seen within the first 48–72 h but may be delayed in some cases for up to 14 days. The main symptoms of delirium tremens involve a series of life-threatening autonomic hypersensitivity. Symptoms include extreme agitation, confusion, hallucinations both visual and auditory, garbled speech, tachycardia, hypertension, hyperpyrexia, diaphoresis, and mydriasis. Generally, ethanol withdrawal lasts from 1 to 6 days and generally peaks at 5 days. Alcohol withdrawal can persist past 5 days.

Treatment usually involves protocols that are hospital-specific and involves assessment tools to grade the severity of withdrawal syndrome and to treat the symptoms. A common scale used is the Clinical Institute Withdrawal Assessment (CIWA), which is based on a grading and scoring system according to which medication doses are administered (Spiegel, Kumari, and Petri, 2012). Generally, treatment is with a short- or long-acting form of benzodiazepine. Antipsychotics may be used such as Haldol, Zyprexa, or Seraquel but caution should be used not to induce seizures. Monitoring of the QTc interval should also be done at initiation and during dosing. An antihypertensive may also be ordered such as metropolol or clonidine for autonomic dysfunction and cardiovascular strain from alcohol withdrawal symptoms.

> **Clinical Pearls**
>
> Caution should be used with lorazepam infusion as the active metabolite contained in the IV form can cause an anion gap acidosis that is attributed to PG toxicity. Midazolam infusion is commonly used with monitoring of infusion generally done in critical care units due to risk of respiratory depression. End-tidal CO_2 should also be monitored.

Anion and non-anion gap acidosis and osmolar anion gap

Certain acidotic states can help the practitioner diagnose what may have been ingested. If an anion gap acidosis is present, an osmolar gap should be measured. The definition of anion gap is the difference between measured cations and anions. In an increased anion gap metabolic acidosis, an anion that is not measured in the electrolyte panel accumulates in the blood. Serum bicarbonate levels decrease as it is consumed during neutralization of this compound or acid, therefore increasing the calculated anion gap. Some causes of elevated anion gap are included in the mnemonic "MUDPILES":

M—methanol, metformin
U—uremia (renal failure), hepatorenal failure
D—diabetic ketoacidosis
P—paraldehyde, propofol, propylene glycol
I—iron, isoniazid, ibuprofen
L—lactic acidosis, which could also be conditions leading to lactic acidosis such as seizure, hyperthermia, hypotension, low perfusion states, carbon monoxide, and hydrogen sulfate
E—ethylene glycol, ethanol
S—salicylates, starvation ketoacidosis (adapted from Levine et al., 2011, p. 799)

Additional substances that may produce mild anion gap include theophylline. Toluene (from glue sniffing) use also produces non-anion gap acidosis.

The calculation is as follows: [serum sodium] – [serum chloride + serum bicarbonate] = anion gap

The normal anion gap is less than 16 mEq/l. Some causes of **decreased** anion gap are hypoalbuminemia, congestive heart failure, multiple myeloma, lithium, iodine toxicity, and administration of aminoglycosides. There are many online calculators that can help you calculate this number.

Non-anion gap acidosis

This can also be called normal anion gap acidosis. It develops from an increased excretion of bicarbonate or increased production of chloride (e.g., hyperchloremic acidosis from excessive normal saline infusion). It presents as an acidosis that is not accompanied by an anion gap. It can easily be remembered by the mnemonic "HARD-UP." Some causes are

hyperalimintation,
acetazolamide,
renal tubular acidosis,
diarrhea, or a
ureteroenteric or
pancreaticoduodenal fistula.

Osmolar gap

Osmolality is the measurement of the number of particles dissolved in a kilogram of solvent. Osmolarity is the actual number of particles per liter of solution. An elevated osmolar gap suggests that there is an unmeasured solute (Levine *et al.*, 2011). Major osmotically active solutes are sodium, glucose, bicarbonate, urea, chloride, and potassium. These are measured in the calculated osmolarity equation:

$$2 \times \left\{ \left[NA\left(mEq/l\right) \right] + \left[BUN\left(mg/dl\right) \right] \right\}/2.8 + glucose\left(mg/dl\right)/18$$

Normal osmolarity is 280–295

To calculate osmolar gap (which is the difference between the measured serum osmolarity and the calculated result), check a serum osmolarity level, calculate the serum osmolarity, then subtract that number from the other to get the osmolar gap. Osmolar gap also needs to be corrected in the setting of a positive ETOH level. To correct for ETOH, take the ETOH level, divide by 4, and add that number to the calculated osmolarity, then subtract this number from the measured osmolarity. For example, the equation would look like this:

Osmolarity corrected for elevated ETOH level

$$Calculated\ osmolarity = \left\{ 2 \times \left[NA\left(mEq/l\right) \right] + \left[BUN\left(mg/dl\right) \right] \right\}/2.8 + glucose\left(mg/dl\right)/18 + ETOH/4.6$$

The calculated osmolarity is then subtracted from the measured serum osmolarity to identify the osmolar gap. The normal osmolar gap is less than 10 mEq/l.

Drug ingestions that cause an increased osmolar gap include ethanol, methanol, isopropyl alcohol, ethylene glycol, and propylene glycol. Nontoxic causes include DKA, renal failure, severe hyperlipidemia, inaccurate testing techniques, mannitol, and glycerol. If an osmolar gap is present without an anion gap, common causes may include isopropyl alcohol ingestion, sickle cell syndrome in multisystem organ failure, absorption of sorbital, and intravenous immunoglobulin (IVIG) infusions.

The monitoring and treatment of drug and substance overdoses is complex and continually changing. This chapter has covered many common overdoses resulting in ICU admissions but continual research is needed for most categories of treatment and conditions. Regional Poison Control Centers are an excellent resource to support strong clinical history and physical assessment skills. Because overdoses may be accidental or intentional, strong patient advocacy and social assessments are paramount in determining type and progression of overdose symptoms as well as meaningful support for those affected by the overdose.

References

Ables, A.Z. and Nagubilli, R. (2010) Prevention, diagnosis, and management of seratonin syndrome. *American Family Physician*, **81** (9), 1139–1142.

Adler, S.G. and Weening, J.J. (2006) A case of acute renal failure. *Clinical Journal of Social Nephrology*, **1**, 156–165.

American Association of Poison Control Centers (2012) https://aapcc.s3.amazonaws.com/files/library/Bath_Salts_Data_for_Website_5.31.2013.pdf (accessed July 27, 2014)

Anderson, A. (2007) Management of beta andrenergic blocker poisoning. *Clinical Pediatric Emergency Medicine*, **9**, 4–16.

Arbour, R. (2003) Propylene glycol toxicity occurs during low-dose infusions of lorazepam. *Critical Care Medicine*, **2** (31), 664–665.

Athuraliya, T.N. and Jones, A.L. (2009) Prolonged N-acetylcysteine therapy in late acetaminophen poisoning associated with acute liver failure-a need to be more cautious? *Critial Care*, **13** (3), 144.

Baud, F.J., Megarbane, B., Deye, N., and Leprince, P. (2007) Clinical review: aggressive management and extracorporeal support for drug-induced cardiotoxicity. *Critical Care*, **11**, 207.

Bebarta, V.S., Maddry, J., Borys, D.J., and Morgan, D.L. (2011) Incidence of tricyclic antidepressant-like complications after cyclobenzaprine overdose. *The American Journal of Emergency Medicine*, **29** (6), 645–649.

Berlin, G., Brodin, B., Hilden J.-O., and Martensson, J. (1985) Acute dapsone intoxication: a case treated with continuous infusion of methylene blue, forced diuresis and plasma exchange. *Clinical Toxicology*, **22**, 537–548.

Boothby, L.A., Doering, M.S., and Hatton, R.C. (2003) Carisoprodol: a marginally effective skeletal muscle relaxant with serious abuse potential. *Hospital Pharmacy*, **38** (4), 337–345.

Boyer, E.W. (2012) Management of opioid analgesic overdose. *New England Journal of Medicine*, **367** (2), 146–155.

Boyer, E.W. and Shannon, M. (2005) The seretonin syndrome. *New England Journal of Medicine*, **352**, 1112–1120.

Britt, G.C. and McCance-Katz, E.F. (2005) A brief overview of the clinical pharmacology of "club drugs". *Substance Use & Misuse*, **40**, 1189–1201.

Brush, D.E. (2005) Antidepressant poisoning, in *Manual of Overdoses and Poisonings* (eds C.H. Linden, J.M. Rippe, and R.S. Irwin), Lippincott Williams and Wilkins, Philadelphia, p. 41.

Buchanan, J.A. and Lavonas, E.J. (2012) Agranulocytosis and other consequences due to use of illicit cocaine contaminated with levamisole. *Current Opinion in Hematology*, **19**, 27–31.

Cave, G. (2011) Intravenous lipid emulsion as antidote: how should we chew the fat in 2011? *Critical Care Medicine*, **39** (4), 919–920.

Cawley, M.J. (2011) Short-term lorazepam infusion and concern for propylene glycol toxicity: case report and review. *Pharmacotherapy*, **21** (9), 1140–1144.

Chabria, S.B. (2006) Rhabdomyolysis: a manifestation of cyclobenzaprine toxicity. *Journal of Occupational Medicine and Toxicology*, **1** (16), 1–2.

Chun, L.J., Tong, M.J., Busuttil, R.W., and Hiatt, J.R. (2009) Acetaminophen hepatoxicity and acute liver failure. *Journal of Clinical Gastroenterology*, **43** (4), 342–349.

Coco, T.J. and Klasner, A.E. (2004) Drug-induced rhabdomyolysis. *Current Opinion Pediatrics*, **16**, 206–210.

Czuchlewski, D.R., Brackney, M., Ewers, C. *et al.* (2010) Clinicopathologic features of agranulocytosis in the setting of levamisole-tainted cocaine. *American Journal of Clinical Pathology*, **133**, 466–472.

Day, L.T. and Jeanmonod, R.K. (2008)Serotonin syndrome in a patient taking Lexapro and Flexeril: a case report. *The American Journal of Emergency Medicine*, **26**, 1069.el–1069.e3.

DeMaria Jr, S. and Weinkauf, J. (2011) Cocaine and the club drugs. *International Anesthesiology Clinics*, **49** (1), 79–101.

DePont, A.C. (2007) Extracoporeal treatment of intoxications. *Current Opinion in Critical Care*, **13**, 668–673.

Devlin, R.J. and Henry, J.A. (2008) Clinical review: major consequences of illicit drug consumption. *Critical Care*, **12** (202), 1–7.

Dunkley, E.J.C., Isbister, G.K., Sibbritt, D. *et al.* (2003) The hunter serotinin toxicity criteria: simple and accurate diagnostic decision rules for serotonin toxicity. *Quarterly Journal of Medicine*, **96**, 635–642.

Engebretsen, K.M., Kaczmarek, K.M., Morgan, J., and Holger, J.S. (2011) High-dose insulin therapy in beta-bocker and calcium channel-blocker poisoning. *Clinical Toxicology*, **49**, 277–283.

Ernst, L., Schiebel, H.M., Theuring, C. *et al.* (2011) Identification and characterization of JWH-122 used as new ingredient in "spice-like" herbal incenses. *Forensic Science International*, **208**, 31–35.

Every-Palmer, S. (2011) Synthetic cannabinoid JWH-018 and psychosis: an explorative study. *Journal of Drug and Alcohol Dependence*, **117** (2), 152–157.

Eyer, F. and Ziker, T. (2007) Bench-to-bedside review: mechanisms and management of hyperthermia due to toxicity. *Critical Care*, **11** (236), 1–8.

Falck, R., Li, L., Carlson, R., and Wang, J. (2006) The prevalence of dextromethorphan abuse among high school students. *Pediatrics*, **118**, 2267–2269.

Farre, M., Torre De La, R. Gonzalez, M.L. *et al.* (1997) Cocaine and alcohol interactions in humans: neuroendocrine effects and cocaethylene metabolism. *Journal of Pharmacology and Experimental Therapeutics*, **283** (1), 164–176.

Filley, C.M. and Kleinschmidt-DeMasters, B.K. (2001) Toxic leukoencephalopathy. *New England Journal of Medicine*, **345** (6), 425–432.

French, L.K. and Tarabar, A. (2010) Antihistamine toxicity follow-up. *Medscape*, http://emedicine.

medscape.com/article/812828-followup (accessed July 27, 2014)

Garg, A.D., Hippargi, R.V., and Gandhare, A.N. (2008) Toad skin-secretions: potent source of pharmacologically and therapeutically significant compounds. *The Internet Journal of Pharmacology*, **5** (2), 17.

Ghosh, A. and Ghosh, T. (2010) Herbal drugs of abuse. *Systematic Reviews in Pharmacy*, **1** (2), 141–145.

Gillman, K. (2011) *Serotonin toxicity, seratonin syndrome*, http://www.psychotropical.com/index.php/serotonin-toxicity

Givens, M., Kalbfleisch, K., and Bryson, S. (2008) Comparison of methanol exposure rates reported to Texas poison control systems. *Western Journal of Emergency Medicine*, **9** (3), 150–153.

Givens, M.L. and O'Connell, E. (2007) Toxicologic issues during cardiopulmonary resuscitation. *Current Opinion in Critical Care*, **13** (3), 287–293.

Gotway, M.B., Marder, S.R., Hanks, D.K. *et al.* (2002) Thoracic complications of illicit drug use: an organ system approach. *Radiographics*, **22** (Supp 1), S1119–S1135.

Gussow, L. (2009) Myths of toxicology: gastric lavage. *Emergency Medicine News*, **31** (11) 7–8.

Hall, A.P. and Henry, J.A. (2006) Acute toxic effects of 'Ecstasy'(MDMA) and related compounds: overview of pathophysiology and clinical management. *British Journal of Anaesthesia*, **96** (6), 678–685.

Hampson, N.B. and Hauff, N.M. (2008) Risk factors for short-term mortality from carbon monoxide poisoning treated with hyperbaric oxygen. *Critical Care Medicine*, **36** (9), 2523–2527.

Harris, C.R. (2006) *The Toxicology Handbook for Clinicians*, Mosby Elsevier, Philadelphia.

Hedges, J., Jeppson, K., and Whitehead, P. (2003) Antipsychotic medication and seizures: a review. *Drugs Today*, **39** (7), 551–557.

Hodgman, M.J. and Garrard, A.R., (2012) A review of acetaminophen poisoning. *Critical Care Clinics*, **28**, 499–516.

Horowitz, B.Z. (2012) Emergent Management of Calcium Channel Blocker Toxicity, http://misc.medscape.com/pi/android/medscapeapp/html/A813485-business.html (accessed July 26, 2014).

Howell, B.A. and Chauhan, A. (2010) Current and emerging detoxification therapies for critical care. *Materials*, **3**, 2483–2505.

Hunter, H. and Taljanovic, M.S. (2003) Foreign bodies. *Radiographics*, **23**, 731–757.

Intelligence Bulletin: Dextrometorphan (n.d.), http://www.justice.gov/archive/ndic/pubs11/11563/11563p.pdf

Iqbal, N. (2001) Neurotoxic effects of inhalants. *Annals of Saudi Medicine*, **21** (3–4), 216–218.

Isbister, G.K., Balit, C.R., Whyte, I.M., and Dawson, A. (2003) Valporate overdose: a comparative cohort study of self poisonings. *Journal of Clinical Pharmacology*, **55**, 398–404.

Jammalamadaka, D. and Raissi, S. (2010) Ethylene glycol, methanol and isopropyl alcohol intoxication. *The American Journal of the Medical Sciences*, **339** (3), 276–281.

Kao, L.W. and Nanagas, K.A. (2004) Carbon monoxide poisoning. *Emergency Medicine Clinics of North America*, **22**, 985–1018.

Kemmerer, D.A. (2007) Anticholinergic syndrome. *Journal of Emergency Nursing*, **33**, 76–78.

Kerr, G.W., McGuffie, A.C., and Wilkie, S. (2001) Tricyclic antidepressant overdose: a review. *Emergency Medicine Journal*, **18** (4), 236–241.

Korioth, T. (2011) Legal substances land teens in emergency departments. *American Academy of Pediatrics*, **32** (7), 22.

Leitch, I.M., Lim, T.H., and Boura, A.L.A. (2000) *Novel Drugs From Toad Skins*, RIDC Publication, Australia.

Lessenger, J.E. and Feinberg, S.D. (2008) Abuse of presciption and over-the-counter medications. *Journal of the American Board of Family Medicine*, **21** (1), 45–54.

Levin, T.T., Cortes-Ladino, A., Weiss, M., and Palomba, M.L. (2008) Life-threatening seratonin toxicity due to a citalopram-fluconazole drug interaction: case reports and discussion. *General Hospital Psychiatry*, **30**, 372–377.

Levine, M., Brooks, D.E., Truitt, C.A. *et al.* (2011) Toxicology in the ICU: part 1: general overview and approach to treatment. *Chest*, **140** (3), 795–806.

Lheureux, P.E., Zahir, S., Penaloza, A., and Gris, M. (2005) Bench-to-bedside review: antidotal treatment of sulfonylurea-induced hypoglycemia with octreotide. *Critical Care*, **9**, 543–549.

Licari, E., Calzavacca, P., Warrillow, S.J., and Bellomo, R. (2009) Life-threatening sodium valproate overdose: a comparison of two approaches to treatment. *Critical Care Medicine*, **37** (12), 3161–3164.

Ling, L. (ed) (2001) *Toxicology Secrets*, Hanley & Belfus, Philadelphia.

Lowes, R. (2011) FDA: avoid methylene blue or linezolid with serotonergics. *Medscape Medical News*, http://www.medscape.com/viewarticle/747076 (accessed July 27, 2014).

Mansouri, A. and Lurie, A.A. (1993) Concise review: methemoglobinemia. *American Journal of Hematology*, **42**, 7–12.

Marsolek, M.R., White, N.C., and Litovitz, T.L. (2010) Inhalant abuse: monitoring trends by using poison control data 1993–2008. *Pediatrics*, **125**, 906–914.

McAllen, K.J. and Schwartz, D.R. (2010) Adverse drug reactions resulting in hyperthermia in the intesive care unit. *Critical Care Medicine*, **38** (6), s244–s252.

McBane, S. and Weigle, N. (2010) Is it time to drug test your chronic pain patient? *The Journal of Family Practice*, **59** (11), 628–633.

Meehan, T.J., Bryant, S.M., and Aks, S.E. (2010) Drugs of abuse: the highs and lows of altered mental states in the emergency department. *Emergency Medicine Clinic*, **28**, 663–682.

Modesto-Lowe, V. and Petry, N.M. (2001) Recognizing and managing "illy" intoxication. *Psychiatric Services*, **52** (12), 1660–1662.

Morrison, B. and Chaudhry, V. (2012) Medication, toxic, and vitamin-related neuropathies. *Continuum*, **18**, 139–160.

Musselman, M.E. and Saely, S. (2013) Diagnosis and treatment of drug-induced hyperthermia. *American Journal of Health-System Pharmacy*, **70** (1), 34–42.

Muzawazi, R. and Manickam, B. (2012) The use of intravenous lipd emulsion as an antidote in drug toxicity-an update. *Darlington and County Durham Medical Journal*, **6** (1), 11–17.

Neale, B.W., Mesler, E.L., Young, M. *et al.* (2005) Propylene glycol-induced lactic acidosis in a patient with normal renal function: a proposed mechanism and monitoring recommendations. *Annals of Pharmacotherapy*, **39** (10), 1732–1735.

Neerman, M.F. and Uzoegwu, C.L. (2010) Is dextromethorphan a concern for causing a false positive during urine drug screening? *Laboratory Medicine*, **41**, 457–460.

Okie, S. (2010) A flood of opioids, a rising tide of deaths. *The New England Journal of Medicine*, **363** (21), 1981–1985.

Olsen, K.M. (2005) *Pharmacologic agents associated with QT interval prolongation*. Journal of Family Practice, June (Suppl), S8–S14.

Olson, K.R. (ed) (2012) *Poisoning and Drug Overdose*, 6th edn, McGraw-Lange, New York.

Ozcan, M.S. and Weinberg, G. (2011) Update on the use of lipid emulsions in local anesthetic systemic toxicity: a focus on differential efficacy and lipid emulsions as part of advanced cardiac life support. *International Anesthesiology Clinics*, **49** (4), 91–103.

Ozhasenekler, A., Gokhan, S., Guloglu, C. *et al.* (2012) Benefit of hemodialysis in carbamazepine intoxications with neurological complications. *European Review for Medical and Pharmaceutical Sciences*, **1**, 43–47.

Page, C.B., Hacket, L.P., and Isbister, G.K. (2009) The use of high-dose insulin-glucose euglycermia in beta-blocker overdose: a case report. *Journal of Medical Toxicology*, **5** (3), 139.

Peces, R., Azorin, S., Peces, C., and Selgas, R. (2010) Prolonged haemoperfusion as treatment for acute carbamazepine poisoning. *Nefrologia*, **30** (1), 127–130.

Plotkin, J.S., Buell, J.F., Njoku, M.J. *et al.* (1997) Methemoglobinemia associated with dapson treatment in solid organ transplant recipients: a two-case report and review. *Liver Transplantation and Surgery*, **3**, 149–152.

Pothiawala, S. and Ponampalam, R. (2011) Tramadol overdose: a case report. *Proceedings of Singapore Healthcare*, **20** (3) 219–223.

Prosser, J.M. and Nelson, L.S. (2011) The toxicology of bath salts: a review of synthetic cathinones. *Journal of Medical Toxicology*, **8** (1), 33–42.

Reilly, E.F. and Stawicki, S.P. (2008) ICU corner: high- yield toxicology: essential facts for the critical care boards. *OPUS 12 Scientist*, **2** (1), 33–38.

Roberge, R.J. and Francis, E.H. (2002) Use of naloxone in valproic acid overdose: case report and review. *The Journal of Emergency Medicine*, **22** (1), 67–70.

Roberts, J.R. (2010) Antidotes you should know: octreotide for sulfonylurea-induced hypoglycemia. *Emergency Medicine News*, **32** (2), 10–12.

Rothschild, L., Bern, S., Oswald, S., and Weinberg, G. (2010) Intravenous lipid emulsion in clinical toxicology. *Journal of Trauma-Resuscitation and Emergency Medicine*, **18**, 51.

Ruth-Sahd, L.A., Zulkosky, K., and Fetter, M.E. (2011) Carbon monoxide poisoning: case studies and review. *Dimensions of Critical Care Nursing*, **30** (6), 303–314.

Scalley, R.D., Ferguson, D.R., Piccaro, J.C. *et al.* (2002) Treatment of ethylene glycol poisoning. *American Family Physician*, **66** (5), 807–813.

Schwartz, B.G., Rezkalla, S., and Kloner, R.A. (2010) Cadiovascular effects of cocaine. *Circulation*, **122**, 2558–2569.

Shadnia, S., Brent, J., Mousavi-Fatemi, K. *et al.* (2012) Recurrent seizures in Tramadol intoxication: implications for therapy based on 100 patients. *Basic & Clinical Pharmacology & Toxicology*, **111**, 133–136.

Siff, J.E., Meldon, S.W., and Tomassoni, A.J. (1999) Usefulness of the total iron binding capacity in the evaluation and treatment of acute iron overdose. *Annals of Emergency Medicine*, **33** (1), 73–76.

Simlai, J. and Khess, C.R.J. (2008) Inhalant abuse in the youth: a reason for concern. *Industrial Psychology Journal*, **17** (1), 55–58.

Simons, F.E.R. (2004) Advances in H1-antihistamines. *The New England Journal of Medicine*, **351** (21), 2203–2217.

Skold, A. and Klein, R. (2013) Symptomatic-low grade methemoglobinemia because of dapsone: a multiple hit hypothesis. *American Journal of Therapeutics*, **20** (6), e729–e732.

Smith, C., Cardile, A.P., and Miller, M. (2011) Bath salts as a "legal high". *The American Journal of Medicine*, **124** (11), 1–2.

Smollin, C.G. (2010) Toxicology: pearls and pitfalls in the use of antidotes. *Emergency Medicine Clinics of North America*, **28**, 149–161.

Spiegel, D.R., Kumari, N., and Petri, J.D. (2012) Safer use of benzodiazepines for alcohol detoxification. *Current Psychiatry*, **11** (10), 10–14.

Spiller, H.A. and Sawyer, T.S. (2006) Toxicology of oral antidiabetic medications. *American Journal of Health-System Pharmacy*, **63** (10), 929–938. doi:10.2146/ajhp050500.

Spiller, H.A., Ryan, M.L., and Weston, R.G. (2011) Clinical experience with and analytical confirmation of "bath salts" and "legal highs" (synthetic cathinones) in the United States. *Clinical Toxicology*, **49**, 499–505.

Sternbach, H. (1991) The serotonin syndrome. *The American Journal of Psychiatry*, **148**, 705–713.

Teker, M., Özdemir, H., Saidoglu, L. *et al.* (2010) Levosimendan as a rescue adjunct in amlodipine intoxication. *Middle East Journal of Anesthesiology*, **20** (6), 869–872.

Traub, S.J., Hoffman, R.S., and Nelson, L.S. (2003) Body packing-the internal concealment of illicit drugs. *New England Journal of Medicine*, **349**, 2519–2526.

Wade, J.F., Dang, C.V., Nelson, L., and Wasserberger, J. (2010) Emergent complications of the newer anticonvulsants. *The Journal of emergency medicine*, **38** (2), 231–237.

Weaver, L.K. (2009) Carbon monoxide poisoning. *New England Journal of Medicine*, **360** (12), 1217–1225. doi:10.1056/NEJMcp0808891.

Wells, D.L. and Ott, C.A. (2011) The "new" marijuana. *The Annals of Pharmacotherapy*, **45** (3), 414–417.

Wimbiscus, M., Kostenko, O., and Malone, D. (2010) MAO inhibitors: risks, benefits, and lore. *Cleveland Clinic Journal of Medicine*, **77** (12), 859–882.

Yang, R., Miki, K., He, X. *et al.* (2009) Prolonged treatment with N-acetylcystine delays liver recovery from acetaminophen hepatotoxicity. *Critical Care*, **13**, 1–7.

Yaucher, N.E., Fish, J.T., Smith, H.W., and Wells, J.A. (2003) Propylene glycol-associated renal toxicity from lorazem infusion. *Pharmacotherapy*, **23** (9), 1094–1099.

Yildiz, T.S., Toprak, D.G., Arisoy, E.S., and Solak, M. (2006) Continous venovenous hemodiafiltration to treat controlled-release carbamazepine overdose in a pediatric patient. *Pediatric Anesthesia*, **16**, 1176–1178.

Index

Note: Page references in *italics* refer to Figures; those in **bold** refer to Tables and Boxes

---

Critical Care Nursing: Monitoring and Treatment for Advanced Nursing Practice, First Edition. Edited by Kathy J. Booker.
© 2015 John Wiley & Sons, Inc. Published 2015 by John Wiley & Sons, Inc.